Measurement Tools in Patient Education

Barbara Klug Redman, PhD, RN, FAAN, is Dean and Professor at the University of Connecticut School of Nursing. She received her Masters and PhD degrees at the University of Minnesota. She received her BSN at South Dakota State University. She has also been a Post Doctoral Fellow at the The John Hopkins University, a Fellow in Medical Ethics at Harvard Medical School, and is a Fellow of the American Academy of Nursing. Dr. Redman's career began as a staff nurse at a hospital in South Dakota. Dr. Redman has been Executive Director of the American Nurses Association, American Nurses Foundation, and American Association of Colleges in Nursing. She has also held professorships at the universities of Washington, Minnesota and Johns Hopkins University. She has received honorary doctorates from Georgetown University and the University of Colorado. Dr. Redman has published numerous works in patient education, including *The Practice of Patient Education* which is now in its 8th edition and has been translated into Japanese, Finish, Dutch, and German.

Measurement Tools in Patient Education

Barbara K. Redman
PhD, RN, FAAN

 Springer Publishing Company

Springer Publishing Company, Inc.
536 Broadway
New York, NY 10012-3955

Cover design by: Margaret Dunin
Acquisitions Editor: Ruth Chasek
Production Editor: Kathleen Kelly

97 98 99 00 01/5 4 3 2 1

Library of Congress Cataloging-in-Publication Data

Measurement tools in patient education / [edited by] Barbara K. Redman.
    p.   cm.
   Includes bibliographical references and index.
   ISBN 0-8261-9860-0
   1. Patient education—Evaluation.   2. Patient education—Statistical method.
I. Redman, Barbara Klug.
   [DNLM: 1. Patient Education—methods.   2. Education Measurement—methods.
W 85 M485 1997]
R727.4.M   1997
615.5'071—dc21
DNLM/DLC
for Library of Congress   97-29477
                                                   CIP

Printed in the United States of America

To my daughter Melissa

Contents

I

An Introduction

Virtually all health professionals teach patients, although few think of it as a potentially full-fledged intervention with measurable outcomes. The time is long passed when the field of patient education should have developed, validated, and regularly used measurement tools in both research and clinical practice. Neither practice nor research will progress without the ability to assess with rigor specific patient and group learning needs, and hone teaching interventions to a known level of effectiveness.

The literature for patient education has always been scattered among disease-specific journals in various health disciplines and social science journals applied to health. Only one journal—*Patient Education and Counseling*—is specific to patient education, and several of the few journals in the field of health education occasionally include materials relevant to patient education. In the author's experience, the formal retrieval systems have never identified more than a small portion of the relevant literature. That portion of the literature that addresses measurement tools in patient education is similarly scattered and not easily identifiable. This becomes particularly difficult when one needs to identify possible choices of tools for a particular application or when one is trying to determine the range of measurement tools available in a field of patient education.

The measurement tools described in this book were collected as part of a search for patient education literature, accomplished by routine searching of approximately 150 journals, indexes, and databases to nursing and medical literature for the past 10 years, and branching through references contained in relevant published articles. Approximately 90 authors were contacted and asked for permission to include their tools. After multiple contacts, nearly 70 responded. Some of these tools were judged to be too unrelated to patient education, too early in their development, or too old so that their content was no longer judged to be useful, or required prohibitively expensive licensing fees. Therefore, the 50 included in this book must be understood to represent an incomplete list. Nevertheless, this collection allows an initial point from which to describe what is available in the field. Because the measurement characteristics of only a few have been studied in more than a preliminary way, work using most should incorporate additional studies of validity and reliability.

TABLE I.1   What Is Measured

	N	%
Theoretical model	1	2
Knowledge	17	34
Beliefs/attitudes/behaviors	8	16
Learning assessment/instructional design/delivery	9	18
Self-efficacy	14	28
Quality of life	1	2

TABLE I.2   Source of Publication

	N	%
Patient education/health education journal	7	14
Medical journal	2	4
Nursing journal	17	34
Disease-, age-, or gender-specific journal	16	32
Social science/health services research journal	7	14
Other	1	2

Tables I.1 and I.2 describe the focus of measurement and the published source for the 50 tools included in this volume. About 30% were developed to measure knowledge. Many self-efficacy (SE) scales were included because this construct has been shown repeatedly to be important to patient execution of behaviors and because SE beliefs are specific to a particular set of tasks. Instruments were most likely to have been published in disease-, age-, or gender-specific journals, or in nursing journals. Clearly, many disciplines are contributing to the development of these tools, and searching for them will require scholars and clinicians to look outside their fields. Eighty-five percent were first published between 1990 and 1995.

What is so striking about the collection of instruments is how few are oriented to the integrated concept of patient self-management, arguably the central outcome from patient education. It is not clear that combinations of these instruments would serve to measure patient self-management. Second, they clearly are not evenly distributed over the disease entities/patient groups for which patient education is considered essential. By far, the largest number were developed to measure diabetes. Third, few others than those that were developed to measure a theoretical model, such as the health belief model, have a theoretical base. Fourth, few are available for children or specifically for the elderly.

Each author was contacted to obtain the most recent version of the tool, scoring guidelines and studies of validity and reliability. Other citations to the work contained in Social Sciences Citation Index were reviewed for additional studies of validity and reliability, and critiques of the tools. This information was used to write the descriptive sections about each instrument. The review of each instrument is organized around common sections: instrument description including readability if available, psychometric properties, summary of studies using the instrument, and a critique summary. Particular attention was paid to the different cultures in which the instrument has been used.

1

Measurement in Patient Education Practice and Research

Patient education is an old idea, but one that has been susceptible to trends of fashion in medical practice. The old paradigm of physicians choosing what, if any, information to share with patients, was first abridged with the legal and ethical doctrine of informed consent and increasingly by the conceptualization that psychosocial interventions are as critical to good health outcomes as are treatments based on the biomedical model.

Perhaps because patient education has been a battleground for the authority of physicians and their model of health care, its research base has developed faster than has a system for reliably delivering it as a service with clear standards of quality. Under the now fading system of fee for service, it has infrequently been reimbursed and, therefore, neglected. But all the trends in health care point to the need to upgrade and universalize the provision of patient education seriously.

1. An impressive body of research, summarized in more than 25 metaanalyses shows conclusively that patient education can contribute significantly to positive health care outcomes (Redman, 1996). In some of these areas, such as diabetes education, enough research has accumulated to provide results that are robust and generalizable across gender, age, and time (Devine, 1992).
2. The rise of evidence-based medicine, translating this research into clinical practice, is necessary to achieve rapidly increasing standards for efficiency and quality in health care.
3. Evidence in various fields that requirements for at least informing patients is steadily evolving, sometimes backed by regulatory sanctions. The provision of written information on prescription drugs through government and voluntary programs is an example. During the 1960s, physicians were viewed as the sole dispensers of such information, and they alone would determine for each patient how much information should be given. Now, both the U.S. Food and Drug Administration (FDA) and other voluntary organizations provide this information, direct-to-consumer advertising of prescription drugs occurs under FDA regulation, pharmacists are required by federal law to offer counseling about medications to patients who receive state-assisted services, and some countries have mandated patient information leaflets for prescription drugs (Nightingale, 1995).

Patient education operates within each field of practice, varying widely in state of development. For example, a system of services with national accreditation standards and with certification for individual providers exists in the diabetes field and, to some extent, in the prenatal education field. Other fields of patient education practice may have model education programs that have been evaluated (asthma), or relatively available programs and educational materials (cardiac rehabilitation), or an active research community and a set of outcomes developed by consensus (arthritis), or only beginning agreement about what an educational program might look like and what it might accomplish (psychoeducation for the mentally ill). Despite this extreme variability, patient education services will face the same pressures for evidence-based practice as do all services. Yet, at this time, the field does not have a tradition of evaluation and especially not of outcome evaluation.

Other trends also support the need for a much more concerted effort in measurement in patient education.

1. The traditional behavioral approach in medicine that compliance is the goal of patient education means that in a field like diabetes, the primary focus of patient education should be glucose management and metabolic control, with patient adherence as the primary measure of the effectiveness of programs. A now rapidly evolving alternative view is that education and care should address the impact of diabetes on the totality of a person's life. Under this model, relevant skills include the integration of diabetes into a healthy life and managing the stress caused by living with diabetes (Anderson, 1995). To date, diabetes education program evaluation has focused narrowly on assessing patient knowledge and glycemic control, to the exclusion of other variables, such as self-efficacy, quality of life, patient functioning, problem solving, and coping skills (Glasgow & Osteen, 1992).
2. The set of theories that attempt to predict or explain why people behave as they do in relation to their health includes the health belief model, health locus of control, attribution theory, theory of reasoned action, and the transtheoretical model of behavior change. In only a few cases has significant effort been invested in developing measures from these models that are sensitive to change and applicable to a variety of health problems, but even here constructs and scales have not been widely or diversely validated. In addition, we are still at a rudimentary stage of understanding whether some of these models are better than others in producing outcomes, in understanding which components of the model are needed to achieve change, and how they actually function to produce health (Clark & McLeroy, 1995).
3. The integration of research results in the metaanalyses shows serious measurement problems in patient education: The content of usual care (which forms the comparison group) is virtually never described. This also means that the effect sizes reflect an increment above care that already includes some patient education (Devine, 1992). In some fields, few studies include direct comparison between different types of psychosocial care (Devine & Reifschneider, 1995), perhaps, in large part, because clear descriptive systems for interventions do not exist.

Although little is known about how patient education is routinely practiced in this country, the author argues that its performance could be improved by routine incorporation of formal assessment and evaluation tools. This change in practice will

1. Clarify outcomes the field recognizes and can attain outside of controlled research settings and establish benchmarks of quality of service that can be attained and surpassed by others.
2. Improve outcomes of learning and instruction through the process of assessment of learning needs, diagnosis of learning problems and possible adverse effects, such as confusion and fear from poor instruction, and feedback to patients about how close they are to reaching their own goals.

3. Accurately predict how much learning is needed to attain important outcomes and what will happen if it is not attained.
4. Relieve documentation problems, which have been rife in the field, although they are now being addressed through incorporation of patient education into critical paths.
5. Facilitate examination of issues of fairness in attainment across various groups, of outcomes patient education can deliver.

The purposes of patient education include

1. Attainment of health outcomes shown to be affected by patient education, including physiological, psychosocial, and functional status; behaviors, such as coping and problem solving; knowledge; symptom control; home maintenance; well-being; quality of life; patient satisfaction (Lang & Marek, 1990); and avoidance of adverse effects of care, such as premature death and return hospitalizations. Optimization of use of resources might be added. All of these classes of outcomes can be affected by patient education, dependent on the efficacy of what is to be taught as well as on the efficacy of the teaching process to help the patient learn the skills. Patients experience natural variation in symptom severity and impact of disease, so observed change may be a product of this natural fluctuation rather than the effects of the care provided.
2. Facilitation of patient decision making.
3. Optimization of patient and family care skills about health, treatment options, and how to manage a regimen.

More specifically, the purposes for the use of formal measurement tools in patient education can include the following:

1. Diagnosis or assessment of the patient's educational needs for various levels of functioning.
2. Establishment of criterion levels of achievement known to be necessary for independent patient or family functioning.
3. Evaluation of the effectiveness of teachers and programs including catching and correcting adverse effects of teaching.
4. Continuous improvement of care by using outcomes to improve interventions and including benchmarking.
5. In the aggregate, tracking of the level of achievement of groups of patients against what is known to be necessary for effective outcomes (i.e., a "report card" on the performance of the health care system in this important area of practice).

The outcomes movement in health is an essential one. Because patient education is important in reaching many outcomes and essential for some, the field must pay serious attention to routinely documenting those outcomes and improving the interventions to reach them. Measurement tools in patient education have been developed in no particularly systematic way but rather through the interests of individuals. For example, the rise of a potent theory can stimulate development of many tools. This is the case with self-efficacy—the topic of chapter 2.

To participate in the modern practice of quality and outcomes improvement, the field will have to develop further instrumentation. For example, a wide range of age-appropriate instruments for pediatrics is needed, and few tools exist to measure the ability of patients to make informed decisions. The problem is perhaps more acute because the quality and accessibility of clinical information about patient education is commonly believed to be poor. Although new practices, such as clinical paths, help to assure some documentation, such approaches rarely document psychometrically based outcomes or enough about the character and length of the intervention to form the basis for improvement. In addition, we know little about whether the tools that exist reflect the outcomes of most importance to patients. The use of health quality-of-life scales is a step in that direction.

Finally, the serious work that must be done to assure culturally relevant measurement tools is hardly begun. Such relevance depends on understanding how different groups define functioning, quality of life and health, and using measurements that reflect these understandings. Lack of such tools seriously affects ability of health professionals to develop interpretations that can prevent disease, reduce disruption, disability, and cost that disease generates in the society as a whole (Clark & McLeroy, 1995).

MEASUREMENT CHARACTERISTICS

Detailed technical discussions of the development and testing of measurement tools is widely available from many sources (DeVellis, 1991; Gable & Wolf, 1993). A brief conceptual review is provided here.

Validity, the central concept in measurement, is an evaluative judgment about whether an interpretation of test scores or actions based on it, are adequately supported. It involves content relevance and representativeness (content validity); generalizability including across time and raters, traditionally thought of as reliability concerns; convergent pattern of correlations between measures of the same construct (convergent validity) and discriminant pattern of distinctness from measures of other constructs (discriminant validity); and lack of negative impact on individuals or groups deriving from a source of test invalidity. Population validity describes the ability to generalize results across subgroups and ecological validity across settings. Validity is, therefore, an integrative summary focused on the relationship between the evidence and the inferences drawn (Messick, 1995).

Thus, establishing validity has a judgmental element in first examining the adequacy of operational and conceptional definitions, and second in expert judging of adequacy of sampling from the content universe the test is meant to represent. This occurs before the test is administered. Validity also has an empirical element, which allows examination of how the items perform when they are administered to many individuals (300 or 5 to 10 subjects per item) representative of those in the target group (Gable & Wolf, 1993). Using too few subjects means that the patterns of covariation among the items may not be stable. Items should be highly intercorrelated, with high item-scale correlations, and show relatively high item variance with means close to the center of the range of possible scores (DeVellis, 1991).

Construct validation is an ongoing process of testing hypotheses about relationships of data from items or scales with other known instruments, with the theory on which the scale is based and with known groups showing that a scale can differentiate members of one group from another. Factor analysis is one method used to identify or verify within a given set of items subsets of those items that are clustered together by shared variation to form constructs or factors. Factor analysis may be exploratory or confirmatory to examine how the factors fit to the theory. The original pool of items is frequently three to four times as large as the final scale, with items removed as their measurement characteristics are known, to improve the final scale.

Cronbach's α is the most commonly used measure of internal consistency reliability; it is an indication of the proportion of variance in the scale scores that is attributable to the true score. A scale is internally consistent to the extent that its items are highly intercorrelated. An α of .65 to .70 is minimally acceptable for research, .70 to .80 is respectable, and .8 to .9 is good. Scales intended for individual diagnosis should have reliabilities in the middle .90s. More reliable scales increase statistical power for a given sample size relative to less reliable measures (DeVellis, 1991). Interrater and stability reliability measure the relationship between scores given by different raters or scores on the instrument at different periods. For knowledge tests, an overrepresentation of easy items will produce a ceiling effect, whereas overinclusion of difficult items will produce a floor effect. Generally, items with means too near to an extreme of the response range will have low variances (DeVellis, 1991).

Of particular importance for interventions such as patient education is the sensitivity of a measure—evidence that it detects an important change as a result of a treatment of known efficacy. Another characteristic, sensibility, refers to characteristics of an instrument that make it usable in a clinical setting (Rowe & Oxman, 1993). Sensibility includes comprehensibility, clarity and simplicity of questions, adequacy of instructions, ease of usage, applicability to the variety of patients with a particular problem, and acceptability to patients.

Cutoff scores are not commonly indicated for the instruments summarized in this book. Yet, for instruments with high enough reliability to influence decisions about individuals, such scores are implicitly used. A cutoff score or standard may be set using a combination of several methods, yet it is frequently finally judged by whether it is credible to the people who will be judged using it. The cutoff score (standard) first is based on the relationship between the test scores and a future criterion. It also may be based on the deliberations of several samples of judges in which they examine each item to identify the response options that a minimally competent examinee should be able to perform. The standard should differentiate masters from nonmasters in the subject matter of the test (Berk, 1986).

Before using instruments, it is always wise to check bibliographical sources for recent updates and revisions.

REFERENCES

Anderson, R. M., Funnell, M. M., Butler, P. M., Arnold, M. S., Fitzgerald, J. T., & Feste, C. C. (1995). Patient empowerment; results of a randomized controlled trial. *Diabetes Care, 18*, 943–949.

Berk, R. A. (1986). A consumer's guide to setting performance standards on criterion-referenced tests. *Review of Educational Research, 56*, 137–172.

Clark, N. M., & McLeroy, K. R. (1995). Creating capacity through health education: What we know and what we don't. *Health Education Quarterly, 22*, 273–289.

DeVellis, R. F. (1991). *Scale development: Theory and applications.* Newbury Park: Sage.

Devine, E. C. (1992). Effects of psychoeducational care with adult surgical patients: A theory-probing meta-analysis of intervention studies. In T. D. Cook et al. (Eds.), *Meta-analysis for explanation.* New York: Russell Sage Foundation.

Devine, E. C., & Reifschneider, E. (1995). A meta-analysis of the effects of psychoeducational care in adults with hypertension. *Nursing Research, 44*, 237–245.

Gable, R. K., & Wolf, M. B. (1993). *Instrument development in the affective domain.* Boston: Kluwer Academic.

Glasgow, R. E., & Osteen, V. L. (1992). Evaluating diabetes education: Are we measuring the most important outcomes? *Diabetes Care, 15*, 1423–1432.

Lang, N. M., & Marek, K. D. (1990). The classification of patient outcomes. *Journal of Professional Nursing, 6*, 158–163.

Messick, S. (1995). Validity of psychological assessment. *American Psychologist, 50*, 741–749.

Nightingale, S. L. (1995). Written patient information on prescription drugs: The evolution of government and voluntary programs in the United States. *International Journal of Technology Assessment in Health Care, 11*, 399–409.

Redman, B. (1996). *The practice of patient education.* St. Louis: Mosby–Year Book.

Rowe, B. H., & Oxman, A. D. (1993). An assessment of the sensibility of a quality-of-life instrument. *American Journal of Emergency Medicine, 11*, 374–380.

2

Measurement of Self-Efficacy and Quality of Life in Patient Education

Self-efficacy and quality of life are nontraditional measures applied to patient education. They represent different measurement issues for this field. Perceived self-efficacy (SE) refers to a belief in one's capability to organize and execute specific courses of action. There are many measures of self-efficacy (SE), some brief, which should be judged for their usefulness in capturing this important outcome for patient education. Although measures of health-related quality of life (HRQOL) are also numerous, many measure domains not likely to be affected by education.

SELF-EFFICACY

Research accumulating over the past 30 thirty years shows that across many behaviors, SE is a potent predictor of important outcomes. Indeed, the total effect of SE on health behaviors is believed to exceed the effects of any single variable (Schwarzer, 1992). Efficacy beliefs influence behavior through their effects on behavioral choice, effort expenditure, distress response to taxing conditions, and persistence in the face of difficulties. Anxiety and stress reactions are low when people cope with tasks in their perceived SE range. People tend to avoid activities they believe exceed their efficacy (Bandura, 1989).

Assessment of SE involves asking individuals to rate their ability to perform a particular behavior along some graded dimension of task difficulty, such as number of repetitions or closeness to an ideal criterion. Although a general SE trait may operate in human behavior, Bandura (1989) maintains that measures of SE must be specific to the stressful event and its attendant behaviors to allow precise study of interventions designed to enhance coping in potentially aversive situations.

Routine use of these measures can help to identify individuals who, even though they are skilled, may lack the confidence to undertake behaviors critical to their treatment. Crippling anxiety that yields avoidant behaviors reflects an assessment that the individual cannot manage threatening events—a lack of SE. It is also important to know how extensive an intervention is necessary to create adequate levels of SE—for example, is a special exercise program important, or will individuals attain adequate SE simply by resumption of usual daily activities?

The elements known to develop SE can be incorporated into patient education interventions. Successfully accomplishing the behavior, positive persuasion informing the patient about his capabilities, helping the patient to accurately interpret the physical feelings that accompany performance activities, and vicarious experiences with others, all provide sources of efficacy information. This information must be selected, weighed, and integrated by the individual into a judgment. Likewise, over time, repeated failure takes an increasing toll on perceived SE and beliefs about how much environmental control is possible.

Two examples may be helpful in understanding how SE may be built into education programs. In a self-management program, Lorig and Gonzalez (1992) used persons with arthritis to teach others and thus to serve as models. Data from clinical studies indicate that more than one half of the variance in early labor pain and about one third of the variance in active labor pain may be explained by the single variable of maternal confidence in the ability to cope. This confidence has been found to be significantly increased by childbirth education (Lowe, 1991). It is also possible for educational programs to be so poorly designed that the conditions necessary to developing strong feelings of SE would not be present.

Ewart (1992) describes the role of SE theory in interventions to aid individuals recovering from acute myocardial infarction or coronary artery bypass graft (CABG). In both instances, many problem behavioral and emotional reactions stem from uncertainties about one's physical capabilities. Patients who have undergone CABG tend to interpret chest wall pain as ischemic; they may abandon prescribed exercises unless they are counseled on how to interpret those exercise-induced sensations that are without cardiac importance. There is remarkably consistent evidence that SE appraisals are superior to functional exercise evaluation in predicting exercise adherence.

Measurement issues discussed in chapter 1 must be applied to SE. Even a short-term measurement of test-retest reliability may be inappropriate because it is theorized that SE is not expected to be a stable trait. Some SE measures also measure outcome expectations based on the notion that such expectations make SE more likely.

SE scales vary on three dimensions: (a) magnitude, referring to the level of difficulty of the behavior and commonly measured on scales of 0 to 10 or 0 to 100; (b) generality, referring to the number of domains of behavior in which individuals judge themselves to be efficacious and over time; and (c) strength, referring to the confidence individuals have in the attainment of a specific task and usually assessed by tasks graded as to level of impediment. Conceptual analysis of the domain of functioning is important to determine the competencies involved and the barriers and challenges one will have to manage. For example, perceptions of efficacy for maintaining a low-calorie diet may decrease when only fast foods are available. Conditions internal to the individual can also challenge perceptions of efficacy—conditions of depression, loneliness, or intoxication. An understanding of these barriers requires interviews with members of the target population. Diagnosis is more useful when efficacy beliefs are measured for each of the competencies involved (Maibach & Murphy, 1995). A threshold of efficacy strength may be required to even attempt a course of action.

Although SE is not the only psychological factor that may impact health outcomes, the importance of this element is underscored by the numerous studies that show its effect on health behavior. It also is alterable.

HEALTH-RELATED QUALITY OF LIFE

All illnesses require adaptation by patients and their families. Although there is a common set of constraints, such as decreased physical and role functioning, each illness has its own specific variations of adaptive challenges. Many HRQOL measures are constructed for a particular disease entity.

Although it is relatively recent that HRQOL has been perceived to have substantial potential as an end point in health, this perception is likely to expand as more toxic treatments are used. HRQOL is an organizing concept that brings together a set of domains related to the physical, functional, psychological, and social health of the individual (Testa & Nackley, 1994). Quality of life (QOL) is best understood as representing the gap between one's actual functional level and one's ideal standard. It is variously described in several domains.

1. *Physical well-being*. Perceived and observed bodily function or disruption—a combination of disease symptoms, treatment side effects, and general physical well-being as perceived by the patient.
2. *Functional well-being*. One's ability to perform the activities related to one's personal needs, ambitions, or social roles.
3. *Emotional well-being*.
4. *Social well-being*. Perceived social support, maintenance of leisure activities, and family functioning (Cella, 1994).

The best understood application of QOL measures is in clinical trials, as evidence of the effects of different interventions including evaluation of pharmaceutical agents and, more controversially, in allocation of resources. Their performance is impressive. For example, QOL measures have been shown in trials to be better than conventional rheumatological measures as predictors of long-term outcomes in rheumatoid arthritis, in terms of both morbidity and mortality. They can, therefore, be used to identify patients needing particular attention, to screen for psychosocial problems, to monitor patients' progress or to determine choice of treatment (Fitzpatrick et al., 1992).

Use of HRQOL as a primary end point is especially important when palliation of disease symptoms or improvement of patient functioning or a sense of patient control is the primary goal of treatment; that is the case, for example, in joint replacement surgery, management of psychiatric disorders, and pharmacological management of asthma and epilepsy. Such use can lead to design of interventions specifically to enhance HRQOL (Fitzpatrick & Albrecht, 1994).

For the most part, HRQOL measures are not currently used in routine individual patient care (Fitzpatrick & Albrecht, 1994), perhaps, in part, because reliability standards for individual assessment are rarely met with HRQOL tools (Hays, Anderson, & Revicki, 1993). Although all HRQOL measures must be evaluated in terms of their ability to capture important clinical changes in patient functioning, this is typically the last property of a scale to be evaluated because it involves longitudinal follow-up.

QOL Measures and Patient Education

Traditionally, evaluation of diabetes education programs, as an example, has focused on knowledge and on physiological outcomes. Tilly (1995) added QOL measures to evaluation of the Diabetes Day Care Program, an educational intervention using an individual education plan, as part of an outcomes management program. The evaluation showed clinically and statistically significant improvement in glycemic control as well as in frequency of diabetes-related symptoms, serving as a measure of diabetes-related QOL. The pre-post design precluded strong evidence that the program was the cause.

In care of persons with cancer (Grant et al., 1990), HRQOL measurements revealed vulnerable periods for those undergoing specific treatments, signaling need for interventions geared toward relief of physical and psychological distress.

Recent research found no correlation between measures of glycemic control and HRQOL at a single point or longitudinally, for patients with non–insulin-dependent diabetes mellitus. Such a finding may help to explain the difficulty some patients have in achieving good glycemic control. Because good control does not enhance HRQOL in the short term, patients may be unwilling to follow complex and intrusive regimens that do not appear to improve their health status (Weinberger et al., 1994).

For this book, the author has chosen from among many HRQOL measures one with domains more directly amenable to impact from patient education. Ingersoll's Diabetes QOL for Youths measures domains of disease impact, disease worries, and life satisfaction, all open to educational effects. Domains such as physical health, mental health, social health, and mobility may be affected by learning how to optimize functioning in these domains but may also be more heavily affected by medical treatment.

Questions About Measurement

There are several measurement problems with HRQOL. For example, little is known about the relative importance of the major dimensions, and it is assumed that by aggregating measures of physical, functional, emotional and social well-being, one can approximate a single index of QOL (Cella, 1994). For many uses of HRQOL measures, sensitivity to change is important. Longer, generic HRQOL instruments that are meant to cross disease entities may include several items not relevant to the particular disease or treatment group for a set of patients. Some items may be static and not a feasible target for the health care intervention, or there may be floor or ceiling effects (Fitzpatrick et al., 1992). Thus, these instruments may not be sensitive to change; yet, sensitivity of a QOL measure to changes in disease state and treatment phase are likely to be important.

HRQOL measures may be specific to a disease; a population of patients, such as the elderly; certain functions, such as sexual; or a given problem, such as pain. General measures have the advantage of picking up unforseen side effects unrelated to the target condition and can be used for comparison across conditions (Guyatt, 1993). Personalized versions, where a person creates his or her own domains, appear to be more sensitive to patients' overall judgment of change than do conventionally formatted questionnaires (Fitzpatrick & Albrecht, 1994). Because many scales are not completely linear, a change of two units on the low end of the scale is rarely equivalent to a change of two units at the high end of the scale (Lydick & Epstein, 1993).

There is no reference standard for HRQOL. Therefore, one looks for evidence that scores bear a close relationship to change in the patient's global ratings of change, and for symptoms, such as dyspnea, to the patient's ability to function (Guyatt, 1993). The minimal important difference is the smallest difference in score that patients perceive as beneficial and would mandate, in the absence of troublesome side effects and excessive costs, a change in the patient's management. Information about the performance of these instruments across cultural groups is usually not available (Juniper, Guyatt, Willan, & Griffith, 1994).

Interrater reliability is not likely to be relevant because a proxy would not know about an individual's well-being. Test-retest reliability also may not be relevant because one expects change in HRQOL over time.

REFERENCES

Bandura, A. (1989). Human agency in social cognitive theory. *American Psychologist, 44*, 1175–1184.

Cella, D. F. (1994). Quality of life: Concepts and definition. *Journal of Pain and Symptom Management, 9*, 186–192.

Ewart, C. K. (1992). Role of physical self-efficacy in recovery from heart attack. In R. Schwarzer (Ed.), *Self-efficacy: Thought control of action.* Washington, DC: Hemisphere.

Fitzpatrick, R., & Albrecht, G. (1994). The plausibility of quality-of-life measures in different domains of health care. In L. Nordenfelt (Ed.), *Concepts and measurement of quality of life in health care.* Boston: Kluwer Academic.

Fitzpatrick, R., Flethcer, A., Gore, S., Jones, D., Spiegelhalter, D., & Cox, D. (1992). Quality of life measures in health care: 1. Applications and issues in assessment. *British Medical Journal, 305*, 1074–1077.

Grant, M., Padilla, G. V., Ferrell, B. R., & Rhiner, M. (1990). Assessment of quality of life with a single instrument. *Seminars in Oncology Nursing, 6*, 260–270.

Guyatt, G. H. (1993). Measurement of health-related quality of life in heart failure. *Journal of the American College of Cardiology, 22*(Suppl. A), 185A–191A.

Hays, R. D., Anderson, R., & Revicki, E. (1993). Psychometric considerations in evaluating health-related quality of life measures. *Quality of Life Research, 2*, 441–449.

Juniper, E. F., Guyatt, G. H., Willan, A., & Griffith, L. E. (1994). Determining a minimal important change in a disease-specific quality of life questionnaire. *Journal of Clinical Epidemiology, 47*, 81–87.

Lorig, K., & Gonzalez, V. (1992). The integration of theory with practice: A 12-year case study. *Health Education Quarterly, 19*, 355–368.

Lowe, N. K. (1991). Maternal confidence in coping with labor: A self-efficacy concept. *Journal of Obstetric, Gynecological, and Neonatal Nursing, 20*, 457–463.

Lydick, E., & Epstein, R. S. (1993). Interpretation of quality of life changes. *Quality of Life Research, 2*, 221–226.

Maibach, E., & Murphy, D. A. (1995). Self-efficacy in health promotion research and practice: Conceptualization and measurement. *Health Education Research, 10*, 37–50.

Schwarzer, R. (1992). *Self-efficacy: Thought control of action.* Washington, DC: Hemisphere.

Testa, M. A., & Nackley, J. F. (1994). Methods for quality-of-life studies. *Annual Review of Public Health, 15*, 535–539.

Tilly, K. F., Belton, A. B., & McLachlan, J. F. C. (1995). Continuous monitoring of health status outcomes: Experience with a diabetes education program. *The Diabetes Educator, 21*, 413–419.

Weinberger, M., Kirkman, M. S., Samsa, G. P., Cowper, P. A., Shortliffe, E. A., Simel, D. L., & Feussner, J. R. (1994). The relationship between glycemic control and health-related quality of life in patients with non-insulin-dependent diabetes mellitus. *Medical Care, 32*, 1173–1181.

II

Description of Tools

Each review is organized around a common framework of (a) description, administration, and scoring guidelines; (b) psychometric properties; and (c) critique and summary, and references. The reader should keep in mind the standards for psychometric properties described in chapter 1: the variety of kinds of evidence about validity including the number of participants used, levels of reliability needed for various kinds of uses for the instrument, and evidence of sensitivity to a patient education intervention.

A

Basic Patient Education Needs

3

Patient Learning Needs Scale

Developed by Susan Galloway, Natalie Bubela, Elizabeth McCay, Ann McKibbon, Eleanor Ross, and Lynn Nagle

INSTRUMENT DESCRIPTION, ADMINISTRATION, AND SCORING GUIDELINES

The Patient Learning Needs Scale (PLNS) is designed to measure patients' perceptions of learning needs to manage their health care at home, at time of discharge from hospital to home for a medical or surgical illness. PLNS requires less than 20 minutes to complete. It yields a total score of 40 to 200, with higher scores indicating more importance placed on having discharge information. Individual factor scores may also be calculated. Because the PLNS subscales are composed of an unequal number of questions, percentage means are calculated for subscale scores. A community version asks people who are at home how important each item was to learn about before discharge (Galloway et al., n.d.). In nearly all of the published work on the PLNS, an earlier version was used, with 50 items scored 0 to 5 and 7 subscales, making numerical comparison of scores and items with the present scale difficult.

PSYCHOMETRIC PROPERTIES

Development and initial evaluation of the scale was based on responses of 301 adults hospitalized with medical or surgical illnesses. Items developed from patient interviews were reviewed by nurses, doctors, patients, and healthy nonhospitalized individuals to check for item clarity, representativeness of what one needed to know to manage their own care at home, and ease or difficulty in completion of the items (Bubela et al., 1990).

Factor analysis showed five clinically meaningful factors.

1. Support and care in the community, defined as knowledge about negotiating the health care system, recognizing and obtaining intrapersonal support, and performing preventive skin care (items 17, 31,13, 32, 12, 27, 22, 10, 33, 29, with a Cronbach's α of .91)
2. Medications, defined as the knowledge required to understand and administer medications (items 35 to 37, 4, 25, 39, 6, 26, with a Cronbach's α of .90)

3. Treatment and activities of living, defined as knowledge about treatment, and guidelines for physical activity, nutrition, and sleep (items 24, 18, 2, 28, 30, 20, 38, 23, with an α of .85)
4. Complications and symptoms, defined as information needed to form expectations about the illness impact, and the specific information needs around recognition and management of symptoms and complications (items 8, 11, 3, 5, 21, 34, 7, 9, with an α of .82)
5. Illness-related concerns, defined as how to communicate about illness and how to manage in areas, such as hygiene, rest, and elimination problems (items 15, 40, 19, 1, 14, 16, with an α of .76). Total scale α is .95 (Galloway et al., n.d.).

In another study, PLNS total scale α was .97, with .80 to .90 for the subscales (Galloway, Bubela, McKibbon, McCay, & Ross, 1993). Convergent validity was supported by the finding that patients who perceived more uncertainty in their illness experience placed more importance on health-related information 48 hours before going home (Galloway & Graydon, 1996). It has not been possible to examine concurrent validity as there has been no parallel instrument available (Galloway et al., n.d.).

CRITIQUE AND SUMMARY

PLNS results can help health professionals focus the scope and content of educational interventions, especially because acutely ill individuals have neither the physiological stability nor the cognitive energy to learn about care at home until near the time of discharge. Length of time spent in the hospital, number of discharge medications, and patient perception of the influence of the illness on his life were positively correlated with information needs at the time of discharge. Number of medications may be an indirect indicator of the severity of problems faced by the individual or may hinder mental processing of information (Bubela & Galloway, 1990). Several studies with different populations in different countries (Bostrom, Crawford-Swent, Lazar, & Helmer, 1994; Bubela et al., 1990; Galloway, Bubela, McKibbon, McCay, & Ross, 1993) have found that medications, treatments and complications, and enhancing quality of life (symptom management) were consistently identified as most important discharge learning needs.

Although the scale will elicit the area of discharge information that is important, it does not delineate the specific content that might satisfy the learning need (Galloway et al., n.d.). For identification of gaps in existing discharge programs, subjects may be asked for each item if the information has been given and the satisfaction with the information provided. It would be useful to study the relationship between timely identification of learning needs by PLNS, adequate meeting of these needs, and the quality of life during recovery. The PLNS has been used to study nurse- and patient-initiated call systems of follow-up after hospitalization. Mean scores for each factor on the PLNS by kind of follow-up may be found in the article by Bostrom, Caldwell, McGuide, and Everson (1996).

REFERENCES

Bostrom, J., Caldwell, J., McGuire, K., & Everson, D. (1996). Telephone follow-up after discharge from the hospital: Does it make a difference? *Applied Nursing Research, 9,* 47–52.

Bostrom, J., Crawford-Swent, C., Lazar, N., & Helmer, D. (1994). Learning needs of hospitalized and recently discharged patients. *Patient Education and Counseling, 23,* 83–89.

Bubela, N., & Galloway, S. (1990). Factors influencing patients' informational needs at time of hospital discharge. *Patient Education and Counseling, 16,* 21–28.

Bubela, N., Galloway, S., McCay, E., McKibbon, A., Nagle, L., Pringle, D., Ross, E., & Shamian, J. (1990). The Patient Learning Needs Scale: Reliability and validity. *Journal of Advanced Nursing, 15,* 1181–1187.

Galloway, S., Bubela, N., McCay, E., McKibbon, A., Ross, E., & Nagle, L. (n.d.). *Patient Learning Need Scale: Description and administration guidelines.* Authors.

Galloway, S. C., Bubela, N., McKibbon, A., McCay, E., & Ross, E. (1993). Perceived information needs and effect of symptoms on activities after surgery for lung cancer. *Canadian Oncology Nursing Journal, 3,* 116–119.

Galloway, S. C., & Graydon, J. E. (1996). Uncertainty, symptom distress, and information needs after surgery for cancer of the colon. *Cancer Nursing, 19,* 112–117.

PATIENT LEARNING NEED SCALE

Introduction for Hospital Administration

At hospital discharge, many people have some questions about how to manage once they are at home. Different people have questions about different things. The following is a list of things which some people like to know in order to care for themselves at home. For each item indicate how important it is for *you* to learn about before going home.

Introduction for Community Administration

Many people who are leaving the hospital have some questions about how to manage their care at home. Different people have questions about different things. The following is a list of things which may be important to know about to be able to care for yourself at home. Now that you are at home, please rate how important you now think each item is to learn about before hospital discharge.

Please rate how important each item is to know about before going home.

1 = not important
2 = slightly important
3 = moderately important
4 = very important
5 = extremely important

In order to manage my care at home it is important for me to know:

1.	What to do if I have trouble urinating.	1 2 3 4 5
2.	How to prepare the foods I am to eat.	1 2 3 4 5
3.	How to prevent a complication from occurring.	1 2 3 4 5
4.	How to take each medication.	1 2 3 4 5
5.	What symptoms I may have related to my illness.	1 2 3 4 5
6.	When to take each medication.	1 2 3 4 5
7.	How this illness will affect my life.	1 2 3 4 5
8.	How to recognize a complication.	1 2 3 4 5
9.	How this illness will affect my future.	1 2 3 4 5
10.	How to care for my feet properly.	1 2 3 4 5
11.	What complications might occur from my illness.	1 2 3 4 5
12.	How to recognize my feelings toward my illness.	1 2 3 4 5
13.	How to contact community groups for my health condition.	1 2 3 4 5
14.	When I can take a bath or a shower.	1 2 3 4 5
15.	How to talk to family/friends about my illness.	1 2 3 4 5
16.	How much rest I should be getting.	1 2 3 4 5
17.	How to get through the ''red tape'' in the health care system.	1 2 3 4 5
18.	What the possible side effects of my treatment are.	1 2 3 4 5
19.	What to do if I have trouble with my bowels.	1 2 3 4 5
20.	What to do if I cannot sleep properly.	1 2 3 4 5
21.	How to manage the symptoms I may experience.	1 2 3 4 5
22.	How I can avoid stress.	1 2 3 4 5
23.	What physical exercise I should be getting.	1 2 3 4 5
24.	What the purposes of my treatment are.	1 2 3 4 5
25.	Why I need to take each medication.	1 2 3 4 5
26.	Where I can get my medication.	1 2 3 4 5
27.	Where I can get help in handling my feelings about my illness.	1 2 3 4 5

1 = not important
2 = slightly important
3 = moderately important
4 = very important
5 = extremely important

28.	Which foods I can and cannot eat.	1 2 3 4 5
29.	How to prevent my skin from getting red.	1 2 3 4 5
30.	Which vitamins and supplements I should take.	1 2 3 4 5
31.	How to get through the "red tape" to get services at home.	1 2 3 4 5
32.	Who to talk to about my concerns about death.	1 2 3 4 5
33.	How to prevent my skin from getting sore.	1 2 3 4 5
34.	How to manage my pain.	1 2 3 4 5
35.	When to stop taking each medication.	1 2 3 4 5
36.	How each medication works.	1 2 3 4 5
37.	What to do if I have a reaction to a medication.	1 2 3 4 5
38.	What physical activities I cannot do such as lifting.	1 2 3 4 5
39.	The possible reactions to each medication.	1 2 3 4 5
40.	Where I can get help for family to deal with my illness.	1 2 3 4 5

Used with permission: Galloway, S., Bubela, N., McCay, E., McKibbon, A., Ross, E., & Nagle, L.

4

Constructed Meaning Scale: Measuring Adaptation to Serious Illness

Developed by Betsy L. Fife

INSTRUMENT DESCRIPTION, ADMINISTRATION, AND SCORING GUIDELINES

The construction of meaning is a central aspect of adaptation to serious illness. The concept of meaning commonly refers to the relationship between individuals and their world as well as to individuals' unique perceptions of their place within that world. It encompasses the individual's perceptions of her ability to accomplish future goals; to maintain the viability of interpersonal relationships; and to sustain a sense of personal vitality, competence, and power. It is these perceptions that give a sense of coherence to life in the face of loss, change, and personal upheaval (Fife, 1994a).

Because serious illness imposes irrevocable change that totally disrupts the continuity of everyday life, individuals are forced to rapidly redefine the meanings they have assumed as fact in the routine of living. Structures of meaning are cumulative learned phenomena; in the case of an event, partially the outcome of an attributional search for the cause of the event; and also a method of obtaining cognitive control. The Constructed Meaning Scale is based in the theoretical framework of symbolic interactionism. Because it is expected that the construction of meaning may influence future behavior, such a scale would be used to assess how the individual's perceptions of identity and social world have been affected by the illness, and would serve as a clinical marker of the quality of adaptation persons will be able to achieve (Fife, 1994a).

The scale is scored using the values on the questionnaire, reversing the scoring of items as necessary so that the most positive response is given a value of 4 (B. L. Fife, personal communication, February, 1996). The highest possible score on the scale, 32, is indicative of the most positive meaning, whereas the lowest score of 8 indicates a negative sense of the meaning.

PSYCHOMETRIC PROPERTIES

Data from which the scale was developed were gathered by interview from 38 White persons diagnosed as having cancer. Three specific changes in self-meaning emerged: loss of personal control, threats to self-esteem or -worth, and changes in body image (Fife, 1994a).

Studies of reliability and validity of the scale have been carried out with 422 persons diagnosed as having cancer. Nine percent were Black, and 12% were of low socioeconomic status. Items were based on and supported by data obtained from persons living with cancer and on symbolic interactionist theory, supporting content validity. Construct validity (extent to which the scale performed in accordance with theoretical expectations) was empirically supported in several ways.

1. Individuals newly diagnosed with nonmetastatic cancer or those in first remission were more likely to construct a positive meaning about their illness than did those with a first recurrence or those with metastatic disease. The scale did distinguish between these groups (mean scores in these groups range from 20.8 to 23.6).
2. Prior research suggests that the construction of meaning and emotional response would be correlated. This was the case with more positive meaning associated with the positive poles of the various emotional response dimensions, such as composed-anxious, elated-depressed, agreeable-hostile, energetic-tired, clearheaded-confused, and confident-unsure.
3. Social support from family, friends and professionals was predictive of meaning—the greater the support, the more positive the meaning about the implications of the illness for patients' lives.
4. Use of denial and positive focusing was associated with development of a more positive meaning about the illness, whereas the use of avoidance was strongly related to the construction of negative meaning.
5. Formulation of meaning was associated with an attempt to develop a sense of control or mastery (Fife, 1995).
6. In a study of 125 men and 206 women with various forms of cancer, the more positive the meaning, the more positive the adjustment (Fife, 1994b).

Item-total correlations ranged from .5 and .72, with all coefficients significant, providing support for the existence of homogeneity within the scale. Cronbach's α was .81. Factor analysis showed that each item in the scale contributed to the primary factor (Fife, 1995).

CRITIQUE AND SUMMARY

So far, use of the tool has been limited to research and those with cancer; this work should be extended to those with other threatening or debilitating diseases. Because construction of meaning is specific to the experience with a particular disease, norms would likely be different for other diseases. Beginning work has also been done on use of the scale within the dyad of patient and partner, showing that communication within the dyad was significantly associated with the development of meaning for partners but not for patients. Extension of this work should prove helpful in understanding how to care for partners as well as for patients (Germino, Fife, & Funk, 1995).

This scale appears to have been developed and used with populations not as diverse as those with which it might be used. Further work is necessary to support validity, increase reliability, and study its sensitivity to interventions. The Constructed Meaning Scale addresses an important construct central to both the theory and practice of health care.

REFERENCES

Fife, B. L. (1994a). The conceptualization of meaning in illness. *Social Science and Medicine, 38,* 309–316.

Fife, B. L. (1994b). Gender differences and adjustment to cancer. *Research in Sociology of Health Care, 11,* 107–125.

Fife, B. L. (1995). The measurement of meaning in illness. *Social Science and Medicine, 40,* 1021–1028.

Germino, B. B., Fife, B. L., & Funk, S. G. (1995). Cancer and the partner relationship: What is its meaning? *Seminars in Oncology Nursing, 11,* 43–50.

CONSTRUCTED MEANING SCALE

Directions:

The items below ask how you see your life being affected by your illness. *Circle* the number that best describes how you have been feeling about your life during the *past two weeks*.

		Strongly Agree	Agree	Disagree	Strongly Disagree
1.	I feel my illness is something I will never recover from.	1	2	3	4
2.	I feel my illness is serious, but I will be able to return to life as it was before my illness.	1	2	3	4
3.	I feel my illness has changed my life permanently so it will never be as good again.	1	2	3	4
4.	I feel I have made a complete recovery from my illness.	1	2	3	4
5.	I feel that I am the same person as I was before my illness.	1	2	3	4
6.	I feel that my relationships with other people have not been negatively affected by my illness.	1	2	3	4
7.	I feel that my illness experience has made me a better or stronger person.	1	2	3	4
8.	I feel my illness has permanently interfered with my achievement of the most important goals I have set for myself.	1	2	3	4

5

Child Attitude Toward Illness Scale

Developed by Joan K. Austin

INSTRUMENT DESCRIPTION, ADMINISTRATION, AND SCORING GUIDELINES

Research has indicated that children with chronic illness are at risk for development of behavior problems, poor self-concept, and social withdrawal. The Child Attitude Toward Illness Scale (CATIS) is designed to provide systematic assessment of how favorably or unfavorably children feel about having a chronic physical condition. Initial items were generated from results of past research. To date, the tool has been used with children of middle-class background, 8 to 12 years of age, with asthma or epilepsy (Austin & Huberty, 1993).

The conceptual framework undergirding CATIS is family stress theory. Negative feelings can contribute to the stressors already placed on the family by the child's illness and positive feelings as a resource to help the family successfully adapt to the illness. Most research on adaptation to childhood chronic illness has focused on parents' perceptions and feelings about their children's illness and has failed to include perceptions from the children. Yet children who have negative feelings are more likely to engage in maladaptive coping behaviors and subsequently have a more negative adaptation to the condition than children who have positive feelings about having a chronic illness. Children's feelings are thought to be especially important when the condition has an attached stigma, such as epilepsy (Austin & Huberty, 1993).

The scale in the form for administration may be seen on the following page. The chronic condition is placed in the blank area (e.g., asthma or seizures). Ratings are on 5-point scales. Items 1, 2, 4, 5, 7, 9, 11, and 13 are reverse scored. Scores on each item are then summed and divided by 13 (Austin & Huberty, 1993). A more positive score reflects a more positive attitude toward the condition (Austin, Smith, Risinger, & McNelis, 1994). Children with epilepsy had a mean score of 3.2, whereas those with asthma had a mean score of 3.4 (Austin & Huberty, 1993).

PSYCHOMETRIC PROPERTIES

Initial studies showed an internal consistency reliability of .8 (coefficient α), with item-total correlations ranging between .27 and .59, and test-retest reliability of .8. Confirmatory factor analysis results supported one unitary construct in the scale. In a follow-up study of 136 children with epilepsy and 133 with asthma, CATIS scores were significantly negatively correlated with school absences, anxiety, intensifying behavior problems, and depression, and significantly positively correlated with happiness, satisfaction, and self-concept scores. Attitude scores and self-concept scores were also positively correlated. These relationships lend support for construct validity of the CATIS for the measurement of children's attitudes toward having a chronic health condition (Austin & Huberty, 1993).

CRITIQUE AND SUMMARY

CATIS is a short self-report scale to be used in the clinical setting to assess children's attitudes about having a chronic condition, as a starting point for discussion of their feelings. It could also be used to evaluate whether educational programs designed to help groups of children cope with chronic conditions change these feelings (Austin & Huberty, 1993). These studies represent initial work in development of the scale. Cross-validation is needed with different samples of chronically ill children to determine if the findings are valid and reliable for these samples. CATIS was originally developed for use in research; with further development, it appears to have potential for use in the clinical setting (Austin & Huberty, 1993).

Traditionally, treatment of childhood epilepsy has emphasized neurological aspects over psychosocial factors, with seizure frequency considered the most important clinical outcome. Yet children with this condition have a high prevalence of behavior and learning problems not strongly correlated with seizure variables. The results of these studies indicate need for programs that prevent development of these problems for children with epilepsy (Austin et al., 1994).

REFERENCES

Austin, J. K., & Huberty, T. J. (1993). Development of the Child Attitude Toward Illness Scale. *Journal of Pediatric Psychology, 18,* 467–480.

Austin, J. K., Smith, M. S., Risinger, M. W., & McNelis, A. M. (1994). Childhood epilepsy and asthma: Comparison of quality of life. *Epilepsia, 35,* 608–615.

CHILD ATTITUDE TOWARD ILLNESS SCALE (CATIS)

Here are 13 questions that ask about you and your feelings. Read each one carefully. If there is anything that you do not understand, please ask us about it. For each question, put a check mark ✓ above the response that best describes your feelings. Answer *every* question even if some are hard to decide, but check only *one* answer. There are no right or wrong answers. Only *you* can tell us how you feel, so we hope that you will mark the way you *really* feel inside.

---

1. How good or bad do you feel it is that you have _____ ?

    | Very Good | A Little Good | Not Sure | A Little Bad | Very Bad | |

2. How fair is it that you have _____ ?

    | Very Fair | A Little Fair | Not Sure | A Little Unfair | Very Unfair | |

3. How happy or sad is it for you to have _____ ?

    | Very Sad | A Little Sad | Not Sure | A Little Happy | Very Happy | |

4. How bad or good do you feel it is to have _____ ?

    | Very Good | A Little Good | Not Sure | A Little Bad | Very Bad | |

5. How often do you feel that your _____ is your fault?

    | Never | Not Often | Sometimes | Often | Very Often | |

6. How often do you feel that your _____ keeps you from doing things you like to do?

    | Very Often | Often | Sometimes | Not Often | Never | |

7. How often do you feel that you will always be sick?

    | Never | Not Often | Sometimes | Often | Very Often | |

8. How often do you feel that your _____ keeps you from starting new things?

    | Very Often | Often | Sometimes | Not Often | Never | |

9.   How often do you feel different from others because of your _____?

| Never | Not Often | Sometimes | Often | Very Often | _____ |

10.   How often do you feel bad because you have _____ ?

| Very Often | Often | Sometimes | Not Often | Never | _____ |

11.   How often do you feel sad about being sick?

| Never | Not Often | Sometimes | Often | Very Often | _____ |

12.   How often do you feel happy even though you have _____ ?

| Never | Not Often | Sometimes | Often | Very Often | _____ |

13.   How often do you feel just as good as other kids your age even though you have _____ ?

| Very Often | Often | Sometimes | Not Often | Never | _____ |

6

Bernier Instructional Design Scale

Developed by Mary Jane Bernier

INSTRUMENT DESCRIPTION, ADMINISTRATION, AND SCORING GUIDELINES

Printed educational materials (PEMS) are among the most economical and frequently used methods for educating individuals about health matters. They are portable, reusable, and permanent. Patient educators are often frustrated by the lack of quality control in PEMS that are available (Bernier, 1993a).

The literature in patient education indicates that little evaluation of actual learning outcomes is carried out by the developers or users of PEMs. So, although congruence between desired outcomes as specified by PEM developers and the actual learning achieved by the target population represents the ultimate measure of quality in a PEM, the author seeks to develop an alternative way to evaluate them—through expert consensus of important characteristics of PEMs. Criteria were selected from the literature, and a convenience sample of 11 individuals with experience in development of patient education materials was used as a consensus group. The criteria include primarily content and format issues, clustered by phase of development (Bernier & Yasko, 1991).

PSYCHOMETRIC PROPERTIES

Results of the pilot study described previously established the basis for evaluating the content validity of an evaluation of a patient education materials instrument. A pilot test of the Bernier Instructional Design Scale (BIDS) was conducted by four master's-prepared nurses who applied the BIDS to a test PEM individually and then met to discuss their ratings. Eighty-nine members of a patient education committee and graduate nursing students at a university medical center established interrater reliability for the BIDS by applying the scale to the test PEM that was used in the pilot study. The interrater agreement was only 40% and on replication 65%, both below desirable levels. Other forms of validity were not addressed, pending achieving more adequate levels of reliability (Bernier, 1993b).

CRITIQUE AND SUMMARY

Work is under way to simplify the measurement scale and to include persons with backgrounds in instructional design and learning theory. Further study is required before the instrument can be used as an empirical referent for exploring relationships between instructional design quality and achievement of patient learning outcomes (Bernier, 1993b).

The assumption that expert opinion about the criteria used in creating PEMs influences the quality of the product and subsequent learning outcomes (Bernier & Yasko, 1991) is open to question. A preferred alternative would be criteria weighted by the balance of the research evidence undergirding them as effective in creating learning outcomes in patients. Such an instrument could be of considerable use if it improved the efficiency and effectiveness of educational materials.

No norms or sample scores were provided. Presumably, scores could be used in a couple of ways: (a) alternative PEMs could be rated and the one with the highest score chosen for use, and (b) the score level most highly related to the best learning outcomes could be established empirically and then used as a basis for choosing a PEM. Because interrater reliability has been a problem, it would be essential to check that and, if low, ask raters to discuss items on which their ratings disagree.

A tool designed for the same purposes as is the PEM (design, use, and level of educational materials) but more focused on a public/community health perspective, may be found in Rice and Valdivia (1991).

REFERENCES

Bernier, M. J., & Yasko, J. (1991). Designing and evaluating printed educational materials: Model and instrument development. *Patient Education and Counseling, 18,* 253–263.

Bernier, M. J. (1993a). Developing and evaluating printed education materials: A prescriptive model for quality. *Orthopaedic Nursing, 12*(6), 39–46.

Bernier, M. J. (1993b). *Patient education in nursing: Development of a scale to evaluate the instructional design quality of printed educational materials.* Pittsburgh: University of Pittsburgh.

Rice, M., & Valdivia, L. (1991). A simple guide for design, use and evaluation of educational materials. *Health Education Quarterly, 18,* 79–85.

THE BERNIER INSTRUCTIONAL DESIGN SCALE (BIDS)
(REVISED, JUNE 1993)

The instructional design principles contained in the BIDS are presented in the format of a rating checklist to facilitate the rating of the printed education materials (PEMs) that are used with patients/families. Please begin the rating procedure by reading each instructional design principle contained on the BIDS. Then read the PEM(s) that you wish to evaluate. Use the BIDS to record your rating of the level of the instructional design principles that are present in the PEM by making a check in the appropriate column. Space is provided at the bottom of each page for rater comments regarding special problems or difficulty in applying the instructional design principles to the PEM.

THE RATING SCALE:
  0   = NOT MET
  1   = PARTIALLY MET
  2   = MET
 NA = NOT APPLICABLE

EXAMPLE: Instructional design principle #2 states, "The font or print size can be read easily by the target group." A PEM that is written in a print size as small as this print (font 9) would not be appropriate for a general target audience since the readers would be of many age groups and some would have difficulty reading this print. The appropriate rating for PEM text written in the 9 font would be 0 = NOT MET if the PEM was intended to be used by a general audience. The 35 instructional design principles of the BIDS are listed below.

PRINCIPLE: *SCALE:*

		0	1	2	NA
1.	There is sufficient contrast between the ink and paper to make reading easy.	—	—	—	—
2.	The font or print size can be read easily by the target audience. (This is an example of a 14-point font; this is a 12-point font which is the minimum font recommended for the general public.)	—	—	—	—
3.	The type style is legible and easy to read.	—	—	—	—
4.	Drawings/illustrations are recognizable to the target group with or without explanatory text.	—	—	—	—
5.	Drawings/illustrations are labeled clearly.	—	—	—	—
6.	Drawings/illustrations represent racial and ethnic groups appropriate to the target audience.	—	—	—	—

COMMENTS:

PRINCIPLE:			*SCALE:*	

		0	1	2	NA
7.	Titles and subtitles are clear and informative.	___	___	___	___
8.	The vocabulary of the PEM is one that reflects words commonly used by the target group.	___	___	___	___
9.	Necessary health terms are defined.	___	___	___	___
10.	Terms are used in a consistent manner throughout the PEM.	___	___	___	___
11.	The writing style is one that will actively engage the reader and stimulate active participation.	___	___	___	___
12.	The active voice is used. (EXAMPLE: The sentence, ''Many persons with colostomies *find it beneficial to be* a member of an ostomy support group'' is better than the passive voice, ''Many persons with colostomies *have found that they benefited* from an ostomy support group.'')	___	___	___	___
13.	The use of double (or multiple negatives) is avoided. (EXAMPLE: This sentence is confusing, ''There is *no* reason why a person with diabetes should *not* exercise when they are *not* ill.'')	___	___	___	___
14.	The purpose of the PEM is made clear to the target group.	___	___	___	___
15.	The relevance of the educational content to the target group is clearly stated.	___	___	___	___
16.	The learning objectives that are stated or implied and the educational content of the PEM relate to one another.	___	___	___	___
17.	The learning objectives that are stated or implied relate to the intended learning outcome that is stated or implied in the PEM.	___	___	___	___
18.	Only the most essential information about the topic is presented using not more than 3–4 main points.	___	___	___	___
19.	The content is accurate.	___	___	___	___
20.	The content is presented in concrete terms rather than as abstract ideas and concepts.	___	___	___	___
21.	The content is written in a style that is patient-centered.	___	___	___	___
22.	The content is presented in a way that relates and integrates the new information to what is already known and understood by the target group.	___	___	___	___

COMMENTS:

PRINCIPLE:		SCALE:		
	0	1	2	NA

23. Examples are used to bridge the gap between what the target group already knows and the content that is to be taught and learned. ___ ___ ___ ___

24. The examples that are used contain the central characteristics of the ideas and concepts under discussion. ___ ___ ___ ___

25. The content is presented in a manner that is respectful of the customs and traditions of the target group. ___ ___ ___ ___

26. The information load of the educational material is appropriate to the target group. (The more unfamiliar the information, the smaller the amount to be presented at one time.) ___ ___ ___ ___

27. The content focuses on what the target group should *do* as well as *know*. ___ ___ ___ ___

28. The main ideas of the PEM are divided into meaningful units of content. ___ ___ ___ ___

29. The educational material moves from simple to more complex content in a manner that is organized and logical. ___ ___ ___ ___

30. The educational content is current. ___ ___ ___ ___

31. Specific, precise instructions are given if the target group is expected to carry out some health or self-care activity. ___ ___ ___ ___

32. Important ideas and points of content are repeated as reinforcement throughout the PEM. ___ ___ ___ ___

33. Sentences are kept in logical order and they present a coherent structure for the information being conveyed in the PEM. ___ ___ ___ ___

34. Summaries/synopses of the educational content being delivered are included throughout the PEM. ___ ___ ___ ___

COMMENTS:

Instructional design principle #35 is concerned with the readability level of the PEM under review. A yes/no evaluation scale is appropriate for this principle. *Materials that are intended for the general public should be written at the 6–8th grade reading level.* You can determine the grade level of a PEM by applying the SMOG formula (Doak, Doak, & Root, 1985), which is described here:

A total of 30 sentences are examined when the SMOG formula is applied:

(1)   Ten consecutive sentences are selected from the beginning of the PEM, 10 from the middle, and 10 near the end.

(2)   The number of syllables for each word in the 30 sentences is determined. For example, the word "cough" contains one syllable, the word "mucus" contains two (mu/cus), the word "polio" contains three (po/li/o), and "pneumonectomy" contains four syllables (pneu/mon/ec/tomy).

(3)   The number of words containing three or more syllables are counted (including repetitions).

(4)   The nearest perfect square root of the total number of words with three or more syllables is determined and the number, 3 (a constant in the formula) is added to the square root to obtain the grade level.

For example, a PEM that had 53 words with three or more syllables included in the 30 sentences selected for evaluation would have a square root of 7 since $7 \times 7 = 49$. By adding the constant 3, the reading level for the PEM would be designated at the 10th grade (7 + 3).

35.   The PEM is written at a readability level that is appropriate to
the target group.   _____YES   _____NO

In your opinion, what is the general quality level of the PEM you have just evaluated? (Please check one)

_____ Good and I would recommend its use

_____ Fair, but I would have some concerns about using it

_____ Not good

7

Hospital Patient Education Survey

Developed by Diedre Degeling, Glenn Salkeld, John Dowsett, and Paul Fahey

INSTRUMENT DESCRIPTION, ADMINISTRATION, AND SCORING GUIDELINES

This survey was designed to establish a baseline of patient education programs conducted in Australian hospitals and to describe how these programs were supported by management. A "planned" patient education program was defined as one designed for a specific patient group with stated goals and objectives. Patient education was defined as a "planned learning experience using a combination of methods such as teaching, counselling and behavior modification techniques which influence patients' knowledge and health behavior." The instrument takes 10 to 15 minutes to complete (Degeling, Salkeld, Dowsett, & Fahey, 1990, p. 129).

PSYCHOMETRIC PROPERTIES

Six administrative components first identified in an American Hospital Association (AHA) survey, formed the conceptual basis and major part of the survey: a written policy, a budget, a patient education committee, a patient education coordinator, documentation in patients' notes and a resource area for patient education materials or activities, and their relationship to the conduct of planned programs. The questionnaire was pilot tested with health educators and research officers from hospitals in the Sydney metropolitan area. Comments were sought on the structure, relevance, applicability, form, and simplicity of the questions. The survey was sent to 320 general medical and surgical hospitals in Australia in 1986. (Degeling et al., 1990).

CRITIQUE AND SUMMARY

Regular surveys to describe the availability of patient education services in health care institutions in a country or other political unit are important to policy makers. The Hospital Patient Education Survey depends for an important part of its content on relationships established during AHA surveys that formal structure implies that a program is relatively permanent or in some way more effective than are programs that do not have such structure. Such an assumption may not be correct. In other words, the relevant content domain is not well established. It may be more important to ask questions about number of patients served, the outcomes they achieved, incidence of avoidable negative effects, such as premature rehospitalization because of inadequate patient or caregiver learning, although institutions may not keep such data.

Since the time of this survey (1986), in the United States anecdotal evidence would suggest that patient education program structures have been altered because of hospital reengineering. Before undertaking a national survey with the Hospital Patient Education Survey, serious pilot work would be advisable. It would be helpful to have a standardized measure by which to describe and assess patient education programs periodically that exist in a particular field or geographical area including their availability to the target group for which they were designed. The Hospital Patient Education Survey is a first attempt, which should be updated and studied.

REFERENCE

Degeling, D., Salkeld, G., Dowsett, J., & Fahey, P. (1990). Patient education policy and practice in Australian hospital. *Patient Education and Counseling, 15,* 127–138.

HOSPITAL PATIENT EDUCATION SURVEY

PLEASE ANSWER BY CROSSING THE NUMBER WHICH CORRESPONDS TO YOUR RESPONSE. ALL REFERENCES TO PATIENT EDUCATION INCLUDE BOTH 'GROUP' SESSIONS AND 'ONE-TO-ONE' TEACHING.

---

1. Does your hospital conduct patient education?
   Yes (1)
   No (2)
   If no, please go to question 2 *only*.
   If yes, please go to question 3.

2. What do you consider to be the main reason for not conducting patient education programs in your hospital? (Please cross one or more boxes)
   Lack of trained patient educators ( )
   Lack of knowledge about patient education ( )
   The hospital is not big enough to warrant programs ( )
   There is no demand for patient education ( )
   It is not considered to be a part of routine patient care ( )
   No funds are available for programs ( )
   Other, please specify ( )

3. Are these programs planned (that is—are they designed for a specific target patient group with written goals and objectives)?
   Yes (1)
   No (2)
   A combination of both (3)

4. Please indicate into which categories your programs would fall. (Please cross one or more boxes)
   Respiratory (e.g., asthma) ( )
   Orthopaedics ( )
   Rheumatology (e.g., arthritis) ( )
   Diabetes ( )
   Cardiology/Cardiac Surgery (e.g., hypertension) ( )
   Cancer ( )
   Renal ( )
   Obstetrics ( )
   Stress Management ( )
   Weight Management ( )
   Nutrition ( )
   Other, please specify ( )

5. Does your hospital have a written policy on patient education? (Please cross one box only)
   Yes (1)
   No (2)
   In the planning stages (3)
   If no, please go to Question 6.
   If yes, go to Question 7. We would be grateful if you could send us a copy of your policy.

6. In the absence of written policy, which of the following would best describe the framework under which programs are developed? (Please cross one box only)

    Informal policy (unwritten) determined by the individual departments coordi-   (1)
    nating the program

    Informal policy (unwritten) determined by the Patient Education officer/Coor-   (2)
    dinator

    Informal policy (unwritten) determined by a Committee   (3)

    A general philosophy guided by the hospital's objectives and approach to   (4)
    patient care

    Other, please specify   (5)

7. Does your hospital have a patient education committee?

    Yes   (1)
    No   (2)
    In the planning stages   (3)
    If no, please go to Question 11.
    Otherwise, go to Question 8.

8. What are the main functions of the committee? (Please cross one or more boxes)

    To advise on the content of the programs   ( )
    To advise on the implementation of the programs   ( )
    To coordinate patient education programs   ( )
    To review programs   ( )
    To appraise health education officers   ( )
    To act as a brainstorming panel   ( )

9. If yes, is your committee multidisciplinary?

    Yes   ( )
    No   ( )
    If no, please go to Question 11.
    Otherwise, go to Question 10.

10. What health disciplines are represented on the committee? (Please cross one or more boxes)

    Occupational Therapy   ( )
    Physiotherapy   ( )
    Speech Pathology   ( )
    Nursing Administration   ( )
    Nursing Education   ( )
    Medical Administration   ( )
    Patient Education Coordinator   ( )
    Health Educators   ( )
    Dietitians   ( )
    Visiting Medical Officers   ( )
    Discharge Planners   ( )
    Social Workers   ( )
    Finance/Administration   ( )
    Pharmacy   ( )
    Consumers/Patient Representatives   ( )
    Other Paramedical   ( )
    Others, please specify   ( )

11. Is there an individual within your institution specially designated to coordinate patient education?
    Yes (1)
    No (2)
    If no, please go to Question 14.
    Otherwise, go to Question 12.

12. Does this person devote all of his/her time to the coordination of patient education?
    Yes (1)
    No (2)
    If yes, please go to Question 14.
    Otherwise, go to Question 13.

13. If the person designated for patient education has other obligations, what percentage of time is spent on the management of patient education within your hospital? (Please cross one box only)
    Up to 20 percent of the work time (1)
    Up to 30 percent of the work time (2)
    Up to 40 percent of the work time (3)
    Up to 50 percent of the work time (4)
    Up to 60 percent of the work time (5)
    Up to 70 percent of the work time (6)
    Up to 80 percent of the work time (7)
    Up to 90 percent of the work time (8)

14. Which of the following health care workers are involved in patient education programs? (Please cross one or more boxes)
    Dietitian ( )
    Doctor ( )
    Occupational Therapist ( )
    Pharmacist ( )
    Physiotherapist ( )
    Nurse ( )
    Social Worker ( )
    Speech Pathologist ( )
    Other, please specify ( )

15. Are funds for patient education (in your hospital) available through (please cross one or more boxes)
    A separate patient education service budget ( )
    Supported by many different budgets in individual departments ( )
    Other, please specify ( )

16. Are patient education programs recorded in the patient's notes?
    Yes (1)
    No (2)

17. Are patient education programs formally evaluated?
    Yes (1)
    No (2)
    Sometimes (3)
    If no, please go to Question 20.
    Otherwise, go to Question 18.

18. How are the activities mainly evaluated? (Please cross one box only)
    Comments from participants about the program during or at the end of the   ( )
    program
    Assessment made of participants before and after the program   ( )
    Assessment made of participants at end of program only   ( )
    Systematic comparison of participant's performance in program with a "con-   ( )
    trol" group or individuals who did not attend the program

19. Program valuation results are reviewed by: (Please cross one or more boxes)
    Patient Education Committee   ( )
    Patient Education Coordinator   ( )
    Programme Workers   ( )
    Patient's Doctor   ( )
    Quality Assurance/Peer Review Committee   ( )
    Do not know if results are reviewed   ( )
    Other, please specify   ( )

20. Is there a special area within your hospital where patient education resources
    are available?
    Yes   ( )
    No   ( )
    If no, please go to Question 23.
    Otherwise, go to Question 21.

21. If yes, this area is available to (Please cross one box only)
    Staff only   (1)
    Restricted to staff and patients   (2)
    Freely available to all users   (3)

22. Are there any staff assigned to this area to assist with enquiries? (Please cross
    one box only)
    Yes   ( )
    No   ( )

23. The statements below give opinions. Please indicate how you feel about them
    by crossing the appropriate box.
    A Patient Education Committee is important to the success and overall quality
    of the programs. (Please cross one box only)
    Strongly agree   (1)
    Agree   (2)
    Neither agree or disagree   (3)
    Disagree   (4)
    Strongly disagree   (5)

24. Patient education is an integral part of patient care. (Please cross one box
    only)
    Strongly agree   (1)
    Agree   (2)
    Neither agree or disagree   (3)
    Disagree   (4)
    Strongly disagree   (5)

25. If you feel that this questionnaire does not adequately describe patient educa-
    tion in your hospital, please tell us why.

From Degeling, D., Salkfeld, G., Dowsett, J., & Fahey, P. (1990). Patient education policy and practice in Australian hospitals. *Patient Education and Counseling, 15,* 127–138.

8

Hopkins Competency Assessment Test: A Measure of Cognitive Capacity

Developed by Jeffrey S. Janofsky, Richard J. McCarthy, and Marshal F. Folstein

INSTRUMENT DESCRIPTION, ADMINISTRATION, AND SCORING GUIDELINES

Caregivers frequently need to determine whether a patient has sufficient cognitive capacity to learn, use, and retain important self-care skills. There is at present no satisfactory assessment tool for this purpose. Perhaps a test, such as the Hopkins Competency Assessment Test (HCAT), used to help the clinician evaluate clinical capacity (or clinical competency) of patients to give informed consent, write advance directives, or make treatment decisions is of use in screening basic ability to understand. This test does not determine legal competency.

HCAT consists of a short essay, written at various reading levels, and a questionnaire for determining patients' understanding of the essay. The questionnaire is written at the 6th-grade reading level. The essay is written at high, middle, and low reading levels because the authors' pilot data showed subjects with high educational attainment had difficulty comprehending the version written for persons with a low reading level. HCAT is printed in 14-point type to minimize effects of visual impairment. It can be read to patients to eliminate illiteracy as a confounding factor. One point is given for each correct answer; possible scores range from 0 to 10. Average administration time is 10 minutes, thus allowing rapid screening of large numbers of patients for the competencies tested (Janofsky, McCarthy, & Folstein, 1992).

PSYCHOMETRIC PROPERTIES

Number of correct answers of medical and psychiatric inpatients ($N = 41$) on HCAT was an accurate predictor of clinical capacity as assessed by a psychiatrist. For this psychiatrist, a cutoff score of 4 on HCAT identified clinically competent patients. Perhaps criteria used by other psychiatrists would be associated with a different HCAT threshold for competency. Interobserver reliability for HCAT was .95. Subjects' scores were distributed over the HCAT range of 0 to 10 (Janofsky, McCarthy, & Folstein, 1992).

CRITIQUE AND SUMMARY

Content for both the essay and the questions is about informed consent and durable power of attorney, of interest for judging ability to give informed consent and write an advance directive. Whether this content would predict ability to understand other clinical decisions is not clear. However, similar tests could be constructed and tested for other common clinical decisions for a particular patient population. In addition, the report of the use of the HCAT for these purposes was based on a limited number of patients and providers at one large teaching hospital.

More than 30% of the subjects in the pilot study were judged incompetent to make treatment decisions. The authors believe that screening every patient for clinical competency is possible and economically feasible. Capability to identify patients not able to make clinical decisions is important because recent court decisions have guaranteed a competent person a right to refuse lifesaving hydration and nutrition (Janofsky, McCarthy, & Folstein, 1992).

Because patient education is intrinsically a part of assisting patients to make treatment decisions, further exploration of HCAT and similar tools are important.

REFERENCE

Janofsky, J. S., McCarthy, R. J., & Folstein, M. F. (1992). The Hopkins Competency Assessment Test: A brief method for evaluating patients' capacity to give informed consent. *Hospital and Community Psychiatry, 43,* 132–136.

ESSAYS AT THREE READING COMPREHENSION LEVELS PRESENTED TO PATIENTS AS PART OF THE HOPKINS COMPETENCY ASSESSMENT TEST

Thirteenth grade	Eighth grade	Sixth grade
Before undergoing a medical procedure, a patient must be informed about the procedure. The patient must understand what the procedure is about, the risks of the procedure, the benefits of the procedure, and alternatives to the procedure. After learning about the procedure the patient then has the option of agreeing to go forth with the procedure or not.	Before a patient has a medical procedure, he must be told about the procedure by the doctor. The patient must know what the procedure is and what could go wrong. The patient should also know what are the good things that could happen as a result of the procedure and what else could be done instead of the procedure. After the patient finds out about the procedure from his doctor the patient then can decide whether to have the procedure done or not.	Before a doctor can do something to a patient, he must tell the patient what he is going to do. The patient must know what the doctor is going to do, what could go wrong, what could go right, and what else the doctor could do instead. After the doctor tells the patient these things, the patient may agree to let the doctor go ahead. Or the patient can tell the doctor not to go ahead.
Patients with chronic disease may lose the ability to understand the information necessary to make responsible decisions regarding their own health care. When that time comes they will not be able to consent to medical treatment and this power must then be delegated to someone else.	Patients who are sick for a long time may not be able to understand what the doctor tells them about what might need to be done. When this happens some patients are not able to give permission to their doctors to have certain tests or procedures done. Then someone else has to make their decisions for them.	Some patients have been sick for a long time. After a while their thinking might not be so good. At that time, the patient might not be able to think well enough to understand what his doctor says. When that time comes he will not be able to let the doctor know what he wants the doctor to do.
Patients can leave formal legal instructions regarding what they would want to have done in specific medical situations and who they would want to make such decisions if they become unable to make them themselves. Such instructions are called a durable power of attorney.	There are two things such patients can do. First, the patient can tell the doctor who he wants to make decisions for him if he is unable. Second, the patient can tell the doctor directly what he wants done if he becomes unable to make decisions himself. These instructions are called a durable power of attorney.	Well patients can tell their doctor what they want the doctor to do. Well patients can also tell their doctor which person they would like for the doctor to talk with when the patient is not able to let the doctor know what he wants done himself. Such things need to be written down on paper. This paper is called a durable power of attorney.
The durable power of attorney allows patients to designate who will make medical decisions for them and what limitations, if any, are placed on the decision making authority.	The durable power of attorney allows patients decide who will make medical decisions for them if they are unable. It also lets the patient decide what the patient himself wants to have done if he is unable to make decisions.	The durable power of attorney lets patients say who will tell the doctor what to do if the patient can't tell the doctor himself. The durable power of attorney also lets a patient say now what he wants to have done and what he doesn't want to have done if he gets sick.

QUESTIONNAIRE ASSESSING RESPONDENT'S UNDERSTANDING OF ESSAY PRESENTED IN THE HOPKINS COMPETENCY ASSESSMENT TEST[1]

Question	Answer
What are the four things a doctor must tell a patient before beginning a procedure?	What the doctor is going to do. What could go right. What could go wrong. What else the doctor could do instead. (1 point for each correct answer)
True or false: After learning about the procedure, the patient can decide not to have the procedure done.	True (1 point for correct answer)
What can sometimes happen to the thinking of a patient who has been sick for a long time?	After a while, the patient's thinking may not be as good as it is now. (1 point for correct answer)
Finish the sentence: A patient whose thinking gets bad may not be able to ⎯⎯⎯⎯⎯.	Tell the doctor what the patient wants done. (1 point for correct answer)
What two things should such patients tell their doctor and family, before their thinking gets bad?	Patients can write down who else the doctor can talk to in order to make medical decisions for them. Patients can write down what medical procedures they want to have done or not have done. (1 point for each correct answer)
What are these instructions to doctors and family called?	They are called durable powers of attorney. (1 point for correct answer)

[1]Possible scores range from 0 to 10.
From Janofsky, J. S., McCarthy, R. J., & Folstein, M. F. (1992). The Hopkins Competency Assessment Test: A brief method for evaluating patients' capacity to give informed consent *Hospital and Community Psychiatry, 43*, 132–136. Copyright 1992, The American Psychiatric Association. Reprinted by permission.

9

Adult and Child Health Behavior Knowledge Scales

Developed by William A. Vega, James F. Sallis,
Thomas Patterson, Joan Rupp, Catherine Atkins,
and Philip R. Nader

INSTRUMENT DESCRIPTION, ADMINISTRATION, AND SCORING GUIDELINES

This set of knowledge scales was developed as part of a project to change dietary fat and sodium and exercise in White and Mexican-American families. Knowledge acquisition is believed to be one step in the process of health behavior change beginning with awareness, knowledge, motivation, and skills before the individual is ready to take health action. Families were the target of intervention because they present an opportunity to change a long-term social environment to support the new behaviors. The particular kind of knowledge judged to be most relevant to this end goal is assessing the particular knowledge necessary to take the behaviors desired (behavioral capability) as opposed to general disease information.

The Adult scale consists of 3 subscales (dietary salt, dietary fat, and exercise), each with 6 items, for a total of 18; the Child scale consists of 3 items for each of the same subscales. Scores are the number of items correctly answered. The Child scales have been used with children in 5th and 6th grades.

PSYCHOMETRIC PROPERTIES

A draft scale of items was developed by the investigators or taken from the Stanford Five-City Project and from the Special Project in Nutrition being conducted in San Francisco. They were pretested at an elementary school in a low- to middle-income neighborhood ($N = 123$ children; 36% White) and in an elementary school in a low-income neighborhood ($N = 68$; 12% White). The Child test-retest reliabilities ranged from .58 to .66 for the subscales and .73 for the full scale, with internal consistency reliability coefficients of .26 to .29 for the subscales and .51 for the total scale. These values were, no doubt, affected by the fact that each subscale was only three items long. Mean scores were dietary salt, 1.1; dietary fat, 1.8; exercise, 1.4; and total, 4.3 (Vega et al., 1987).

The Adult test-retest reliabilities range from .57 to .61 for the subscales and .76 for the full scale, with an internal consistency reliability coefficients of .55 to .59 for subscales and .8 for total scale. Mean scores were dietary salt, 3.4; dietary fat, 2.5; exercise, 3.5; and total, 9.4. Both scales showed an ideal difficulty level in that the mean score was about 50% of the possible score, indicating that although most individuals got some items correct, there was room for improvement. Reliabilities of the subscales, especially for the Child scale, suggest caution in their use separate from total score. Total scale score means for adults were White American males, 12.24; females, 12.19; Mexican-American males, 7.45; females, 6.96. Total scale score means for children were Anglo-American males, 4.31; females, 4.22; Mexican-American males, 3.21; and females, 3.24 (Vega et al., 1987).

Both child and adult knowledge scales went through a rigorous translation process. After being translated into Spanish by two bilingual staff members, they were back translated by two bilingual community residents with limited educational attainment. Finally, a panel of bilingual research staff eliminated inconsistencies and produced the final version (Vega et al., 1987).

The scales were initially tested on family units in Southern California, with 294 adults and 270 children participating. Most Mexican-American adults were monolingual Spanish speakers. A subsequent intervention study (Nader et al., 1989) found a large increase in scale scores and improved diets occurring in the intervention group, but not in the control group. Participants were 206 healthy volunteer, low- to middle-income Mexican-American and White American families (623 individuals), each with a 5th- or 6th-grade child. The intervention families, grouped by ethnic homogeneity, received 3 months of intensive weekly sessions experientially oriented and including families meeting together to review progress, engage in group problem solving, set behavior change and support goals, and mutually encourage progress in dietary and exercise changes for cardiovascular risk reduction. This was followed by 9 months of monthly or bimonthly maintenance sessions. Specifics of the intervention are well described in Nader et al. (1989).

There was evidence that behavior change persisted to 2 and 4 years beyond the completion of the program for some groups and that those who attended more regularly learned more health facts (Atkins et al., 1990; Nader et al., 1992). Thus, the instruments showed sensitivity to interventions.

CRITIQUE AND SUMMARY

Although knowledge is useful in and of itself to patients, and many would see it as their right to have knowledge about their own health, this set of tools looks at knowledge as one of the first steps in behavior change. It is one of the few scales that could be located developed to test minority populations even though the burden of chronic illness is greater overall for these groups. Indeed, studies cited in this review found marginally acculturated Mexican Americans as least aware of health behavior knowledge. Yet this group was responsive to interventions to raise their knowledge.

Little information about content validity of the scales could be located. The authors caution that knowledge of health behaviors is only one of several important determinants of actual behavior change (Vega et al., 1987); for most work, these knowledge scales would, therefore, be only one of several measures used.

REFERENCES

Atkins, C. J., Senn, K., Rupp, J., Kaplan, R. M., Patterson, T. L., Sallis, J. F., & Nader, P. R. (1990). Attendance at health promotion programs: Baseline predictors and program outcomes. *Health Education Quarterly, 17,* 417–428.

Nader, P. R., Sallis, J. F., Patterson, T. L., Abramson, I. S., Rupp, J. W., Senn, K. L., Atkins, C. J., Roppe, B. E., Morris, J. A., Wallace, J. P., & Vega, W. A. (1989). A family approach to cardiovascular risk reduction: Results from the San Diego Family Health Project. *Health Education Quarterly, 16,* 229–244.

Nader, P. R., Sallis, J. F., Abramson, I. S., Broyles, S. L., Patterson, T. L., Senn, K. L., Rupp, J. W., & Nelson, J. A. (1992). Family-based cardiovascular risk reduction education among Mexican- and Anglo-Americans. *Family and Community Health, 15,* 57–74.

Vega, W. M., Sallis, J. F., Patterson, T., Rupp, J., Atkins, C., & Nader, P. R. (1987). Assessing knowledge of cardiovascular health-related diet and exercise behaviors in Anglo- and Mexican-Americans. *Preventive Medicine, 16,* 696–709.

ADULT HEALTH KNOWLEDGE BEHAVIOR SCALE

INSTRUCTIONS: These questions are about diet and exercise. There are some answers you won't know, but answer the questions as best as you can. If you need to guess, that's okay. For each question, check (✓) the correct answer. You are to choose only the one best answer for each question.

SAMPLE:

A.   Walking is good for your health.
  ❐ 1.   True
  ❐ 2.   False
  ❐ 8.   Don't know

---

1.   The best way to reduce blood pressure without medication is to:
  ❐ 1.   Reduce cholesterol intake
  ❐ 2.   Lose weight
  ❐ 3.   Restrict salt
  ❐ 4.   1 and 3 above
  ❐ 5.   2 and 3 above
  ❐ 8.   Don't know

2.   Which of the following foods is highest in saturated fat?
  ❐ 1.   Peanuts
  ❐ 2.   Beef liver
  ❐ 3.   Frankfurters
  ❐ 4.   Roast beef
  ❐ 8.   Don't know

3.   How are the ingredients listed on the label of a food product?
  ❐ 1.   In order of their nutritional content, from the most to the least nutritious
  ❐ 2.   In order of their amount in the product, from the most to the least
  ❐ 3.   In order of how expensive the ingredients are, from most expensive to least expensive
  ❐ 4.   There is no standard order of ingredient labeling, each manufacturer sets its own policy on this matter
  ❐ 8.   Don't know

4.   A good way to reduce saturated fat intake is to:
  ❐ 1.   Use more cheese
  ❐ 2.   Decrease the use of vegetable oil
  ❐ 3.   Cut down on bacon, sausage, and luncheon meat
  ❐ 4.   Use fewer nuts and beans
  ❐ 8.   Don't know

5.   How long and how often do you need to exercise to improve the fitness of your heart and lungs?
  ❐ 1.   1 hour each time, once per week
  ❐ 2.   20 minutes each time, 2 times per week
  ❐ 3.   20 minutes each time, 3 times per week

    ❐ 4. 10 minutes each time, 6 times per week
    ❐ 8. Don't know

6. Below are the ingredient labels from 3 brands of margarine, check the one that is *best* for your heart.
    ❐ 1. Contains partially hydrogenated soybean and cottonseed oils
    ❐ 2. Contains liquid safflower oil, partially hydrogenated soy oil
    ❐ 3. Contains palm oil, partially hydrogenated soy oil
    ❐ 8. Don't know

7. Exercises that are the best for preventing heart disease are:
    ❐ 1. Short, energetic hard bursts of physical exercise
    ❐ 2. Physical activity in which breathing pure air is important
    ❐ 3. Physical activity which causes hard and rapid breathing for a sustained period of time
    ❐ 4. Exercise involving specially designed equipment
    ❐ 8. Don't know

8. The best way to reduce the amount of cholesterol in the blood is to:
    ❐ 1. Avoid tension and stress
    ❐ 2. Decrease the amount of fat you eat
    ❐ 3. Quit smoking and drink less alcohol
    ❐ 4. Decrease the amount of starchy foods in diet
    ❐ 8. Don't know

9. Hydrogenated vegetable fats are:
    ❐ 1. Mainly saturated fat
    ❐ 2. Mainly polyunsaturated fats
    ❐ 3. Solid at room temperature
    ❐ 4. 1 and 2 above
    ❐ 5. 2 and 3 above
    ❐ 8. Don't know

The following statements about health are either true or false. Please read each one and check (✓) "True" if the statement is true or check (✓) "False" if it is false. Please mark only one response for each statement.

10. Soy sauce and steak sauce are low in sodium.
    ❐ 1. True
    ❐ 2. False
    ❐ 8. Don't know

11. Mechanical devices like sauna belts make it easier for you to develop physical fitness.
    ❐ 1. True
    ❐ 2. False
    ❐ 8. Don't know

12. Exercising for 2 hours on the weekend is just as good as exercising for 30 minutes on 4 different days.
    ❐ 1. True
    ❐ 2. False
    ❐ 8. Don't know

13. Seasoned salt, garlic salt, and onion salt should be avoided on a low sodium diet.
    ❐ 1. True
    ❐ 2. False
    ❐ 8. Don't know

14. White cheese is lower in fat than yellow cheese.
    ❐ 1. True
    ❐ 2. False
    ❐ 8. Don't know

15. If you're in good physical condition, your pulse should return to normal within 15 minutes after exercising.
    ❐ 1. True
    ❐ 2. False
    ❐ 8. Don't know

16. Most frozen convenience foods, like T.V. dinners, have large amounts of salt added.
    ❐ 1. True
    ❐ 2. False
    ❐ 8. Don't know

17. Riding your bicycle for 10 minutes twice a day will give you the same results as riding your bicycle for 20 minutes once a day.
    ❐ 1. True
    ❐ 2. False
    ❐ 8. Don't know

18. Fresh pork has as much salt as ham.
    ❐ 1. True
    ❐ 2. False
    ❐ 8. Don't know

Answer Key:

1. (5)   4. (3)   7. (3)   10. (2)   13. (1)   16. (1)
2. (2)   5. (3)   8. (2)   11. (2)   14. (2)   17. (2)
3. (2)   6. (2)   9. (2)   12. (2)   15. (1)   18. (2)

From Vega, W. A., Sallis, J. F., Patterson, T., Rupp, J., Atkins, C., & Nader, P. R. (1987). Assessing knowledge of cardiovascular health-related diet and exercise behaviors in Anglo- and Mexican-Americans, Appendix A, Adult Health Knowledge Behavior Scale. *Preventive Medicine, 26*, 696–709. Reprinted with permission.

CHILD HEALTH BEHAVIOR KNOWLEDGE SCALE

INSTRUCTIONS: These questions are about diet and exercise. There are some answers you won't know, so if you need to guess, that's okay. For each question, check (✓) the one best answer.

SAMPLE:

A. Walking is good for your health
    ❐ 1. True
    ❐ 2. False
    ❐ 8. Don't know

1. A saturated fat is:
    ❐ 1. Butter
    ❐ 2. Corn oil
    ❐ 3. Walnuts
    ❐ 8. I don't know

2. Which of these types of exercise is good for your heart?
    ❐ 1. Four square
    ❐ 2. Baseball
    ❐ 3. Aerobic dance
    ❐ 8. I don't know

3. A good low sodium snack is:
    ❐ 1. Fresh fruit
    ❐ 2. Pickles
    ❐ 3. Tortilla chips
    ❐ 8. I don't know

4. A lunch that is healthy for the heart is:
    ❐ 1. Bologna sandwich, milk, potato chips, cookies
    ❐ 2. Peanut butter sandwich, cheese cubes, celery sticks, milk, apple
    ❐ 3. Lowfat yogurt with fruit, carrot sticks, homemade banana nut bread, nonfat milk
    ❐ 8. I don't know

5. To help your heart, how many minutes should you exercise at a time?
    ❐ 1. At least 5 minutes at a time
    ❐ 2. At least 10 minutes at a time
    ❐ 3. At least 20 minutes at a time
    ❐ 8. I don't know

6. Which of these foods are highest in salt?
    ❐ 1. Hamburger and chicken
    ❐ 2. Fresh vegetables and fruits
    ❐ 3. TV dinners and canned tuna
    ❐ 8. I don't know

7. Some foods that have "hidden" fat are:
    ❐ 1. Corn, bananas, and potatoes
    ❐ 2. Olives, avocados, coconut
    ❐ 3. Broccoli, green beans, and lettuce
    ❐ 8. I don't know

8.   The least amount of aerobic exercise you should do for a healthy heart is?
       ❐ 1.   Three times a week
       ❐ 2.   Two times a week
       ❐ 3.   Once a week
       ❐ 8.   I don't know

9.   Most people eat:
       ❐ 1.   Half as much sodium as they need
       ❐ 2.   As much sodium as they need
       ❐ 3.   Thirty times as much sodium as they need
       ❐ 8.   I don't know

Answer Key:
1. (1)   4. (3)   7. (2)
2. (3)   5. (3)   8. (1)
3. (1)   6. (3)   9. (3)

From Vega, W. A., Sallis, J. F., Patterson, T., Rupp, J., Atkins, C., & Nader, P. R. (1987). Assessing knowledge of cardiovascular health-related diet and exercise behaviors in Anglo- and Mexican-Americans, Appendix B, Child Health Knowledge Behavior Scale. *Preventive Medicine, 26,* 696–709. Reprinted with permission.

B

Diabetes

10

Diabetes Attitude Scale

Developed by Robert M. Anderson, Michael B. Donnelly, and Robert F. Dedrick

INSTRUMENT DESCRIPTION, ADMINISTRATION, AND SCORING GUIDELINES

Some of the major theories of health behavior, such as the health belief model and the theory of reasoned action, emphasize that attitudes and beliefs are a major component of health behavior. The theory of reasoned action also posits the importance of how other people whom the patient views as important feel about the action. The Diabetes Attitude Scale (DAS) is not intended to be or to replace a diabetes attitude scale focusing exclusively on the concerns of persons with diabetes. Rather, its special purpose as expressed by its authors is to allow identification of differences in opinion that could interfere with the quality of the patient–health care provider relationship and ultimately affect the management and treatment of the disease.

The DAS was originally designed to measure the attitudes of health care professionals and was revised to make items less technical for use with patients. The rewording lowered the reading level from 12th to 10th grade. Items are scored with 5 for strongly agree; 4, agree; 3, neither agree nor disagree; 2, disagree; and 1, strongly disagree. Scores for each scale are averaged by the number of items. Positive attitudes are defined as those over 3 and negative as those less than 3.

Findings from the comparison suggest that a significant number of young and well-educated patients do not wish to be told what they should do to care for their diabetes; health care professionals tend to underestimate the perceived negative impact diabetes has on the lives of patients who are required to take insulin; a significant number of older patients do not desire an independent self-care role, although nurses and dietitians indicate strong value on patient autonomy (Anderson, Donnelly, & Dedrick, 1990; Anderson, Fitzgerald, Gorenflo, & Oh, 1993).

DAS can also be used to assess the impact of diabetes education programs on the attitudes of patients and to explore the relationship between attitudes and behavior (Anderson et al., 1990). Mean scores for each item and each scale may be found in Anderson et al. (1990). Mean scale scores range from 3.45 for seriousness of non–insulin-dependent diabetes mellitus (NIDDM) to 4.28 for special training.

PSYCHOMETRIC PROPERTIES

The DAS was tested on a convenience sample of 1,202 persons with diabetes in Michigan. A factor analysis yielded seven subscales.

1. Special training, defined as the extent to which respondents believe health care profession-als need special training to care for persons with diabetes (items 21, 12, 13, 2, 38, 45, 42)
2. Patient compliance, defined as the extent to which respondents support the idea that patients should do as they are told by health care professionals (items 28, 4, 41, 43, 32, 24)
3. Seriousness of NIDDM, defined as the extent to which respondents view NIDDM as a serious disease (items 10, 18, 6)
4. Relationship between blood glucose levels and complications, defined as the extent to which respondents perceive a relationship between blood glucose levels and the onset of the complications of diabetes (items 25, 4, 49, 35)
5. Impact of diabetes on the patient's life, defined as the extent to which respondents believe that diabetes has a significant negative impact on their lives (items 22, 27, 2, 15, 30)
6. Patient autonomy, defined as the extent to which respondents agree the patient should be the primary decision maker about daily self-care of diabetes (items 46, 11, 48, 3, 37)
7. Team care, defined as the extent to which respondents are supportive of the need for nurses and dietitians in the care of diabetes (items 34, 25, 29, 47)

Cronbach's α for the subscales ranged from .63 to .71. These reliabilities were viewed as adequate only for making group comparisons (Anderson et al., 1990).

In general, most respondents believed that health care professionals need special training to care for persons with diabetes, good blood glucose control reduces the likelihood that complica-tions will develop, diabetes has a significant negative impact on the patient's life, and a team approach is essential to diabetes care. Although the respondents generally agreed that NIDDM is a serious disease and were supportive of patients being in charge of their diabetes management, these issues generated the widest differences of opinion (Anderson et al., 1990).

A study of self-reported adherence to 10 diabetes self-care behaviors showed that patients in the high-adherence group had more positive attitudes on the DAS than did patients in the low-adherence group. This finding is believed to provide evidence of construct validity for the DAS (Anderson, Fitzgerald, & Oh, 1993). Differences in the DAS by gender have been investi-gated. Similarities across gender were common, although men were more passive than were women in their diabetes care (Fitzgerald, Anderson, & Davis, 1995).

CRITIQUE AND SUMMARY

The reading level is high for a number of persons with diabetes. Race and socioeconomic class of patients was not reported.

Additional validity studies would be useful. Although the authors report that content validity was assured through the use of a Delphi process for item construction and selection, this process involved only health professionals and not patients. Thus, it is unknown whether the comparisons that can be obtained with the DAS are with attitudes and beliefs held primarily by health professionals. Construct validity support cited previously depends on self-reported adherence to the self-care components as well as the assumption that compliance with self-care is directly related to each subscale.

It is expected that differences in attitudes among patients with diabetes will affect how they receive and act on the content from educational sessions and that it is useful to compare the attitudes of patients and health professionals (Anderson et al., 1990). Further evidence exploring these two expectations would be useful.

REFERENCES

Anderson, R. M., Donnelly, M. B., & Dedrick, R. F. (1990). Measuring the attitudes of patients toward diabetes and its treatment. *Patient Education and Counseling, 16,* 231–245.

Anderson, R. M., Fitzgerald, J. T., Gorenflo, D. W., & Oh, M.S. (1993). A comparison of the diabetes-related attitudes of health care professionals and patients. *Patient Education and Counseling, 21,* 41–50.

Anderson, R. M., Fitzgerald, J. T., & Oh, M. S. (1993). The relationship between diabetes-related attitudes and patients' self-reported adherence. *The Diabetes Educator, 19,* 287–292.

Fitzgerald, J. T., Anderson, R. M., & Davis, W. K. (1995). Gender differences in diabetes attitudes and adherence. *The Diabetes Educator, 21,* 523–529.

FOR PATIENTS AND/OR PROFESSIONALS
DIABETES ATTITUDE SURVEY

Below are some statements about diabetes. Each numbered statement finishes the sentence "In general, I believe that...." You may believe that a statement is true for one person but not for another person or may be true one time but not be true another time. Your answer for that statement should show what you believe is true most of the time or is true for most people. Place a check mark in the parentheses below the word or phrase which is closest to your opinion about each statement. It is important that you answer *every* statement.
*Note—The term "health care professionals" in this survey refers to doctors, nurses, and dietitians.

In general, I believe that:	Strongly Agree	Agree	Neither Agree Nor Disagree	Disagree	Strongly Disagree
1. ... health care professionals need to have special training to provide effective treatment of diabetes.	( )	( )	( )	( )	( )
2. ... having diabetes changes a person's outlook on life.	( )	( )	( )	( )	( )
3. ... people with diabetes should be taught how to choose their own self-care methods (for example, type of diet, type of blood sugar monitoring, number of daily insulin injections).	( )	( )	( )	( )	( )
4. ... controlling their diabetes should be the most important thing in the lives of people with diabetes.	( )	( )	( )	( )	( )
5. ... health care professionals can make a big difference in how well people with diabetes learn to control their disease.	( )	( )	( )	( )	( )
6. ... diabetes that can be controlled by just being on a diet is a pretty mild disease.	( )	( )	( )	( )	( )
7. ... health care professionals should be very concerned about how diabetes affects people emotionally.	( )	( )	( )	( )	( )
8. ... people with diabetes should not have children because of the risk that they may inherit the disease.	( )	( )	( )	( )	( )

In general, I believe that:	Strongly Agree	Agree	Neither Agree Nor Disagree	Disagree	Strongly Disagree
9. ... the nurses and dietitians who teach people to care for their diabetes are good teachers.	( )	( )	( )	( )	( )
10. ... non–insulin-dependent diabetes is a less serious disease than insulin-dependent diabetes.	( )	( )	( )	( )	( )
11. ... people with diabetes should choose their own goals for diabetes treatment.	( )	( )	( )	( )	( )
12. ... it is important for the nurses and dietitians who teach people to care for their diabetes to learn counseling skills.	( )	( )	( )	( )	( )
13. ... health care professionals should be required to continue to learn about diabetes because diabetes care is changing fast.	( )	( )	( )	( )	( )
14. ... people with diabetes who have poor blood sugar control are more likely to have diabetes complications than people who have good blood sugar control.	( )	( )	( )	( )	( )
15. ... it is frustrating to treat diabetes.	( )	( )	( )	( )	( )
16. ... following the recommended diabetes treatment plan will improve blood sugar control.	( )	( )	( )	( )	( )
17. ... doctors do *not* know enough about the diabetic diet.	( )	( )	( )	( )	( )
18. ... people whose diabetes is treated by just a diet do not have to worry about getting many long-term complications of diabetes.	( )	( )	( )	( )	( )
19. ... for many people getting good control of their blood sugar is not worth the effort.	( )	( )	( )	( )	( )
20. ... people with diabetes and their health care professionals should be equally responsible for setting treatment goals.	( )	( )	( )	( )	( )

In general, I believe that:	Strongly Agree	Agree	Neither Agree Nor Disagree	Disagree	Strongly Disagree
21. . . . health care professionals who treat people with diabetes should be trained to communicate well with their patients.	( )	( )	( )	( )	( )
22. . . . diabetes affects almost every part of a diabetic person's life.	( )	( )	( )	( )	( )
23. . . . people who have insulin-dependent diabetes need to go into the hospital when they first get it so they can learn about diabetes.	( )	( )	( )	( )	( )
24. . . . if people with diabetes do not cooperate and follow their recommended treatment there is not much that health care professionals can do for them.	( )	( )	( )	( )	( )
25. . . . to provide enough information about diabetes care to patients, physicians need the help of nurses and dietitians.	( )	( )	( )	( )	( )
26. . . . good blood sugar control will reduce the long-term complications of diabetes.	( )	( )	( )	( )	( )
27. . . . the emotional effect of diabetes is pretty small.	( )	( )	( )	( )	( )
28. . . . people who do not follow their recommended diabetes treatment don't really care about controlling their diabetes.	( )	( )	( )	( )	( )
29. . . . doctors should send people with diabetes to a dietitian to help them with their diet.	( )	( )	( )	( )	( )
30. . . . diabetes is a very serious disease.	( )	( )	( )	( )	( )
31. . . . blood sugar monitoring is *not* much help in treating non–insulin-dependent diabetes.	( )	( )	( )	( )	( )
32. . . . telling patients about the complications of diabetes will scare them into following their recommended treatment.	( )	( )	( )	( )	( )

In general, I believe that:	Strongly Agree	Agree	Neither Agree Nor Disagree	Disagree	Strongly Disagree
33. ...people with diabetes do not follow their recommended treatment as much as they should.	( )	( )	( )	( )	( )
34. ...doctors do *not* need help from nurses and dietitians to treat patients with diabetes.	( )	( )	( )	( )	( )
35. ...there is *not* much use in trying to have good blood sugar control because the complications of diabetes will happen anyway.	( )	( )	( )	( )	( )
36. ...using the food exchange list is the best way to teach people with diabetes about their diet.	( )	( )	( )	( )	( )
37. ...people with diabetes have the right to decide how hard they will work to control their blood sugar.	( )	( )	( )	( )	( )
38. ...nurses and dietitians who have special training in diabetes will give better care to patients.	( )	( )	( )	( )	( )
39. ...it is easier for people to learn about diabetes in clinics and doctors' offices than while they are in the hospital.	( )	( )	( )	( )	( )
40. ...it is hard for health care professionals to convince people to take better care of their diabetes.	( )	( )	( )	( )	( )
41. ...the parents of diabetic teenagers should be in charge of how their children take care of their diabetes.	( )	( )	( )	( )	( )
42. ...to do a good job, diabetes educators should learn a lot about being teachers.	( )	( )	( )	( )	( )
43. ...decisions about caring for diabetes should be made by the doctor.	( )	( )	( )	( )	( )
44. ...there is a basic diabetic personality type.	( )	( )	( )	( )	( )
45. ...diabetes education for health care professionals should cover diabetes in the elderly.	( )	( )	( )	( )	( )

In general, I believe that:	Strongly Agree	Agree	Neither Agree Nor Disagree	Disagree	Strongly Disagree
46. . . . the important decisions regarding daily diabetes care should be made by the person with diabetes.	( )	( )	( )	( )	( )
47. . . . doctors should send people with diabetes to a nurse educator to help them learn about their diabetes.	( )	( )	( )	( )	( )
48. . . . people with diabetes should learn a lot about the disease so they can be in charge of their own diabetes care.	( )	( )	( )	( )	( )
49. . . . having high blood sugar over a long period of time is linked to getting long-term diabetic complications.	( )	( )	( )	( )	( )
50. . . . health care professionals do *not* have much control over how healthy their diabetic patients are.	( )	( )	( )	( )	( )

Reprinted from Anderson, R., Donnelly, M., & Dedrick, R. (1990). Measuring the attitudes of patients toward diabetes and its treatment. *Patient Education & Counseling, 16*: 231–245, with permission from Elsevier Science Ireland Ltd., Bay 15K, Shannon Industrial Estate, Co. Clare, Ireland.

11

Problem Areas in Diabetes Survey

Developed by William H. Polonsky, Barbara J. Anderson, Patricia A. Lohrer, Garry Welch, Alan M. Jacobson, Jennifer E. Aponte, and Carolyn E. Schwartz

INSTRUMENT DESCRIPTION, ADMINISTRATION, AND SCORING GUIDELINES

For those living with diabetes, illness-related emotional distress may not be uncommon, stemming from the self-care demands and worry about long-term complications and frustrations of the regimen and illness. In the complex adjustment to life with diabetes, patients may feel defeated, becoming unmotivated to adhere to the diabetes regimen. Anger, guilt, frustration, denial, fear of hypoglycemia, and loneliness have also been observed. Recent evidence suggests that emotional distress as represented by the presence of affective disorders or poor coping skills may be linked to poor adherence to the self-care regimen, especially among adolescents with insulin-dependent diabetes mellitus. The primary aims of the Problem Areas in Diabetes Survey (PAID) are to serve as a screening measure for clinical and research purposes, and to help clinicians identify patients experiencing high levels of diabetes related distress, so that treatment interventions may be developed around specific problem areas (Polonsky et al., 1995).

Each item represents an aspect of emotional distress in the psychosocial adjustment to diabetes. Summing the item responses creates a total score hypothesized to reflect the overall level of distress, which can range from 20 to 120.

PSYCHOMETRIC PROPERTIES

Items for the tool were solicited from 10 health care providers at the Joslin Clinic and patient comments that focused on the range of difficulties encountered by persons living with diabetes. Early drafts of the items were piloted and then the tool was tested on 451 female patients, all of whom required insulin and had had diabetes for at least 1 year. Approximately 60% of the sample reported at least one serious diabetes-related concern, most frequently worrying about the future and the possibility of serious complications (42%). The mean score was 55, with a standard deviation of 23 and a range of 20 to 115. The percentage of participants who reported serious problems with each item may be found in Polonsky et al. (1995).

There is no absolute criterion or gold standard for emotional adjustment to diabetes. PAID scores were positively associated with measures of general emotional distress, and fear of hypoglycemia and disordered eating attitudes and behaviors; and negatively associated with adherence to recommendations for blood glucose testing, insulin usage, meal planning, and reported self-care behaviors. Greater distress was associated with poorer glycemic control and more frequent short- and long-term complications of diabetes. Cronbach's α (measure of internal consistency) was .95, with item-total correlations ranging from .32 to .84 and a mean of .68 (Polonsky et al., 1995).

CRITIQUE AND SUMMARY

These results are preliminary, in part, because the instrument has been used only with well-educated women who take insulin. Further testing will be necessary to see if scores are sensitive to clinically important changes in patient status and in response to appropriate education or psychosocial interventions believed to promote significant decrease in diabetes-related emotional distress. Retesting of PAID's ability to predict glycemic control in the future will clarify initial findings. It also will be important to establish a score indicative of a pathological level of distress.

Although explicit domains of emotional adjustment were apparently not established, the inclusion of patient comments as a source of items is helpful. Evidence of validity for a variety of interpretations was well accomplished for a survey still in initial stages of development.

Until the work described previously has been accomplished, PAID may serve as a useful clinical tool to identify high levels of diabetes-related distress and a catalyst in initiating dialogue with patients about the specific details of their diabetes-related concern. The data presented are consistent with the hypothesis that diabetes-related emotional distress is an independent major contributor to poor adherence, separate from the contribution of general emotional distress (Polonsky et al., 1995).

REFERENCE

Polonsky, W. H., Anderson, B. J., Lohrer, P. A., Welch, G., Jacobson, A. M., Aponte, J. E., & Schwartz, C. E. (1995). Assessment of diabetes-related distress. *Diabetes Care, 18,* 754–760.

IDENTIFYING YOUR PROBLEM AREAS IN DIABETES (PAID-1)

Name: _____ Age: _____ Sex: M _____ F _____

Diabetes type: Type I (insulin-dependent) _____

Type II (non–insulin-dependent) _____ Taking Insulin? y __ n __

How many years since your diabetes was diagnosed? _____ Today's date _____

DIRECTIONS: Living with diabetes can sometimes be difficult. In day-to-day life, there may be numerous problems and hassles concerning diabetes and they can vary greatly in severity. Problems may range from minor hassles to major life difficulties. Listed below are a variety of potential problem areas which people with diabetes may experience. Consider the degree to which each of the items may have distressed or bothered you *during the past month* and circle the appropriate number.

Please note that we are asking you to indicate the degree to which each item may be bothering you in your life, *not* whether the item is merely true for you. If you feel that a particular item is not a bother or a problem for you, you would circle "1." If it is very bothersome to you, you might circle "6."

		Not a Problem		Moderate Problem		Serious Problem	
1.	Not having clear and concrete goals for your diabetes care?	1	2	3	4	5	6
2.	Feeling discouraged with your diabetes regimen?	1	2	3	4	5	6
3.	Feeling scared when you think about having and living with diabetes?	1	2	3	4	5	6
4.	Uncomfortable interactions around diabetes with family, friends, or acquaintances who do not have diabetes (e.g., a friend advising you on what to eat)?	1	2	3	4	5	6
5.	Feelings of deprivation regarding food and meals?	1	2	3	4	5	6
6.	Feeling depressed when you think about having and living with diabetes?	1	2	3	4	5	6
7.	Not knowing if the moods or feelings you are experiencing are related to your blood sugar levels?	1	2	3	4	5	6
8.	Feeling overwhelmed by your diabetes regimen?	1	2	3	4	5	6
9.	Worrying about reactions?	1	2	3	4	5	6
10.	Feeling angry when you think about having and living with diabetes?	1	2	3	4	5	6
11.	Feeling constantly concerned about food and eating?	1	2	3	4	5	6
12.	Worrying about the future and the possibility of serious complications?	1	2	3	4	5	6

		Not a Problem		Moderate Problem		Serious Problem	
13.	Feelings of guilt or anxiety when you get off track with your diabetes management?	1	2	3	4	5	6
14.	Not "accepting" your diabetes?	1	2	3	4	5	6
15.	Feeling unsatisfied with your relationship with your diabetes physician?	1	2	3	4	5	6
16.	Feeling that diabetes is taking up too much of your mental and physical energy every day?	1	2	3	4	5	6
17.	Feeling alone with diabetes?	1	2	3	4	5	6
18.	Feeling that your friends and family are not supportive of your diabetes management efforts?	1	2	3	4	5	6
19.	Coping with complications of diabetes?	1	2	3	4	5	6
20.	Feeling "burned out" by the constant effort to manage diabetes?	1	2	3	4	5	6

12

Diabetes Pictorial Scale: Assessing Diabetes Knowledge in Children

Developed by Darlene Biggs and William Garrison

INSTRUMENT DESCRIPTION, ADMINISTRATION, AND SCORING GUIDELINES

The Diabetes Pictorial Scale (DPS) is an entirely pictorial scale, intended to allow the diabetes clinician or researcher to assess knowledge, attitudes, and disease-relevant behaviors in the preliterate or marginally literate child, and in older children with cognitive-developmental delays. (It appears at the end of this chapter.) The pictorial approach facilitates a dialogue between the adult and the child, around insulin-dependent diabetes mellitus (IDDM) and its management. The DPS presents forced choice between two pictorially presented polar exemplars, with follow-up probe questions to request greater discrimination. Administration requires 20 minutes with additional time for the follow-up questions. Directions appear on page 75, with a scoring form on page 118 (Garrison & Biggs, 1990a).

The 20 items can be summed, with a higher score purportedly representing better overall adherence and adjustment, although this approach is not advised until more extensive reliability and validity studies are completed. Rather, the child's response to individual items or to clusters of items can be used as an assessment base for clinical or educational interventions. Score statistics for the initial test group used to study validity may be seen in Table 12.1 below. Norms are revised periodically to incorporate new data and are available from the authors[*] (Garrison & Biggs, 1990b).

PSYCHOMETRIC PROPERTIES

DPS has been used for several years in a clinical research project, with 39 children ages 4 to 10, with minority children accounting for about 15% of the sample. Preliminary data show that

[*]Dr. William Garrison, Chief Psychologist, Children's National Medical Center, 111 Michigan Avenue NW, Washington, DC 20010-2970.

TABLE 12.1 Means and Standard Deviations by Whole Sample and Glycemic Control Groupings

Item no.	Description	Poor		Adequate		Whole Sample	
		Mean	SD	Mean	SD	Mean	SD
1.	Amount of exercise	3.1	1.10	2.9	0.88	2.9	0.93
2.	Regularity of insulin injections*	3.8	1.10	3.0	0.42	3.2	1.00
3.	Follows meal plan†	2.7	1.10	3.4	0.68	3.2	0.87
4.	Blood testing regularity	2.8	0.91	2.9	0.98	2.9	0.95
5.	Meals/snacking regularity‡	3.1	0.99	3.5	0.62	3.4	0.75
6.	Exercise regularity	2.3	1.10	2.2	1.20	2.2	1.20

Note: Groupings are based on 4-point, forced-choice items. Example: 4 = *always/a lot*; 3 = *pretty much*; 2 = *sometimes/ sort of*; 1 = *hardly ever/never*.
*Student's $t = 2.16$, df = 37, $P < .03$.
†Student's $t = -2.36$, df = 37, $P < .02$.
‡Student's $t = -1.81$, df = 37, $P < .07$.

From Garrison, W. T., & Biggs, D. (1990). Young children's subjective reports about their diabetes mellitus: A validation of the Diabetes Pictorial Scale. *The Diabetes Educator, 16,* 304–308.

children in poor control as measured by glycosylated hemoglobin assays were more likely to report lower adherence to their meal plan, to report eating their meals and snacks less regularly, and to monitor their blood glucose less regularly. This is evidence of validity (Garrison & Biggs, 1990b).

Because this is a new measurement technique, its authors view DPS as a structured interview rather than as a psychological or medical test. Because the instrument is open to socially desirable responses, caution must be exercised in interpretation of scores and responses. However, sizable variation between and within respondents was still apparent. It has proved useful in eliciting the verbalizations of children (Garrison & Biggs, 1990a).

CRITIQUE AND SUMMARY

The DPS should currently be viewed as largely experimental in nature. In particular, more extensive assessment of psychometric characteristics including test-retest reliability and internal consistency, and sufficient normative data from larger samples of children are needed. Specifically, the scale may help identify outcomes in children as they grow and develop (predictive validity). Aspects of the IDDM regimen and psychosocial aspects of the child's life that are presumably important have been included (Garrison & Biggs, 1990a); more systematic assessment of content validity would be helpful.

The DPS does have the potential to fill a need for a direct and developmentally sensitive measure of younger children's IDDM-specific attitudes, behaviors, and knowledge, and can be used with more objective measures of disease control and patient adherence. This is a group that has largely been neglected in the scientific literature on psychosocial aspects of the disease (Garrison & Biggs, 1990a).

REFERENCES

Garrison, W. T., & Biggs, D. (1990a). The Diabetes Pictorial Scale: A direct measure of young children's knowledge, attitudes, and behavior relevant to their insulin-dependent diabetes mellitus. *The Diabetes Educator, 16,* 21–24.

Garrison, W. T., & Biggs, D. (1990b). Young children's subjective reports about their diabetes mellitus: A validation of the Diabetes Pictorial Scale. *The Diabetes Educator, 16,* 304–308.

The Diabetes Pictorial Scale

Background

This booklet has been designed specifically to allow the diabetes clinician or researcher to assess knowledge, attitudes and disease-relevant behaviors in the younger child. The pictorial approach facilitates a dialogue between the adult and child around diabetes and its management. Because of similarities in format, the scale can be used in conjunction with pictorial versions of the Perceived Competence and Social Acceptance scales, available from Susan Harter, Ph.D. Norms for the measure will be available from the authors periodically as they are revised through continuing data collection.

Directions

The pictures in the booklet are oriented towards the child who will be interviewed. The text is oriented to the examiner. The examiner should introduce the child to the session in the following manner:

"This is a book about children who have diabetes. Each picture shows different children doing different things. Let's see if any of these children are like you."

Then turn to the first picture (exercise) and say:

"This boy (pointing to the picture on the examiner's left) doesn't get very much exercise. This boy (pointing to the picture on the examiner's right) gets a lot of exercise every day."

WHICH ONE IS MORE LIKE YOU?"

The child should point to one picture or the other. Then the examiner should attempt to get a more specific response by giving the child a choice between the two circles below the chosen picture. For example, if the child points at the picture with the boy on the bicycle the examiner would ask:

"Do you get pretty much exercise (pointing to the smaller circle under that picture) or a whole lot of exercise" (pointing to the larger circle under that picture)?

Record the child's response numerically by referring to the number in the appropriate circle on the examiner's page. Then move to the next item and use the same basic wording for the initial and follow-up questions. It is recommended that additional probe questions regarding the child's specific answers to the items be asked AFTER administration of the entire scale so that future items are not influenced by previous discussions about diabetes-related behaviors, attitudes and knowledge.

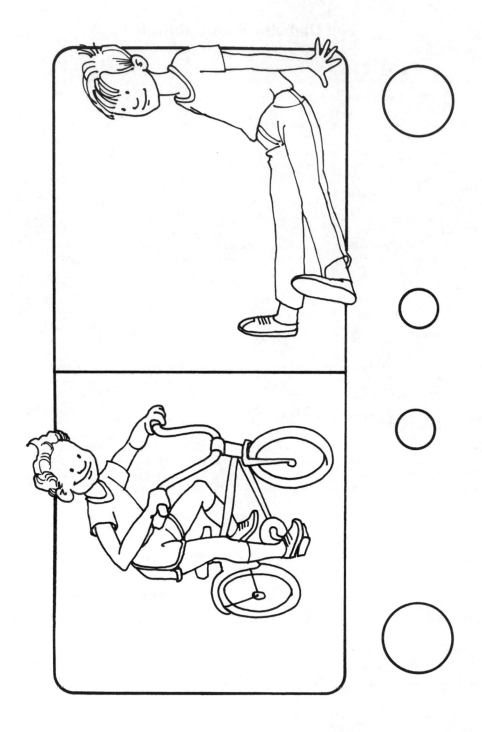

This boy doesn't get very much exercise.

Do you get:

This boy gets lots of exercise every day.

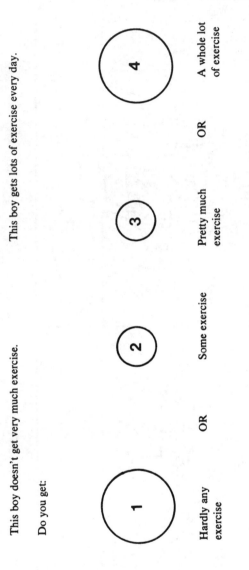

| ① | | ② | | ③ | | ④ |

Hardly any exercise OR Some exercise Pretty much exercise OR A whole lot of exercise

What do you do for exercise?
Why should you exercise?

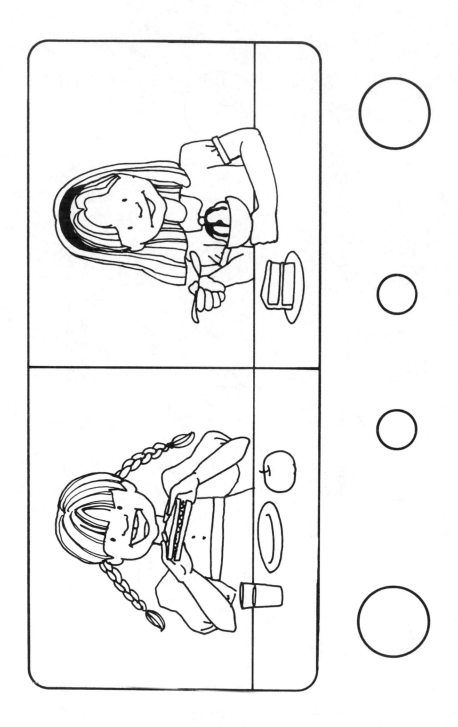

This girl eats whatever she wants.

Do you:

This girl eats only those things she knows she can and should eat.

Do you:

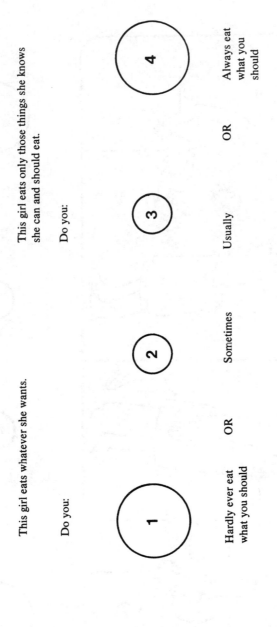

| 1 | 2 | 3 | 4 |

Hardly ever eat what you should OR Sometimes Usually OR Always eat what you should

What does extra food do?

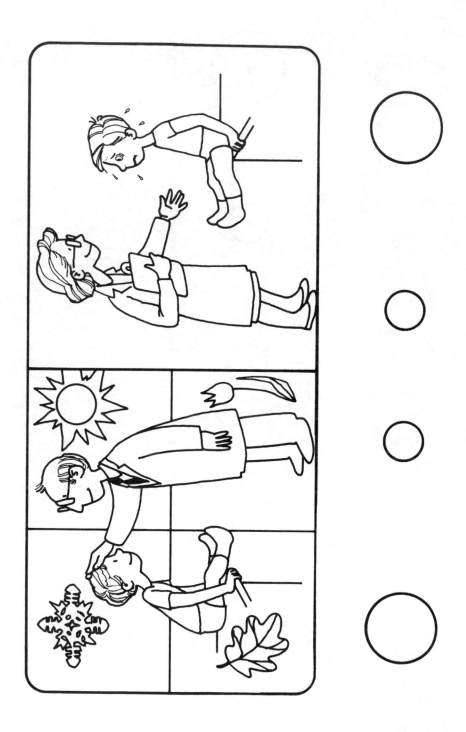

This boy goes to see the diabetes doctor just when he is sick.

Do you go to see the diabetes doctor?

This boy goes to see the diabetes doctor regularly.

(1) (2) (3) (4)

Whenever you want   OR   Once in a while   Whenever you remember   OR   Regularly

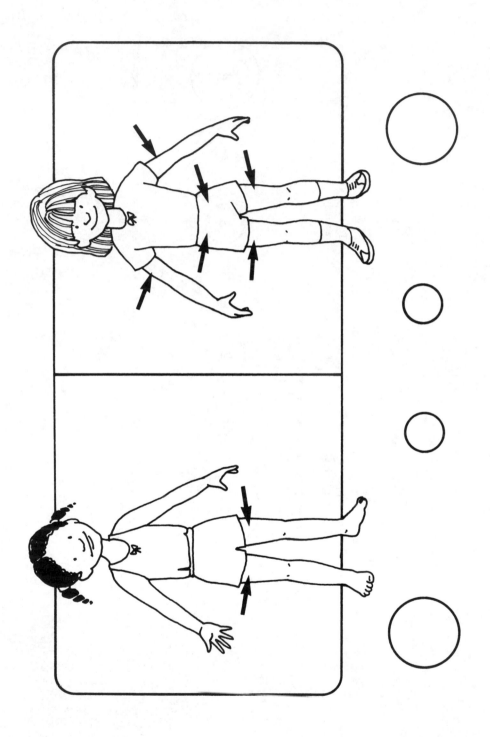

This girl has her insulin shot in different places.

This girl has her insulin shot only in one place.

Do you have your insulin shot?

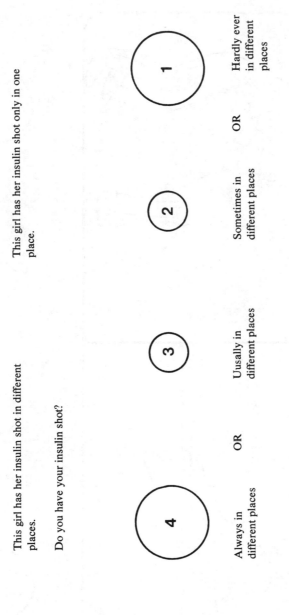

| 4 | OR | 3 | 2 | OR | 1 |

Always in
different places

Uusally in
different places

Sometimes in
different places

Hardly ever
in different
places

Which places do you get your shot?

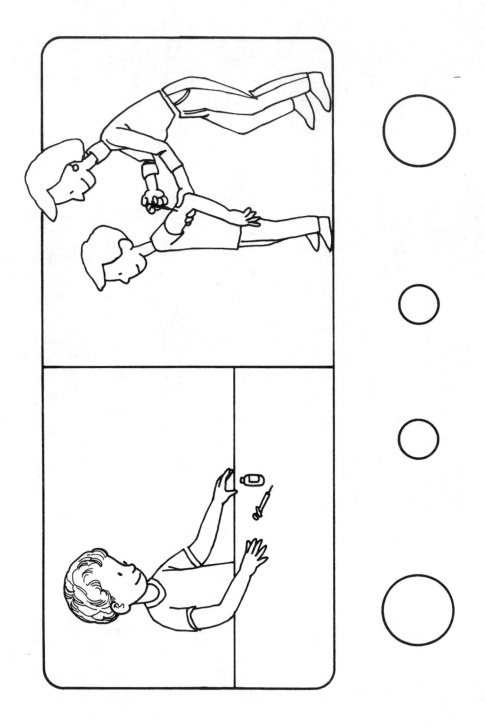

This boy has his mother give him shots.

Do you:

This boy always gives his own shots.

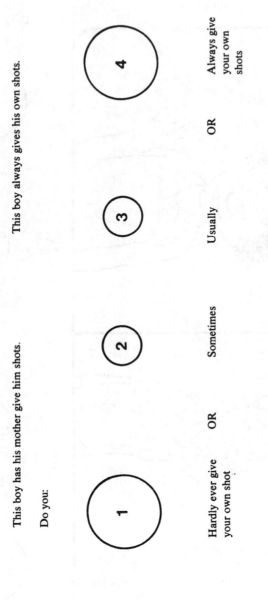

1	2	3	4
Hardly ever give your own shot	Sometimes	Usually	Always give your own shots
OR		OR	

Who gives your shots?

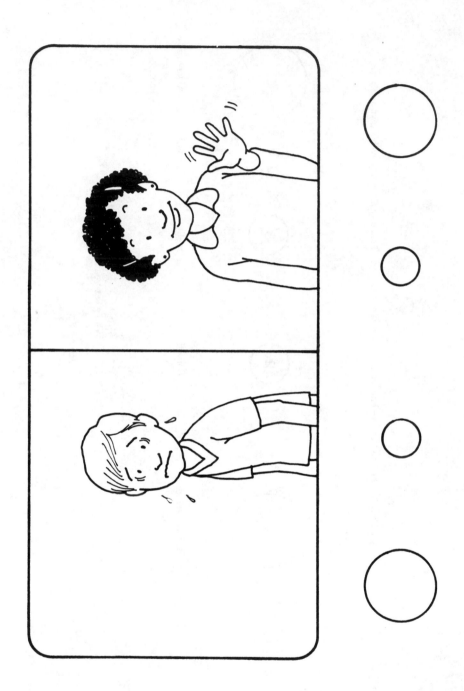

This child doesn't have insulin reactions often.

Do you have:

This child has lots of insulin reactions.

(4)   (3)   (2)   (1)

Some reactions   OR   A Few   Many   OR   Lots of reactions

When do you have reactions?
What do you do about them?

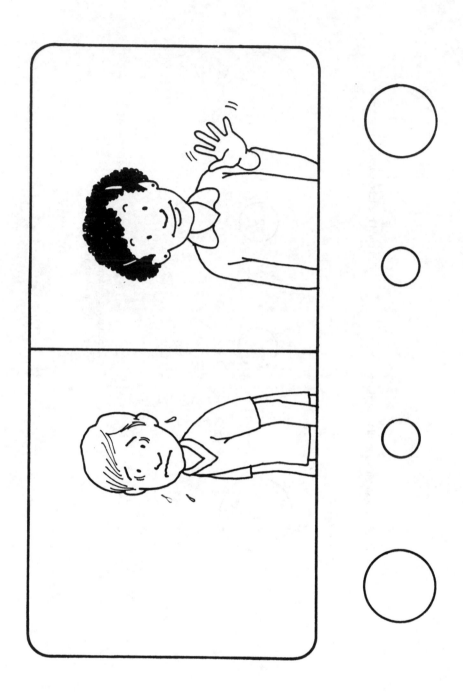

This boy eats his meals and snacks
anytime he wants.

Do your

This boys eats his meals and snacks at the
same time every day.

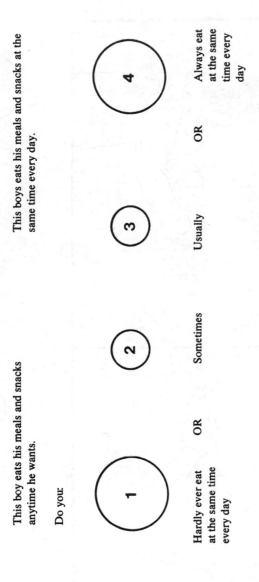

Hardly ever eat
at the same time
every day

OR

Sometimes

Usually

OR

Always eat
at the same
time every
day

When do you eat?
Who chooses your snacks?

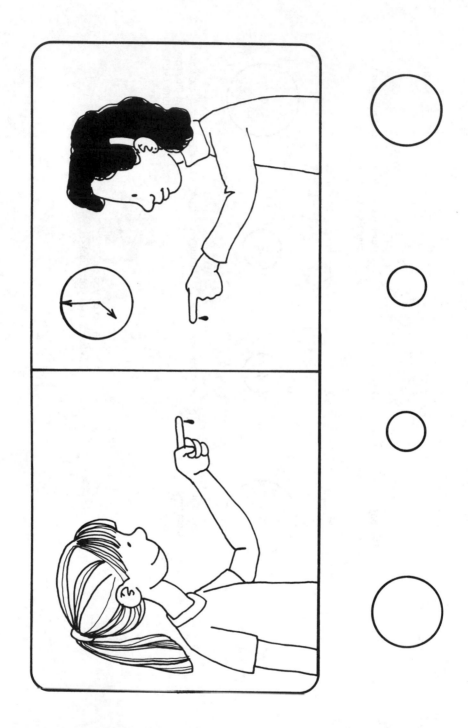

This girl checks her blood glucose level at the same time every day.

This girl checks her blood glucose level whenever she wants.

Do you check your blood glucose level at the same time every day?

(4)   (3)   (2)   (1)

Always   OR   Usually   Sometimes   OR   Hardly ever

When do you check your blood glucose level?
Why do you check it?

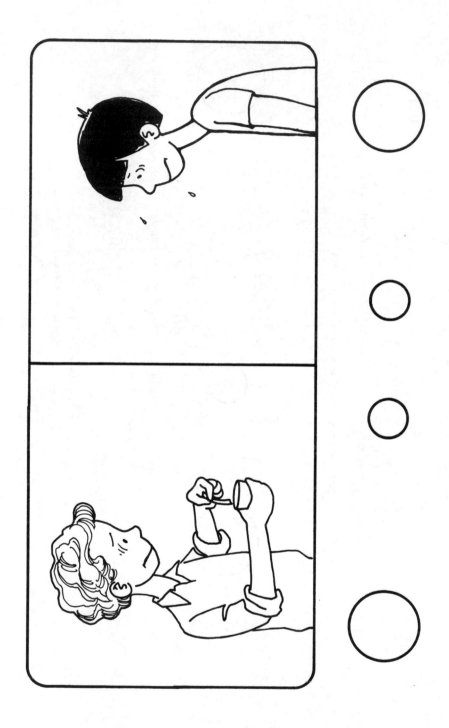

This boy checks his urine whenever he wants.

This boy checks his urine when he is sick.

Do you check your urine at the same time every day?

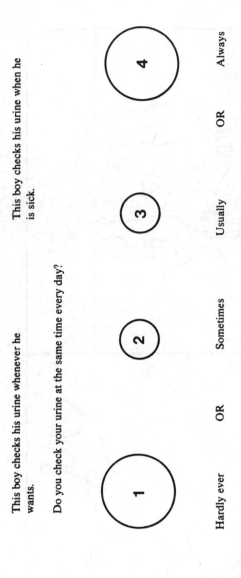

| Hardly ever | OR | Sometimes | Usually | OR | Always |

Why do you check your urine?

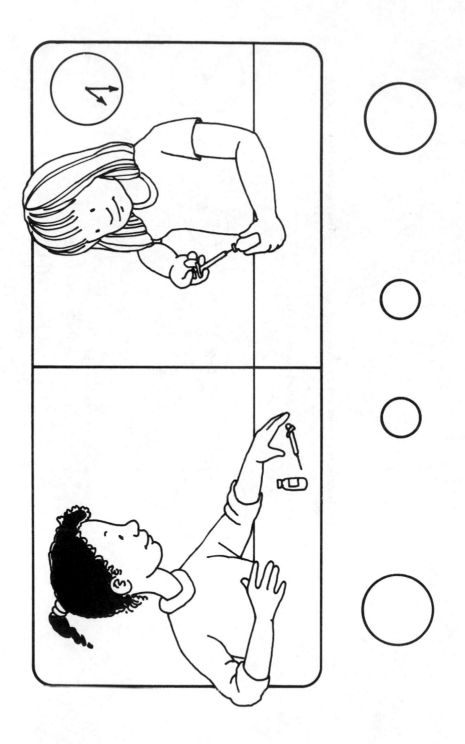

This girl gets her insulin at different times every day.

This girl takes her insulin at the same time every day.

Do you:

4   OR   **3**   **2**   OR   **1**

Always take   Usually   Sometimes   Hardly ever
your insulin at   take your
the same time   insulin at
                                                         the same time

When do you take your insulin?
Do you wait between shots and eating?
How long?

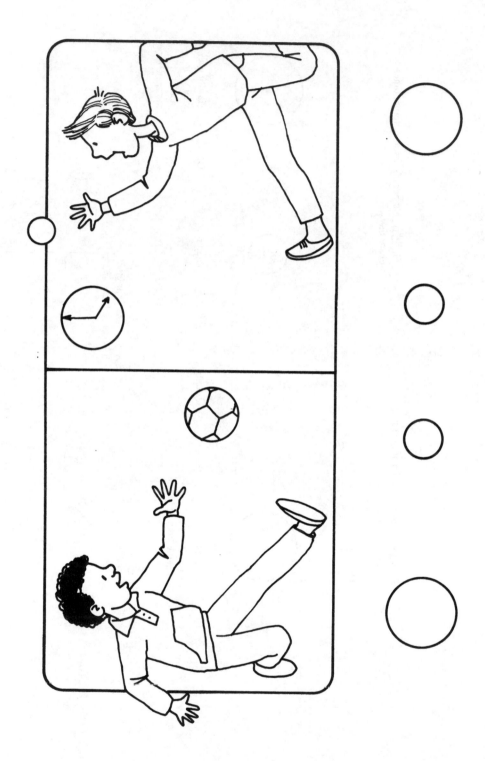

This boy exercises at the same time every day.

Do you exercise?

This boy exercises whenever he wants.

| 4 | OR | 3 | 2 | OR | 1 |

Always at the same time every day

Uusally at the same time

Sometimes at the same time every day

Whenever you want

When do you exercise?
What does exercise do to your blood sugar?

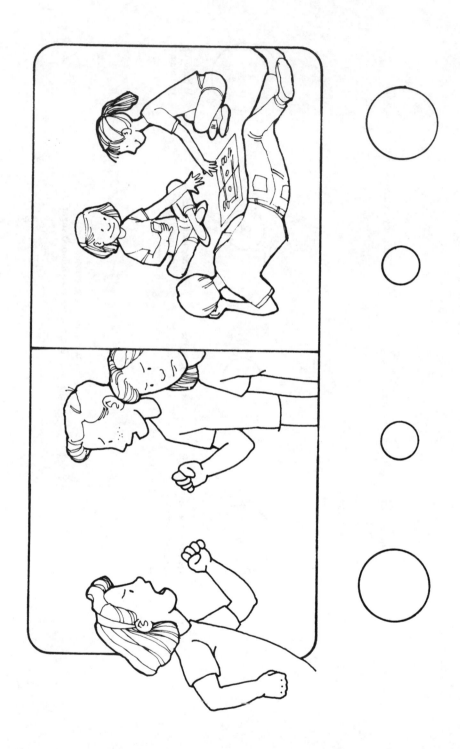

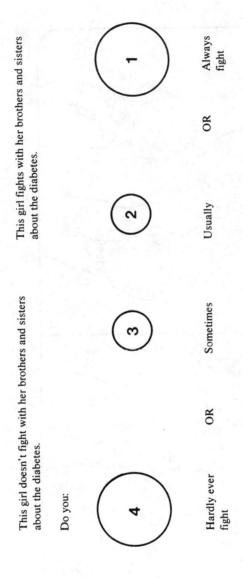

This girl fights with her brothers and sisters about the diabetes.

This girl doesn't fight with her brothers and sisters about the diabetes.

Do you:

4		3		2		1
Hardly ever fight	OR	Sometimes		Usually	OR	Always fight

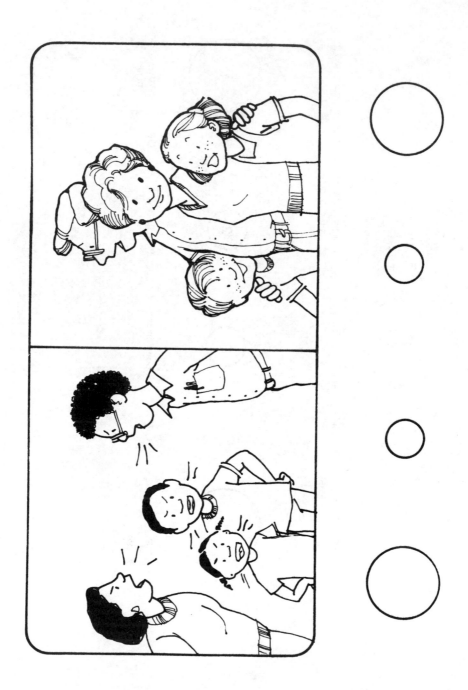

This family doesn't yell
at each other very much.

This family yells alot
and is angry with each other.

Does your family:

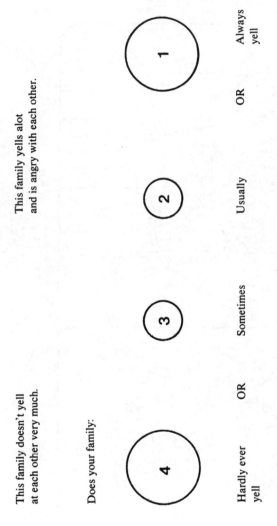

Hardly ever yell	OR	Sometimes	Usually	OR	Always yell
4		3	2		1

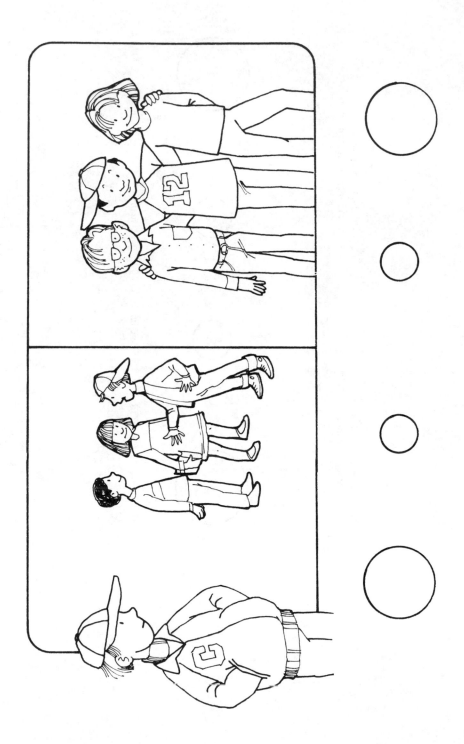

This boy doesn't feel different from other kids.

This boy feels different from other kids.

Do you:

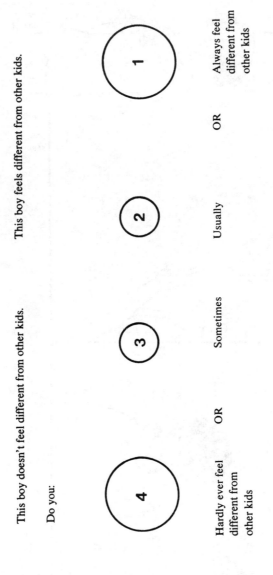

| Hardly ever feel different from other kids | OR | Sometimes | Usually | OR | Always feel different from other kids |

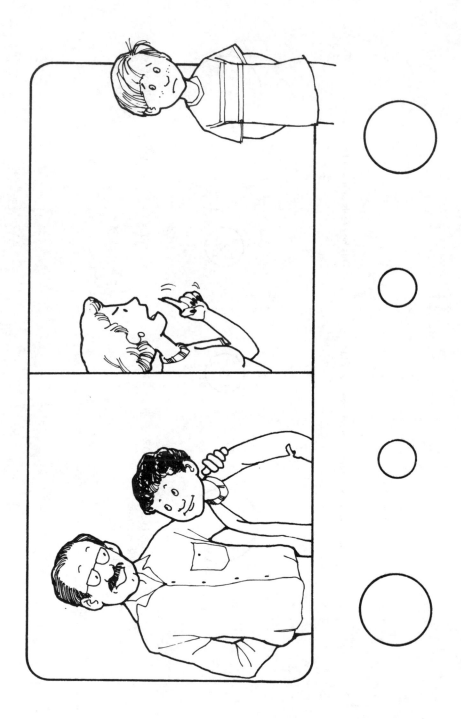

This child's parents yell at him about his diabetes.

Do your parents:

This child's parents don't yell at him about his diabetes.

(1)   (2)   (3)   (4)

Always   OR   Usually   Sometimes   OR   Hardly ever
yell   yell

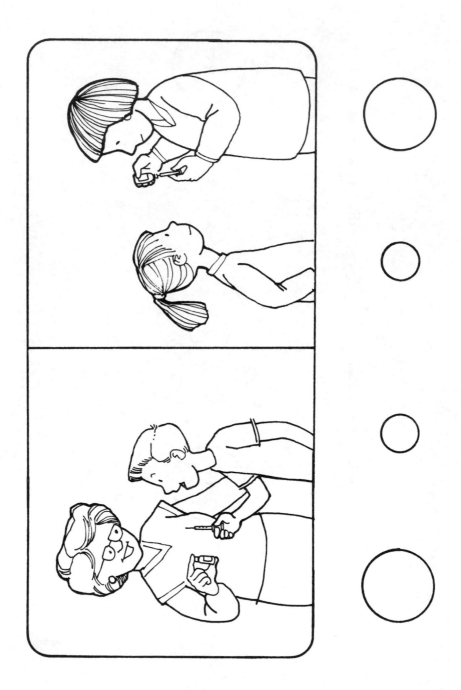

This family doesn't talk about how much insulin to give.

This family talks about how much insulin to give.

Does your family:

(1)   (2)   (3)   (4)

Hardly ever   OR   Sometimes   Usually   OR   Always
talk about   talk about
how much   how much
insulin to give   insulin to give

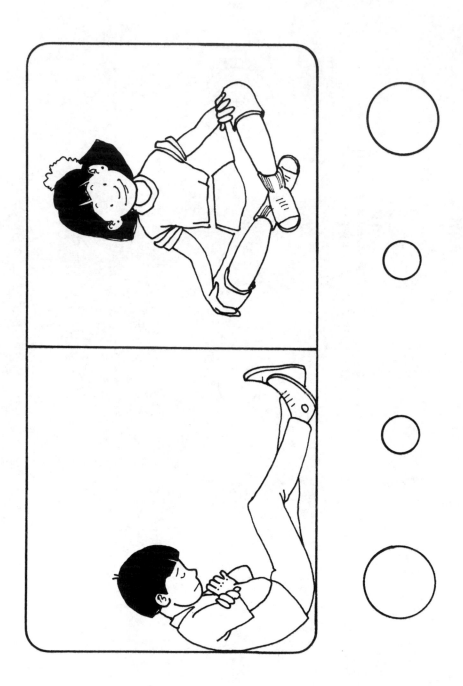

Diabetes doesn't bother this child alot.

Diabetes bothers this child alot.

Does your diabetes:

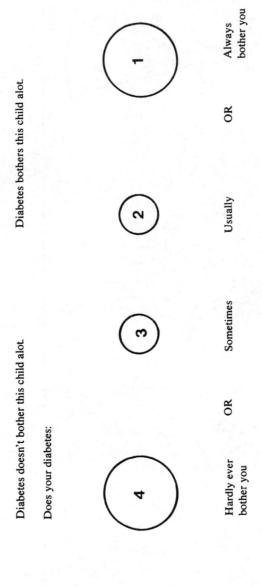

| Hardly ever bother you | OR | Sometimes | Usually | OR | Always bother you |

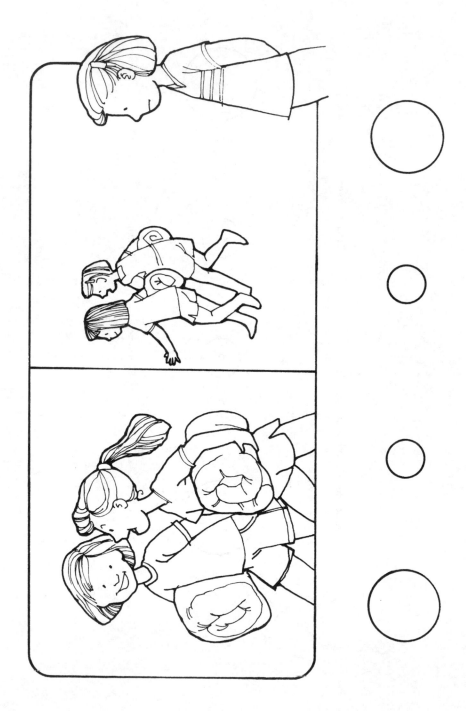

This girl can't do what she likes
because she has diabetes.

Do you:

This girl gets to do what she likes,
even though she has diabetes.

(1) OR (2) (3) OR (4)

Hardly ever   Sometimes   Usually   Always
get to do   get to do
what you want   what you want

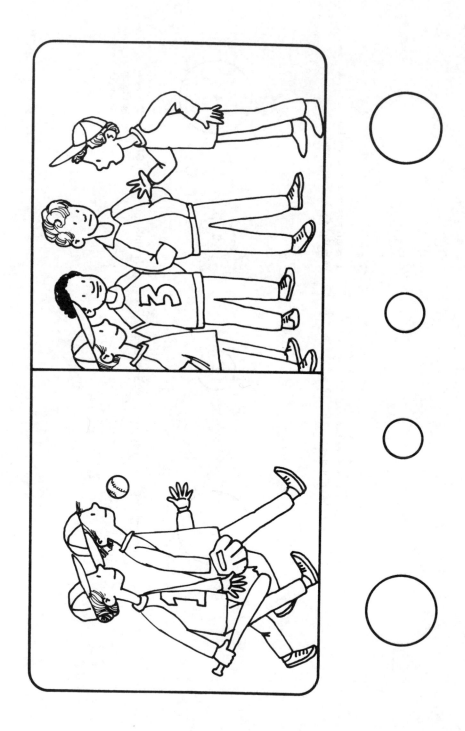

This boy tells all his friends about his diabetes.

This boy doesn't tell anyone about his diabetes.

Do you tell:

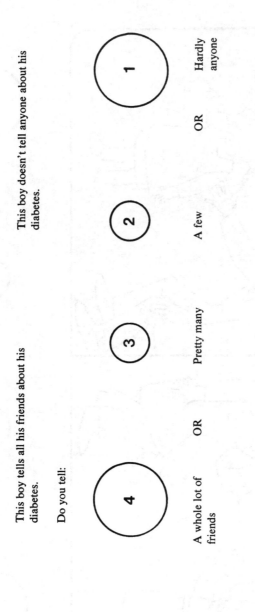

| A whole lot of friends | OR | Pretty many | A few | OR | Hardly anyone |

What did you tell your friends about your diabetes?

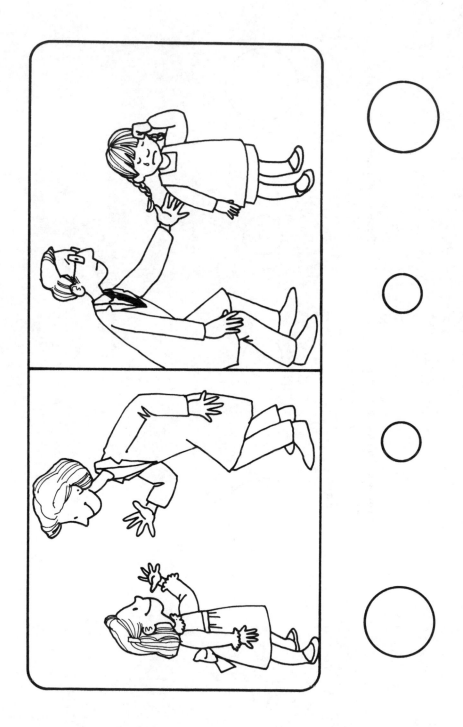

This girl doesn't like to go to see the doctor.

Do you:

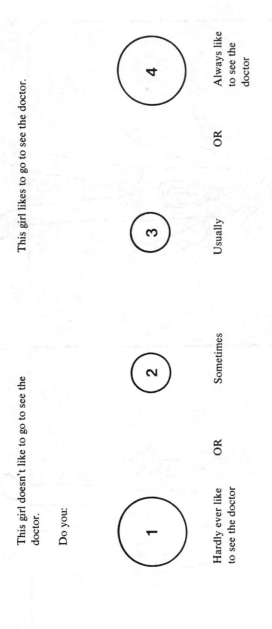

This girl likes to go to see the doctor.

| 1 | | 2 | 3 | | 4 |

Hardly ever like to see the doctor   OR   Sometimes   Usually   OR   Always like to see the doctor

What happens when you go to the doctor?

115

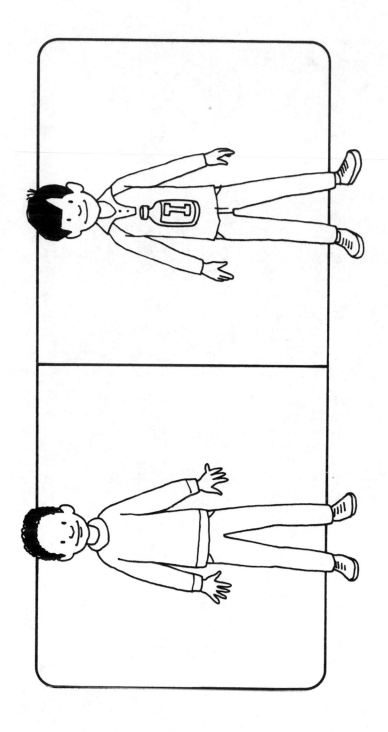

This boy has diabetes and he has enough insulin in his body.

This boy has diabetes but he doesn't have enough insulin in his body.

What does insulin do for this boy?
(point to boy on examiner's left)

What will happen to this boy if there is no insulin?
(point to boy on examiner's right)

Why don't other kids need to take insulin?

DPS Scoring Form

Child's Name: _____ Date _____

Age: _____ Sex: _____ Examiner: _____

Other Pertinent Information: _____

_____

****

ITEM	DESCRIPTION	RESPONSE (circle one)			
1	Frequency of exercise	1	2	3	4
2	Range of diet	1	2	3	4
3	Visits doctor	1	2	3	4
4	Injection sites	1	2	3	4
5	Who gives injections	1	2	3	4
6	Insulin reactions	1	2	3	4
7	Snacks	1	2	3	4
8	Blood glucose monitoring	1	2	3	4
9	Urine checks	1	2	3	4
10	Insulin timing	1	2	3	4
11	Exercise regularity	1	2	3	4
12	Sibling conflict	1	2	3	4
13	Family conflict	1	2	3	4
14	Feeling different	1	2	3	4
15	Parent-child conflict	1	2	3	4
16	How much insulin to give	1	2	3	4
17	Diabetes bothers me	1	2	3	4
18	Do what I like	1	2	3	4
19	Tells friends	1	2	3	4
20	Likes to see doctor	1	2	3	4

TOTAL SCORE: _____

21 Role of insulin:

_____

_____

_____

Additional Notes:

13

Diabetes Quality of Life for Youths

Developed by Gary M. Ingersoll and Davis G. Marrero

INSTRUMENT DESCRIPTION, ADMINISTRATION, AND SCORING GUIDELINES

The Diabetes Quality of Life (DQOL) measure was developed to assess the psychosocial impact of intensified regimens in the Diabetes Control and Complication Trial, which excluded children and adolescents. The Diabetes Quality of Life for Youths (DQOLY) is a modification of the DQOL for specific use in young diabetes populations (older children and adolescents). Self-perceived quality of life is an important, although relatively new, outcome for diabetes management and education programs. Scores for scales are obtained by summing those for items.

PSYCHOMETRIC PROPERTIES

Before field testing, the instrument was reviewed by four health professional specialists in pediatric diabetes care, who recommended dropping DQOL items of limited value for children and adolescents, and adding items relating to school life and peers. Items were then field tested with 15 youths ages 11 to 18, which led to simplification of wording of the questions and response format. The DQOLY was then administered to 74 children and adolescents with insulin-dependent diabetes mellitus and a mean age of 16 years. It is composed of three intercorrelated scales: a Diabetes Life Satisfaction scale (17 items; Cronbach α, .85; mean score, 83.9), a Disease Impact scale (23 items; Cronbach α, .83; mean score, 46.5), and a Disease-Related Worries scale (11 items; Cronbach α, .82; mean score, 29.1), and a self-rating of overall health. Girls were more likely than were boys to report disease-related worries (Ingersoll & Marrero, 1991).

All three scales were predictive of adolescents' self-rated health status with disease-related worries and perceived disease impact inversely related, and diabetes life satisfaction positively related. In combination, the scales accounted for 29% of the variance. DQOLY scales did not correlate with metabolic control as measured by glycosylated hemoglobin values but did so with self-perceived health status in self-reported health status. These data suggest that self-perceived quality of life holds a different meaning to adolescents than it may to clinicians, who frequently equate good metabolic control with quality of life (Ingersoll & Marrero, 1991).

CRITIQUE AND SUMMARY

Because practitioners have a tendency to equate good metabolic control with quality of life, an instrument like the DQOLY should be helpful in seeing them as two different but important health care outcomes against which interventions should be evaluated. This clear distinction is especially important for adolescents because the developmental demands of a restructured body image, new cognitive abilities, a revised value system, new peer and intimate relationships, and establishment of a sense of adult independence may conflict with the task demands for adherence to a diabetes regimen (Ingersoll & Marrero, 1991).

Additional studies of the validity of DQOLY with diverse populations will be helpful to its further development and usefulness. This should include studies of the areas children and adolescents perceive affect their quality of life; alteration of content from a tool for adults may not be sufficient. Unlike some other quality-of-life measures, the DQOLY includes many items that could be affected by self-management education. It would be helpful to know its sensitivity to such interventions.

REFERENCE

Ingersoll, G. M., & Marrero, D. G. (1991). A modified quality-of-life measure for youths: Psychometric properties. *The Diabetes Educator, 17,* 114–118.

DIABETES QUALITY OF LIFE QUESTIONNAIRE: YOUTHS

Please do not place your name on this or any subsequent sheet of paper in this questionnaire. Please answer each question by filling in the blanks or by circling the answer that best reflects your choice.

What is your sex?   [M] Male   [F] Female

What is your ethnic group?   [B] Black   [W] White
                               [H] Hispanic   [A] Asian American
                               [I] American Indian
                               [O] Other

When were you born?   _____/_____
                               Month Year

How old were you when you were first told you had diabetes? _____

In what grade are you currently enrolled? _____

How many days of school did you miss in the last year because of your diabetes? _____

A: **DIRECTIONS:** Read each statement carefully. Please indicate how satisfied or dissatisfied you currently are with the aspect of your life described in the statement. Mark [X] the box that matches how satisfied or dissatisfied you feel: 1 = Very Satisfied, 2 = Moderately Satisfied, 3 = Neither Satisfied nor Dissatisfied, 4 = Moderately Dissatisfied, 5 = Very Dissatisfied. There are no right or wrong answers to these questions. We want your opinion.

	Very Satisfied				Very Dissatisfied
A1: How satisfied are you with the amount of time it takes to manage your diabetes?	[1]	[2]	[3]	[4]	[5]
A2: How satisfied are you with the amount of time you spend getting checkups?	[1]	[2]	[3]	[4]	[5]
A3: How satisfied are you with the time it takes to determine your blood sugar?	[1]	[2]	[3]	[4]	[5]
A4: How satisfied are you with your current treatment?	[1]	[2]	[3]	[4]	[5]
A5: How satisfied are you with the flexibility you have with your diet?	[1]	[2]	[3]	[4]	[5]
A6: How satisfied are you with the burden your diabetes is placing on your family?	[1]	[2]	[3]	[4]	[5]
A7: How satisfied are you with your knowledge about your diabetes?	[1]	[2]	[3]	[4]	[5]

	Very Satisfied				Very Dissatisfied

SPEAKING GENERALLY:

A8: How satisfied are you with your sleep?	[1]	[2]	[3]	[4]	[5]
A9: How satisfied are you with your friendships?	[1]	[2]	[3]	[4]	[5]
A10: How satisfied are you with your work, school, and household activities?	[1]	[2]	[3]	[4]	[5]
A11: How satisfied are you with the appearance of your body?	[1]	[2]	[3]	[4]	[5]
A12: How satisfied are you with the time you spend exercising?	[1]	[2]	[3]	[4]	[5]
A13: How satisfied are you with your leisure time?	[1]	[2]	[3]	[4]	[5]
A14: How satisfied are you with life in general?	[1]	[2]	[3]	[4]	[5]
A15: How satisfied are you with performance in school?	[1]	[2]	[3]	[4]	[5]
A16: How satisfied are you with how your class-mates treat you?	[1]	[2]	[3]	[4]	[5]
A17: How satisfied are you with your attendance at school?	[1]	[2]	[3]	[4]	[5]

Compared with others your age, would you say your health is:

- ❏ Excellent
- ❏ Good
- ❏ Fair
- ❏ Poor

DIRECTIONS: Read each statement carefully. Please indicate *How Often* the following events happen to you. Mark [X] the box that matches how satisfied or dissatisfied you feel: 1 = Never, 2 = Very Seldom, 3 = Sometimes, 4 = Very Often, 5 = All the Time. There are no right or wrong answers to these questions. We are interested in your honest opinion.

	Never	Very Seldom	Some-times	Often	All the Time
B1: How often do you feel pain associated with the treatment of your diabetes?	[1]	[2]	[3]	[4]	[5]
B2: How often are you embarrassed by having to deal with your diabetes in public?	[1]	[2]	[3]	[4]	[5]

	Never	Very Seldom	Some-times	Often	All the Time
B3: How often do you feel physically ill?	[1]	[2]	[3]	[4]	[5]
B4: How often does your diabetes interfere with your family life?	[1]	[2]	[3]	[4]	[5]
B5: How often do you have a bad night's sleep?	[1]	[2]	[3]	[4]	[5]
B6: How often do you find your diabetes limiting your social relationships and friendships?	[1]	[2]	[3]	[4]	[5]
B7: How often do you feel good about yourself?	[1]	[2]	[3]	[4]	[5]
B8: How often do you feel restricted by your diet?	[1]	[2]	[3]	[4]	[5]
B9: How often does your diabetes keep you from driving a car?	[1]	[2]	[3]	[4]	[5]
B10: How often does your diabetes interfere with your exercising?	[1]	[2]	[3]	[4]	[5]
B11: How often do you miss work, school, or household duties because of your diabetes?	[1]	[2]	[3]	[4]	[5]
B12: How often do you find yourself explaining what it means to have diabetes?	[1]	[2]	[3]	[4]	[5]
B13: How often do you find that your diabetes interrupts your leisure time activities?	[1]	[2]	[3]	[4]	[5]
B14: How often are you teased because you have diabetes?	[1]	[2]	[3]	[4]	[5]
B15: How often do you feel that because of your diabetes you go to the bathroom more than others?	[1]	[2]	[3]	[4]	[5]
B16: How often do you find you eat something you shouldn't rather than tell someone that you have diabetes?	[1]	[2]	[3]	[4]	[5]
B17: How often do you hide from others the fact that you are having an insulin reaction?	[1]	[2]	[3]	[4]	[5]
B18: How often do you find that your diabetes prevents you from participating in school activities (for example, a school play, playing a sport)?	[1]	[2]	[3]	[4]	[5]
B19: How often do you find that your diabetes prevents you from going out to eat with your friends?	[1]	[2]	[3]	[4]	[5]
B20: How often do you feel that your diabetes will limit what job you will have in the future?	[1]	[2]	[3]	[4]	[5]

	Never	Very Seldom	Some-times	Often	All the Time
B21: How often do you find that your parents are too protective of you?	[1]	[2]	[3]	[4]	[5]
B22: How often do you find that your parents worry too much about your diabetes?	[1]	[2]	[3]	[4]	[5]
B23: How often do you find that your parents act like diabetes is their disease, not yours?	[1]	[2]	[3]	[4]	[5]

DIRECTIONS: Read each statement carefully. Please indicate how often the following events happen to you. Check [X] the appropriate box. There are no right or wrong answers to these questions. If the question is not relevant to you, check "Does Not Apply."

	Does Not Apply	Never	Seldom	Some-times	Often	All the Time
C1: How often do you worry about whether you will get married?	[0]	[1]	[2]	[3]	[4]	[5]
C2: How often do you worry about whether you will have children?	[0]	[1]	[2]	[3]	[4]	[5]
C3: How often do you worry about whether you will not get a job you want?	[0]	[1]	[2]	[3]	[4]	[5]
C4: How often do you worry about whether you will pass out?	[0]	[1]	[2]	[3]	[4]	[5]
C5: How often do you worry about whether you will be able to complete your education?	[0]	[1]	[2]	[3]	[4]	[5]
C6: How often do you worry that your body looks different because you have diabetes?	[0]	[1]	[2]	[3]	[4]	[5]
C7: How often do you worry that you will get complications from your diabetes?	[0]	[1]	[2]	[3]	[4]	[5]
C8: How often do you worry whether someone will not go out with you because you have diabetes?	[0]	[1]	[2]	[3]	[4]	[5]

	Does Not Apply	Never	Seldom	Some-times	Often	All the Time
C9: How often do you worry that teachers treat you differently because of your diabetes?	[0]	[1]	[2]	[3]	[4]	[5]
C10: How often do you worry that your diabetes will interfere with things that you do in school (sports, music, drama)?	[0]	[1]	[2]	[3]	[4]	[5]
C11: How often do you worry that your diabetes causes you to do things with friends like going on dates or going to parties?	[0]	[1]	[2]	[3]	[4]	[5]

From the Indiana University Diabetes Research and Training Center.

The Diabetes Educator, copyright 1991, the American Association of Diabetes Education.

C

Arthritis

14

Rheumatology Attitudes Index

Developed by Leigh Callahan, Health Report Services

INSTRUMENT DESCRIPTION, ADMINISTRATION, AND SCORING GUIDELINES

The Rheumatology Attitudes Index (RAI) is a revision of the Arthritis Helplessness Index (AHI), originally established to measure motivational, cognitive, and emotional deficits found in individuals who are forced to deal with stressful situations, in this case rheumatic disease. The largely unpredictable nature of the remissions and exacerbations in rheumatic disease may contribute to uncertainty, feelings of helplessness, and passive resignation—a sense of loss of control. Helplessness generally refers to a psychological state in which individuals expect that their efforts will be ineffective (DeVellis & Callahan, 1993).

Although the constructs of learned helplessness, health locus of control (expectation about whether one's health is controlled by one's own behavior or by external forces), self-esteem (evaluation of self-worth), and self-efficacy (beliefs regarding one's own capabilities in specific situations) appear related in most patients, they are, in part, independent. Further research is needed to understand distinctions among them and associations of specific constructs with specific disease status measures better (Callahan, Brooks, & Pincus, 1988).

The RAI is a modification on the AHI in which the items have been reworded to be applicable to rheumatic diseases more generally instead of rheumatoid arthritis specifically and a fifth, neutral response option added to the original four options. The RAI consists of 15 belief statements, scored on a 5-point Likert scale: strongly disagree (= 1), disagree (= 2), do not agree or disagree (= 3), agree (= 4), or strongly agree (= 5). Scores are reversed for items 2, 3, 5, 6, 8, 9, 11, 13, and 15 and summed. A higher score indicates a greater sense of control (Callahan et al., 1988). Sample scores could not be located in published reports using the RAI.

PSYCHOMETRIC PROPERTIES

The original development study of the AHI showed a Cronbach's α of .69, a test-retest reliability of .52 over a 1-year period, and a unidimensional scale. It was later shown to be composed of two relatively independent subscales of internality and personal helplessness. Tests of the AHI found greater perceived helplessness correlated with greater age, lesser education, lower self-esteem, lower internal health locus of control, higher anxiety, depression, and impairment in performing activities of daily living. Changes in AHI scores were strongly correlated with changes in difficulty scores in individual patients, reflecting overall disease severity. The AHI was thought to be useful in clinical evaluation and screening of patients who might benefit from psychosocial interventions, such as education to promote independence and better coping skills (Nicassio, Wallston, Callahan, Herbert, & Pincus, 1985).

In yet another study, perceived helplessness as measured by the AHI and disease severity were the two best predictors of physical functioning cross-sectionally and longitudinally, accounting for 35% to 59% of the variance in physical functioning (Lorish, Abraham, Austin, Bradley, & Alarcon, 1991).

The modified renamed scale (RAI) was found to have an α reliability coefficient of .68, and indication that the RAI and the AHI provide similar information. There was support for external criterion validity in significant correlations between RAI scores and physical measures of disease status including joint count, grip strength, walking time and button test, and self-report scores for difficulty, dissatisfaction, and pain in activities of daily living (Callahan et al., 1998).

A study of the factor structure of the RAI was based on 1,420 individuals with rheumatoid arthritis in 11 cities, with a mean formal education of 12.5 years. The study found two relatively independent scales, which tap separate constructs. One scale measures more of an arthritis specific internal locus of control dimension (items 2, 3, 5, 6, 8, and 9, with a Cronbach α of .75 and a stability coefficient of .59 over 6 months) and a helplessness scale (items 1, 10, 12, 13 reverse scored, and 14, with a Cronbach α of .63 and a stability coefficient of .64 over 6 months). The helplessness subscale is the more clinically useful, associated with greater adjustment difficulties including measures of noncompliance with recommended treatment regimens, greater use of passive pain coping behaviors, and higher impairment in functional status. This scale also appears to be sensitive to changes over time, showing distinct differences in psychological functioning, and behavior and symptom severity 2 years after the original assessment (Stein, Wallston, & Nicassio, 1988).

The helplessness scale by itself has been found to be more significantly related to grip strength; button-test time; 25-foot walking time; joint tenderness, swelling, limited motion, deformity, and total joint count; and erythrocyte sedimentation rate than was the entire RAI. The authors believe this scale constitutes an acceptable measure of helplessness, for research and for screening purposes. Because there is no widely accepted measure of general helplessness, it is difficult to show concurrent validity between the general concept and the rheumatology-specific measures (DeVellis & Callahan, 1993).

Although development of the RAI was accomplished with patients with rheumatoid arthritis, subsequent studies have provided information about its measurement characteristics with patients with systemic lupus erythematosis. As with studies cited previously, Cronbach's α was .70, and there were significant correlations with self-reported physical disability, dissatisfaction, and pain scores (Engle, Callahan, Pincus, & Hochberg, 1990).

Finally, Burckhardt, Mannerkorpi, Hedenberg, and Bjelle (1994) used RAI in a trial of education and education with physical training for women with fibromyalgia (FMS). Classes included information on FMS, the role of stress in the development and maintenance of symptoms, coping strategies, problem-solving techniques, assertiveness training, relaxation strategies, and the importance of physical conditioning. After each educational session, the second experimental group was given an additional hour of physical training. Although the control group did not change significantly on the index, the education group changed significantly in a positive direction.

CRITIQUE AND SUMMARY

Although considerable study of the RAI's psychometric characteristics has been accomplished, more work remains. One potential use of the RAI would be to identify patient subgroups who are more likely to benefit from patient education. Because the reliabilities are at the low end of the acceptable range, the scales may be adequate, at present, for research or general screening purposes but should not be used by themselves for making individual clinical judgments. In addition, the items did not factor as clearly as one might hope, raising concerns about validity (DeVellis & Callahan, 1993).

REFERENCES

Burckhardt, C. S., Mannerkorpi, K., Hedenberg, L., & Bjelle, A. (1994). A randomized controlled clinical trial of education and physical training for women with fibromyalgia. *Journal of Rheumatology, 21,* 714–720.

Callahan, L. F., Brooks, R. H., & Pincus, T. (1988). Further analysis of learned helplessness in rheumatoid arthritis using a "Rheumatology Attitudes Index." *Journal of Rheumatology, 15,* 418–425.

DeVellis, R. F., & Callahan, L. F. (1993). A brief measure of helplessness in rheumatic disease: The helplessness subscale of the Rheumatology Attitudes Index. *Journal of Rheumatology, 20,* 866–869.

Engle, E. W., Callahan, L. F., Pincus, T., & Hochberg, M.C. (1990). Learned helplessness in systemic lupus erythematosus: Analysis using the Rheumatology Attitudes Index. *Arthritis and Rheumatism, 33,* 281–286.

Lorish, C. D., Abraham, N., Austin, J., Bradley, L. A., & Alarcon, G. S. (1991). Disease and psychosocial factors related to physical functioning in rheumatoid arthritis. *Journal of Rheumatology, 18,* 1150–1157.

Nicassio, P. M., Wallston, K. A., Callahan, L. F., Herbert M., & Pincus, T. (1985). The measurement of helplessness in rheumatoid arthritis: The development of the Arthritis Helplessness Index. *Journal of Rheumatology, 12,* 462–467.

Stein, M. J., Wallston, K. A., & Nicassio, P. M. (1988). Factor structure of the Arthritis Helplessness Index. *Journal of Rheumatology, 15,* 427–432.

RHEUMATOLOGY ATTITUDES INDEX

Question	Strongly disagree	Disagree	Do not agree or disagree	Agree	Strongly agree
1.* My condition is controlling my life.	1	2	3	4	5
2.* Managing my condition is largely my own responsibility.	1	2	3	4	5
3.† I can reduce my pain by staying calm and relaxed.	1	2	3	4	5
4.† Too often, my pain just seems to hit me from out of the blue.	1	2	3	4	5
5.* If I do all the right things, I can successfully manage my condition.	1	2	3	4	5
6.* I can do a lot of things myself to cope with my condition.	1	2	3	4	5
7.* When it comes to managing my condition, I feel I can only do what my doctor tells me to do.	1	2	3	4	5
8.* When I manage my personal life well, my condition does not flare as much.	1	2	3	4	5
9.† I have considerable ability to control my pain.	1	2	3	4	5
10.* I would feel helpless if I couldn't rely on other people for help with my condition.	1	2	3	4	5
11.* Usually, I can tell when my condition will flare.	1	2	3	4	5
12.† No matter what I do, or how hard I try, I just can't seem to get relief from my pain.	1	2	3	4	5
13.* I am coping effectively with my condition.	1	2	3	4	5
14.* It seems as though fate and other factors beyond my control affect my condition.	1	2	3	4	5
15.* I want to learn as much as I can about my condition.	1	2	3	4	5

Total Score

*The word "condition" is used in the RAI in lieu of "arthritis" in the Arthritis Helplessness Index.
†The statement is identical in the RAI and Arthritis Helplessness Index.
From Callahan, L. F., Brooks, R. H., & Pincus, T. (1988). Further analysis of learned helplessness in rheumatoid arthritis using a "Rheumatology Attitudes Index." *Journal of Rheumatology, 15*, 418–425.
Used with permission: Health Services Report.

15

Arthritis Knowledge Questionnaire

Developed by Steven M. Edworthy, Gerald M. Devins, and Margaret M. Watson

INSTRUMENT DESCRIPTION, ADMINISTRATION, AND SCORING GUIDELINES

Patient education has long been well accepted in management of arthritis, with development of self-management skills being the principal focus. Patients must have the ability to adjust daily exercise regimens, rest/activity periods, and drug regimens according to the changing activity of their disease. Five other previously reported arthritis knowledge tests are cited in the report describing the Arthritis Knowledge Questionnaire (AKQ) (Edworthy, Devins, & Watson, 1995).

The AKQ consists of two parallel forms, each comprising three subtests: self-management (15 items), arthritis in general (15 items), and rheumatoid arthritis (11 items). These forms are equivalent in item difficulty, content, and internal consistency. Reading level is approximately grade 8 (Edworthy, Devins, & Watson, 1995). It is assumed that scoring involves counting the number of correct responses for each subscale and form.

PSYCHOMETRIC PROPERTIES

Domains identified as important to include in the instrument, based on the Stanford Arthritis Self-Management Program, include diagnosis of disease, medications, use of exercise, control of pain and depression, improvement of sleep, and communication with health care professionals. A rheumatologist, psychologist, physiotherapist, and several lay individuals assessed the questions for content validity, breadth of coverage, and face validity. Patients assessed the questions for comprehensibility (Edworthy et al., 1995).

Coefficient α ranged from .72 to .84 for the subtests and .90 on each of Forms A and B. AKQ scores differed significantly in the hypothesized pattern across four groups of health professionals who should have different knowledge levels about this content. Preliminary data from 37 participants showed significant increases for two of the three subtests before and after arthritis education (Edworthy et al., 1995).

CRITIQUE AND SUMMARY

The AKQ can be used to identify patients who lack understanding of arthritis-related knowledge and can be used to evaluate effectiveness of education efforts. It was carefully developed but includes potential problems with reading level that is too high for some patients. The authors also indicate a possible overemphasis on content relevant to rheumatoid arthritis. The domains of knowledge measured in the AKQ are believed to underlie effective adaptation and arthritis self-management. The authors note that the AKQ does not assess behavioral repertoires of relevant skills, such as problem-solving, energy conservation, and so forth, or the competence of an individual to apply these appropriately in response to situational demands (Edworthy et al., 1995). Thus, it is important to remember that acquisition of relevant knowledge will not be sufficient to meet important patient education goals. There is little description of scores obtained by patients or the level of patient knowledge associated with particular patient outcomes, or patients from a variety of social and educational backgrounds.

REFERENCE

Edworthy, S. M., Devins, G. M., & Watson, M. M. (1995). The Arthritis Knowledge Questionnaire. *Arthritis and Rheumatism, 5,* 590–600.

SCORING GUIDELINES—ARTHRITIS
KNOWLEDGE QUESTIONNAIRE

The Arthritis Knowledge Questionnaire is a two-part questionnaire with 41 questions each. It covers three domains: Arthritis General (G) (yellow), RA-Specific (RA) (pink), and Self-Management (SM) (blue). Part A is completed by the patient before the intervention instruments (e.g., Arthritis Self-Management Program).

Each question has one correct response (indicated by the asterisk). If the patient chooses more than one response to a question, or indicates "Don't Know," the answer should be coded as incorrect. The total score is the sum of correct answers for each domain (Arthritis General, RA-Specific, and Self-Management).

A total score can also be computed overall. The order of the tests can be randomly assigned if you are doing a pre-post study. The total set of 82 questions can be administered at one period if you wish (e.g., in the setting of a cross-sectional survey).

ARTHRITIS KNOWLEDGE QUESTIONNAIRE—PART "A"

RA   1.   In Sjögren's syndrome, a common problem is

A.   too much saliva and other secretions.
B.   dryness of the eyes and mouth.*
C.   cold white fingers.
D.   nausea when you eat fish and some seafood.
E.   Don't know

RA   2.   Methotrexate is

A.   an antimalarial medication.
B.   an anti-inflammatory medication.
C.   an immunosuppressant.*
D.   an anxiolytic.
E.   Don't know

RA   3.   Synovitis is

A.   an inflammation of the sinuses.
B.   another name for tendon.
C.   an inflammation of the joint lining.*
D.   fluid in the joint.
E.   Don't know

RA   4.   Surgery is often used in the treatment of rheumatoid arthritis. This is usually only done when

A.   the disability and pain from a joint cannot be managed with drugs.
B.   one joint (or a few joints) are causing most of your problems.
C.   you are paying particular care to all other parts of your treatment program.
D.   All of the above*
E.   Don't know

RA   5.   If you have a hot or inflamed joint, you should

A.   try to exercise as usual.
B.   give it deep massage to get rid of waste products.
C.   take more medication so it doesn't hurt as much.
D.   None of the above*
E.   Don't know

RA   6.   Gold and penicillamine are two examples of drugs that can

A.   only help reduce symptoms of arthritis.
B.   slow down the progress of arthritis.*
C.   cure arthritis.
D.   make arthritis worse.
E.   Don't know

RA　7.　More women than men are reported to have rheumatoid arthritis; this is thought to be mainly because

  A. women actually do get rheumatoid arthritis more often than men do.[*]
  B. more women complain about their health problems than men.
  C. doctors don't like to tell a man he has rheumatoid arthritis.
  D. men are not aware of their joint problems.
  E. Don't know

RA　8.　Penicillamine usually begins to act

  A. right away.
  B. with the second or third dose.
  C. after about 6 weeks.
  D. in about 3 to 6 months.[*]
  E. Don't know

RA　9.　A Baker's cyst is

  A. swelling of the calf from knee fluid.[*]
  B. a sign you are getting old.
  C. what bakers get after years of kneading bread.
  D. another name for bunion.
  E. Don't know

RA　10.　A disease such as rheumatoid arthritis is called a systemic disease because

  A. a physician must be systemic in order to diagnose it.
  B. it involves the whole body.[*]
  C. it involves a particular system of the body.
  D. it is one of a group of diseases that work as a system.
  E. Don't know

RA　11.　Medications that are used to slow the progress of arthritis

  A. work right away to reduce symptoms of arthritis.
  B. have a slow onset of action.[*]
  C. have very few side affects.
  D. can be stopped once arthritis is in remission.
  E. Don't know

SM　12.　"Progressive relaxation" means

  A. relaxing for longer periods of time each day.
  B. accepting that relaxing takes time to do.
  C. relaxing more completely every day.
  D. tensing and relaxing all the muscle groups in the body.[*]
  E. Don't know

SM　13.　Which food has the highest amount of sodium?

  A. Ten large potato chips.
  B. 3/4 cup of tuna fish packed in oil.
  C. One medium dill pickle.[*]
  D. Two ounces of cheddar cheese.
  E. Don't know

SM 14. The best sleeping position for someone with arthritis largely depends upon

  A. how they have slept all their life.
  B. which joints are involved.*
  C. the number of pillows they have available.
  D. nothing in particular.
  E. Don't know

SM 15. The best time of day to do exercises for arthritis is usually

  A. the first thing in the morning.
  B. in the evening.
  C. when you are relaxed and not tired.*
  D. anytime; it doesn't make any difference.
  E. Don't know

SM 16. To maintain and improve the function of arthritic joints and surrounding muscles, stretching exercise sessions should be done

  A. 2–4 times a day depending on pain.*
  B. once a day every day.
  C. 10 times a day.
  D. as many times as possible every second day.
  E. Don't know

SM 17. If your goals are to increase your endurance, maintain a strong heart, and reduce fatigue, endurance exercises should be done for

  A. one hour every day.
  B. half an hour every day.
  C. twenty minutes 3–4 times a week.*
  D. every time you have a chance.
  E. Don't know

SM 18. If you are often tired because of your arthritis, you should

  A. force yourself to carry on in spite of it.
  B. recognize your limitations and share your problem with others.*
  C. alter your medications because they can be the cause of tiredness.
  D. stay in bed until you feel better.
  E. Don't know

SM 19. If you wish to lose weight safely, one of the best ways is to

  A. try to eat only one well-balanced meal in the evening.
  B. avoid all carbohydrates.
  C. avoid all fats.
  D. become more active.*
  E. Don't know

SM 20. If you have problems communicating with the doctor, the best way(s) to help improve this is to

  A. ask for additional time when you make an appointment.
  B. tell your doctor when you really don't know what is going on.

C.   keep your clothes on when you want to discuss something.
D.   All of the above.[*]
E.   Don't know

SM   21.   The ''relaxation response'' is what people feel

A.   after they have been frightened.[*]
B.   after a good night's sleep.
C.   when they sit down after being on their feet too long.
D.   after they have a hot bath.
E.   Don't know

SM   22.   An exercise program

A.   is similar for all people with arthritis.
B.   is similar for individual age groups.
C.   is designed to meet special needs.[*]
D.   is not needed for people with arthritis.
E.   Don't know

SM   23.   If you have stomach problems while you are taking aspirin, what you could do before
calling your doctor is to try to

A.   spread out the dose and always take it with food.[*]
B.   switch to Tylenol because it causes less stomach problems.
C.   stop taking aspirin.
D.   stop drinking water and milk.
E.   Don't know

SM   24.   The best time to exercise is

A.   when you have the least pain and stiffness.
B.   your medication is having its greatest effect.
C.   you are not tired.
D.   All of the above.[*]
E.   Don't know

SM   25.   If you have discomfort longer than 2 hours after exercise, you should

A.   cut back on the number of times you do the exercises.[*]
B.   stop exercising until you feel better.
C.   do more of this exercise as it obviously is doing some good.
D.   take a little more medication and continue as before.
E.   Don't know

SM   26.   If you are frequently tired because of your arthritis, you should

A.   force yourself to carry on in spite of it.
B.   let people know the problem and rest when you can.[*]
C.   alter your medications as they may be causing the fatigue.
D.   stay in bed until you feel better.
E.   Don't know

G   27.   Tendons are

       A.   fibrous cords that attach muscles to bones.*
       B.   the cover at the end of bones.
       C.   fibrous cords that attach bone to bone.
       D.   bone chips.
       E.   Don't know

G   28.   The most important goal of physicians caring for people with arthritis is

       A.   to keep or improve the present level of functioning.*
       B.   to do everything they can to cure the person.
       C.   to give patients enough medication to stand the pain.
       D.   to keep patients quiet and uncomplaining.
       E.   Don't know

G   29.   The most realistic treatment for arthritis is

       A.   one which gives immediate relief.
       B.   one which helps you keep up a near normal life.*
       C.   one with no unpleasant side affects.
       D.   one which cures the disease.
       E.   Don't know

G   30.   Which of the following is known to be true

       A.   some foods are bad for people with arthritis.
       B.   food allergies can make people with arthritis feel worse.*
       C.   the timing of eating is important to people with arthritis.
       D.   All of the above.
       E.   Don't know

G   31.   Constipation is often a problem for many people who have arthritis. This is because

       A.   they are not as physically active.
       B.   their medications tend to be constipating.
       C.   people with arthritis are often under stress.
       D.   All of the above.*
       E.   Don't know

G   32.   Acetaminophen (Tylenol)

       A.   helps reduce inflammation in arthritis.
       B.   only provides temporary relief of mild pain.*
       C.   should be used regularly with your other arthritis medications.
       D.   can be used as a substitute for aspirin in arthritis.
       E.   Don't know

G   33.   Allergies to medications

       A.   are very common.
       B.   will happen to anyone who takes too much of a medication.
       C.   are the same thing as side effects.
       D.   are rare reactions that mean you should not use that drug again.*
       E.   Don't know

G   34.   Prednisone

    A.   can stop the progress of arthritis.
    B.   is a steroid like the ones athletes use.
    C.   helps reduce inflammation in arthritis.[*]
    D.   is a very safe drug with few side effects.
    E.   Don't know

G   35.   The synovial membrane (or sac)

    A.   secretes a fluid that oils the joint.[*]
    B.   protects the nerve endings.
    C.   covers the muscles like a sheath.
    D.   lies between the tendons and the bursa.
    E.   Don't know

G   36.   Side effects of prednisone

    A.   can include cataracts, brittle bones, muscle wasting.
    B.   can be reduced by keeping the dose low.
    C.   are most common with long-term use (more than a month).
    D.   All of the above.[*]
    E.   Don't know

G   37.   Pain is one of the biggest problems in arthritis. This can

    A.   never be completely controlled.
    B.   only can be controlled with some type of medication.
    C.   be controlled by a very few people using a combination of medication and other methods.
    D.   be controlled by most people using a combination of medications and other methods.[*]
    E.   Don't know

G   38.   If an arthritis medication doesn't work within a few days, you should

    A.   keep taking it as the prescription says.[*]
    B.   probably be taking more of it.
    C.   probably be taking something else with it.
    D.   consider exercising to help speed up your system.
    E.   Don't know

G   39.   To a physician "diagnostic certainty" means

    A.   your guess is as good as mine.
    B.   I am certain you have this diagnosis.
    C.   how certain I am that you have this disease.[*]
    D.   how certain I am that I can diagnose a disease.
    E.   Don't know

G   40.   Medications are used in arthritis to

    A.   reduce inflammation.
    B.   slow down the progress of arthritis.
    C.   help control symptoms of arthritis.
    D.   All of the above are correct.[*]
    E.   Don't know

G   41.   Two to four tablets of aspirin a day can

          A.   only reduce mild pain.*
          B.   reduce inflammation.
          C.   fight infection.
          D.   help both pain and inflammation.
          E.   Don't know

ARTHRITIS KNOWLEDGE QUESTIONNAIRE—"B"

RA   1.   The "sedimentation rate" is used to help determine

A.   a diagnosis.
B.   a measure of disease activity.*
C.   a measure of how thick your blood is.
D.   a measure of how much gunk there is in your blood.
E.   Don't know

RA   2.   Plaquenil usually begins to act

A.   right away.
B.   with the second or third dose.
C.   after about 6 weeks.*
D.   in about 3–6 months.
E.   Don't know

RA   3.   Over a long period of time, rheumatoid arthritis *usually*

A.   becomes less active.*
B.   gets worse and worse.
C.   becomes more active.
D.   stays pretty much the same.
E.   Don't know

RA   4.   People with rheumatoid arthritis should

A.   restrict their diet to certain foods.
B.   always pay special attention to their weight.*
C.   eat only those foods that appeal to them.
D.   only eat foods grown in their own part of the country.
E.   Don't know

RA   5.   What is the *least* likely cause of rheumatoid arthritis?

A.   Weather changes.*
B.   The stresses of living.
C.   Infection.
D.   Genetic factors.
E.   Don't know

RA   6.   Prednisone is used in arthritis to

A.   help reduce symptoms of arthritis.*
B.   slow down the progress of arthritis.
C.   cure arthritis.
D.   make arthritis worse.
E.   Don't know

RA   7.   What do rheumatoid arthritis, ankylosing spondylitis, gout and systemic lupus erythematosus have in common?

A.   They all cause heart problems.

B.   They all require the same medication.
C.   They all can be diagnosed with the same tests.
D.   They are all forms of arthritis.*
E.   Don't know

RA   8.   Imuran is a/an

A.   antimalarial medication.
B.   anti-inflammatory medication.
C.   immunosuppressant.*
D.   tranquilizer.
E.   Don't know

RA   9.   Rheumatoid arthritis (RA) and osteoarthritis (OA)

A.   are just different names for the same disease.
B.   differ only in the parts of the body that are affected.
C.   are different arthritis conditions with few similarities.*
D.   differ because RA causes deformities.
E.   Don't know

RA   10.   Rheumatoid arthritis is the result of

A.   wear and tear on the body.
B.   the aging process.
C.   too much or too little of some kind of food.
D.   a disorder of the immune system.*
E.   Don't know

RA   11.   Treatment for rheumatoid arthritis should normally be started

A.   in the early stages of the disease.*
B.   after a couple of years if it keeps on.
C.   when the tiredness and pain get too much.
D.   only when people are older.
E.   Don't know

SM   12.   If you use "relabelling" to help control your pain you

A.   concentrate on the sensation and analyze it.*
B.   focus on something else.
C.   imagine that the pain is not part of you.
D.   use another word for arthritis.
E.   Don't know

SM   13.   If you need to reduce your salt intake, which of these should *also* be avoided?

A.   Baking powder.
B.   Sodium benzoate.
C.   MSG (monosodium glutamate).
D.   All of the above.*
E.   Don't know

SM   14.   The best sleeping position for people with hip or knee problems is likely

    A.   with knees straight and hips not rotated.[*]
    B.   on back with pillows under the knees.
    C.   side-lying position with knees bent.
    D.   All of the above.
    E.   Don't know

SM   15.   What is the best way to prepare for exercise?

    A.   Warm-up stretches.
    B.   Apply heat or cold to joints.
    C.   Massage muscles.
    D.   All of the above.[*]
    E.   Don't know

SM   16.   The exercises that people with arthritis should do are

    A.   range-of-motion or stretching exercises.
    B.   strengthening exercises.
    C.   endurance exercises like walking or swimming.
    D.   All of the above.[*]
    E.   Don't know

SM   17.   You have exercised too much if

    A.   you have pain that lasts more than 2 hours after the exercise.[*]
    B.   you have any pain or discomfort at all after exercise.
    C.   you can't sleep after exercising.
    D.   you feel stiff the next day.
    E.   Don't know

SM   18.   The first time an activity seems to cause a problem, a person with arthritis should

    A.   avoid the activity in the future.
    B.   repeat the activity at a later date to make sure that it caused the problem.[*]
    C.   go to the emergency room for a doctor's assessment.
    D.   accept that you have to live with the pain and do the activity anyway.
    E.   Don't know

SM   19.   The best diet for someone with arthritis who wishes to lose weight is

    A.   all protein.
    B.   no carbohydrates.
    C.   grapefruit and lecithin.
    D.   None of the above.[*]
    E.   Don't know

SM   20.   What is the *best* way to respond to a new report of a cure for arthritis?

    A.   Learn how to evaluate the claim yourself.[*]
    B.   Give it a fair try.
    C.   Tell your doctor about it.
    D.   Write to the publisher.
    E.   Don't know

SM 21.   To do breathing exercises in order to relax, you

    A.   take a deep breath and hold it for 60 seconds.
    B.   breathe in and out as deeply as possible.
    C.   exhale as much air as you can and inhale as you raise your stomach.
    D.   take a long, slow breath through your nose and exhale through your mouth.*
    E.   Don't know

SM 22.   To help ensure a good night's sleep, you should try to

    A.   take mild sedatives on a regular basis.
    B.   get in the habit of taking a small amount of brandy or wine at bedtime.
    C.   take more painkillers.
    D.   None of the above.*
    E.   Don't know

SM 23.   Medications that you can buy without a prescription

    A.   can sometimes interact with other medicines you may be taking.*
    B.   do not need to be mentioned to your doctor.
    C.   must be harmless because they don't need a prescription.
    D.   are never to be taken with prescribed medications.
    E.   Don't know

SM 24.   Which of the items listed below is a good reason for someone with arthritis *not* to exercise?

    A.   I can't even walk a block.
    B.   The weather affects my joints.
    C.   I'm afraid I'll get too tired and won't be able to get back.
    D.   None of the above.*
    E.   Don't know

SM 25.   Which of the exercises below is *not* an endurance exercise?

    A.   Weight lifting.*
    B.   Stair climbing.
    C.   Stationary bicycling.
    D.   Swimming.
    E.   Don't know

SM 26.   The depression and anxiety that can occur in arthritis is caused by

    A.   fear about the future.
    B.   the pain and poor sleeping.
    C.   unknown causes.
    D.   All of the above.*
    E.   Don't know

G   27.   A symptom is

    A.   something you experience.*
    B.   something the doctor finds on examination.
    C.   the result of a blood test.
    D.   something that looks like something else.
    E.   Don't know

G   28.   In arthritis the usual treatment goal is one which will

    A.   cure you.
    B.   reduce synovitis.
    C.   reduce pain.
    D.   not interfere with your lifestyle.[*]
    E.   Don't know

G   29.   The best type of heat to use for arthritic pain is

    A.   a hot bath.
    B.   a sauna.
    C.   a hot pad.
    D.   All types are about the same.[*]
    E.   Don't know

G   30.   The most common abnormality of an articular joint is

    A.   osteoarthritis.[*]
    B.   synovitis.
    C.   rheumatoid arthritis.
    D.   inflammation.
    E.   Don't know

G   31.   The unusual tiredness often experienced in arthritis is caused by

    A.   the extra energy needed to deal with pain.
    B.   biochemical processes.
    C.   not being able to sleep.
    D.   All of the above.[*]
    E.   Don't know

G   32.   If you are taking nonsteroidal anti-inflammatory (NSAID) medication

    A.   you should not take aspirin in most situations.[*]
    B.   you should take aspirin when things get bad.
    C.   you can substitute aspirin for the NSAID any time you want.
    D.   aspirin should always be taken with the NSAID.
    E.   Don't know

G   33.   Which of the following exercises is *least* helpful to prevent osteoporosis?

    A.   Swimming.[*]
    B.   Running.
    C.   Walking.
    D.   Aerobics.
    E.   Don't know

G   34.   Osteoarthritis generally affects

    A.   the same joints in everyone.
    B.   only the hips and the knees.
    C.   only the spine.
    D.   different joints in different people.[*]
    E.   Don't know

G   35.   Autoimmunity is

     A.   a natural defense against certain diseases.
     B.   a process by which the body works against itself.*
     C.   an unnatural fear of explosives.
     D.   a feeling that the world is against you.
     E.   Don't know

G   36.   The anti-inflammatory effect of aspirin

     A.   is present with doses of one to two tablets a day.
     B.   requires high and continuous levels of aspirin in the blood.*
     C.   lasts for days after a single dose of aspirin.
     D.   is due to the pain-killing effects of aspirin.
     E.   Don't know

G   37.   Medications are *always*

     A.   better absorbed on an empty stomach.
     B.   best taken with meals, or a glass of milk.
     C.   unrelated to food.
     D.   None of the above.*
     E.   Don't know

G   38.   Anti-inflammatory drugs that are used as substitutes for aspirin

     A.   have fewer side effects than aspirin.
     B.   may work better than aspirin for some people.
     C.   usually cost more than aspirin.
     D.   All of the above.*
     E.   Don't know

G   39.   An inflammatory process is one which

     A.   burns up the molecules.
     B.   gives you a fever.
     C.   causes heat and redness.*
     D.   causes people to feel angry.
     E.   Don't know

G   40.   The term "blood level" refers to

     A.   how much blood someone has.
     B.   how many red blood cells float on the serum.
     C.   the amount of something in the blood.*
     D.   the blood pressure level.
     E.   Don't know

G   41.   Which is the best source of calcium? 100 milligrams of
            A.   calcium carbonate.[*]
            B.   calcium chloride.
            C.   calcium gluconate.
            D.   calcium lactate.
            E.   Don't know

From Edworthy, S. M., Devins, G. M., & Watson, M. M. (1995). The Arthritis Knowledge Questionnaire. *Arthritis and Rheumatism, 5,* 590–600.

16

Patient Knowledge Questionnaire in Rheumatoid Arthritis

Developed by J. Hill, H. A. Bird, R. Hopkins, C. Lawton, and V. Wright

INSTRUMENT DESCRIPTION, ADMINISTRATION, AND SCORING GUIDELINES

In therapy of rheumatoid arthritis (RA), patients must adjust daily exercise regimens, rest/activity periods, and drug regimens according to the changing activity of their disease. The authors believe that knowledge of the disease and its treatment is necessary to carry out these self-care tasks. Scoring is indicated on the test. Total score is 30, with a maximum score of 9 on the general knowledge section, of 7 for questions on drugs, and of 7 for questions on exercise (Hill, Bird, Harmer, Wright, & Lawton, 1994).

In one administration (Hill, Bird, Hopkins, Lawton, & Wright, 1991), some patients thought that nonsteroidal anti-inflammatory drugs (NSAIDs) stopped the disease from progressing, two people thought exercise could cure RA, and patients had difficulty in distinguishing between joint protection and energy conservation.

PSYCHOMETRIC PROPERTIES

Topics in the Patient Knowledge Questionnaire in Rheumatoid Arthritis (PKQ) included which patients had identified as important: general knowledge including etiology, symptoms, and tests; drugs and how to take them; exercise regimens; joint protection; and pacing and priorities. After three revisions, the PKQ was considered suitable for piloting with 40 patients, after which items with index of difficulty more than .75 were removed or altered to avoid ceiling effects. It was then repiloted with 29 patients, with a mean score of 15.2 and range of 5 to 24. The

Kuder Richardson for internal consistency was .72 and for test-retest reliability .81, with a 4-week interval (Hill et al., 1994).

Seventy randomly selected patients with RA in the outpatient clinical of a large teaching hospital completed the PKQ. There was a wide variation in total scores ranging from 3 to 28 out of 30, with a mean of 16 (Hill et al., 1991). A later study (Hill et al., 1994) showed a significant increase in PKQ scores after instruction, especially for those cared for by a rheumatology nurse practitioner (mean score = 22) as opposed to those cared for in a clinic (mean score = 16.2).

CRITIQUE AND SUMMARY

More explicit establishment of the content of the domains of knowledge to be tested and expert and patient judgment about the representativeness of the items would be helpful. It would also be helpful to test the notion that this knowledge is important for carrying out self-care regimens. Theory would suggest that items that test problem-solving skills in using the knowledge would be more predictive than would the factual knowledge tested in the PKQ.

REFERENCES

Hill, J., Bird, H. A., Harmer, R., Wright, V., & Lawton, C. (1994). An evaluation of the effectiveness, safety and acceptability of a nurse practitioner in a rheumatology outpatient clinic. *British Journal of Rheumatology, 33,* 283–288.

Hill, J., Bird, H. A., Hopkins, R., Lawton, C., & Wright, V. (1991). The development and use of a patient knowledge questionnaire in rheumatoid arthritis. *British Journal of Rheumatology, 30,* 45–49.

RHEUMATISM RESEARCH UNIT
UNIVERSITY OF LEEDS
KNOWLEDGE QUESTIONNAIRE

This questionnaire has been devised to help us find out how arthritis affects your life.
All your answers will remain strictly confidential.
Could you please answer the questions by circling the letter opposite your answer as in the example below.

1.   What is the name of the type of arthritis you have?
   A.   Ankylosing Spondylitis
   Ⓑ.   Rheumatoid Arthritis
   C.   Fibrositis
   D.   Osteoarthritis

IT IS IMPORTANT TO TRY TO ANSWER ALL THE QUESTIONS

1.   Can you choose TWO true statements from the following list?

   Rheumatoid Arthritis

   A.   is inherited from your parents.
   B.   starts after a joint has been damaged.
   C.   is caused by cold damp weather.
   D.   the cause is not known.
   E.   may be triggered by a bacteria or virus.
   F.   Don't know

2.   Can you choose TWO true statements from the following list?
   Rheumatoid Arthritis

   A.   affects only the bones of the body.
   B.   occasionally affects the lungs, eyes, or other tissues.
   C.   is most common in old age.
   D.   is a long-term disease.
   E.   is curable.
   F.   Don't know

3.   Can you choose THREE symptoms which can be caused by Rheumatoid Arthritis?

   A   Anaemia.
   B.   Nodules.
   C.   Overweight.
   D.   Hair loss.
   E.   High blood pressure.
   F.   Fatigue.
   G.   Don't know

4. Can you choose TWO blood tests which are used to assess how active your arthritis is?

   A. Cholesterol level (CL).
   B. Erythrocyte sedimentation rate (ESR).
   C. Blood group.
   D. Plasma viscosity (PV).
   E. Plasma protein.
   F. Don't know

5. Can you choose TWO true statements about non-steroidal anti-inflammatory drugs?

   A. They stop the disease from progressing.
   B. They take many weeks to start working.
   C. They reduce pain, swelling, and stiffness.
   D. They need only be taken when the pain is bad.
   E. They should be taken with food.
   F. Don't know

6. Can you choose the ONE most common side effect that non-steroidal anti-inflammatory tablets can cause?

   A. Itching of the skin.
   B. Indigestion.
   C. Bruising.
   D. Dry mouth.
   E. Loss of taste.
   F. Don't know

7. Can you choose TWO "long-term drugs" which can put the disease into remission?

   A. D-penicillamine also called Distamine, Pendramine.
   B. Diclofenac also called Voltarol.
   C. Indomethacin also called Indocid, Indocid "R," Imbrilon.
   D. Sulphasalazine also called Salazopyrin, E/C Salazopyrin.
   E. Ibuprofen also called Brufen, Fenbid, Nurofen.
   F. Don't know

8. Can you choose TWO true statements about pain killing tablets?

   Pain killers

   A. are not addictive.
   B. should only be taken when pain is severe.
   C. should be taken before carrying out an activity which you know causes you pain.
   D. should be taken when pain starts to build up.
   E. should always be taken with food.
   F. Don't know

9. Can you choose TWO correct answers about exercise and Rheumatoid Arthritis?

   A. It is unnecessary to exercise if you are normally active.
   B. Exercise will cure rheumatoid arthritis.
   C. Exercise weakens damaged joints.

D. Move your joint to the point of pain and then a bit further.
E. Exercise can reduce the chance of a joint deforming.
F. Don't know

10. Can you choose the TWO most suitable ways for someone with Rheumatoid Arthritis to take regular exercise?

A. Muscle tightening exercises.
B. Gentle jogging.
C. Walking.
D. Yoga.
E. Shopping trips.
F. Don't know

11. Can you choose ONE activity which you should carry out when all your joints are painful and stiff?

A. Refrain from all exercise.
B. Rest in bed for most of the day.
C. Carry out your usual range of movement exercises.
D. Exercise quite vigorously.
E. Don't know

12. Can you choose TWO treatments which would be most suitable if your wrists are becoming more than usually painful, swollen, and stiff?

A. Rest them by putting on wrist splints.
B. Reduce the stiffness by vigorous exercise.
C. Use them as much as possible.
D. Avoid movement by keeping them in one position as much as possible.
E. Put the joints through a full range of movement several times a day.
F. Don't know

13. Can you choose TWO sentences from this list?

The most practical way to protect your joints from strain is to

A. use them quickly.
B. use the larger joints rather than the smaller ones where possible.
C. slide objects rather than lift them.
D. do as little as possible.
E. carry on as though you did not have arthritis.
F. Don't know

14. Can you choose the ONE most suitable activity when you have a busy day planned but realize you're feeling tired?

A. Take the day off and do more tomorrow.
B. Do everything you had planned to do.
C. Take a short rest and then do all the things you had planned.
D. Do essentials and leave the rest.
E. Spend the day resting in bed.
F. Don't know

15. Can you choose TWO suitable methods of conserving your energy?

    A.   Sit down whilst ironing.
    B.   Plan activities to balance work and rest periods.
    C.   Wear splints.
    D.   Use the strongest and largest muscles possible.
    E.   Use both hands to carry objects such as full saucepans.
    F.   Don't know

16. Can you choose TWO methods of joint protection?

    A.   Grip objects tightly.
    B.   Use a dish cloth rather than a sponge.
    C.   Use the palm of your hands not your fingers when opening a jar.
    D.   Apply heat or ice to the joint.
    E.   Having power assisted steering on your car.
    F.   Don't know

THANK YOU FOR ANSWERING THIS QUESTIONNAIRE

CORRECT ANSWERS

1.   d e
2.   b d
3.   a b f
4.   b d
5.   c e
6.   b
7.   a d
8.   c d
9.   d e
10.   a c
11.   c
12.   a e
13.   b c
14.   d
15.   a b
16.   c e

From Hill, J., Bird, H. A., Hopkins, R., Lawton, C., & Wright, V. (1994). An evaluation of the effectiveness, safety and acceptability of a nurse practitioner in a rheumatology outpatient clinic. *British Journal of Rheumatology, 30,* 45–49. Used with permission of Oxford University Press.

17

Arthritis Self-Efficacy Scale

Developed by Kate Lorig, Robert L. Chastain, Elaine Ung, Stanford Shoor, and Halsted R. Holman

INSTRUMENT DESCRIPTION, ADMINISTRATION, AND SCORING GUIDELINES

This scale was developed to measure patient perceived self-efficacy (SE) to cope with the consequences of chronic arthritis. SE appears to be particularly important for patients with rheumatoid arthritis (RA) because the unpredictable fluctuations of RA symptoms may contribute to feelings of helplessness. Patients who feel helpless report more psychological distress and pain than do their less helpless counterparts (Buescher et al., 1991). Patients rate the strength of their perceived ability to perform each item on a scale ranging from 10 to 100 in steps in 10. Item scores are then summed, with a higher score indicating greater SE.

PSYCHOMETRIC PROPERTIES

Steps in the development of this scale may be seen subsequently and are summarized in Table 17.1. Based on a national conference on outcomes measures, specific behaviors of controlling pain and disability were identified as important, translated into items and refined in patient groups through item analysis.

Patients were recruited for the Arthritis Self-Management Course (ASMC) ($N = 97$) by means of public service announcements and referrals from health professionals. Subjects for the concurrent validation and reliability group were past ASMC participants who had not previously completed the efficacy scale questionnaire. Two factors were identified through factor analysis: self-efficacy for physical function (FSE) and self-efficacy for controlling other arthritis symptoms (OSE) (Lorig, Chastain, Ung, Shoor, & Holman, 1989).

Construct validity was upheld by finding of significant correlations between baseline SE and baseline health status, between baseline SE and health status 4 months later, and between 4-month SE and 4-month health status, congruent with SE theory. FSE was most highly related to function (disability); OSE was most highly related to depression. A test of concurrent validity

TABLE 17.1 Steps in the Development of the Self-Efficacy Scale

I. Item generation
   1. 23 items generated by a rheumatologist
   2. 20 items refined in patient focus group
II. Initial instrument development study ($n = 97$)
   1. Baseline and 4-month values
   2. Factor analysis
   3. Function self-efficacy
   4. Other symptom self-efficacy
   5. Alpha coefficient (measure of internal reliability)
   6. Tests of construct validity
III. Concurrent validity test ($n = 43$)
IV. Replication study ($n = 144$)
   1. Baseline and 4-month values
   2. Factor analysis
   3. Pain self-efficacy
   4. Function self-efficacy
   5. Other symptom self-efficacy
   6. Alpha coefficient (measure of internal reliability)
V. Confirmatory analysis ($n = 144$ and $n = 97$)[*]
   1. Factor analysis
   2. Alpha coefficient (measure of internal reliability)
VI. Test-retest reliability study ($n = 91$)

[*]Scales generated on replication sample, then applied to original development sample.
From Lorig, K., Chastain, R. L., Ung, E., Shoor, S., & Holman, H. R. (1989). Development and evaluation of a scale to measure perceived self-efficacy in people with arthritis. *Arthritis and Rheumatism, 32,* 37–44. Copyright, American College of Rheumatology. Used with permission.

of the FSE showed a moderately high correlation (.61) between performance as perceived by patients and actual performance as measured by blinded trained observers. Such findings are consistent with self-efficacy theory (Lorig et al., 1989).

A factor analysis from a replication study ($N = 144$ new subjects) showed three SE subscales: an FSE scale of 9 items (coefficient $\alpha = .89$), an OSE scale of 6 items (coefficient $\alpha = .87$), and a pain-management self-efficacy scale (PSE) of 5 items (coefficient $\alpha = .76$), presented at the end of this description. The three subscales were then applied to data from the initial 97-person sample used for development of the instrument. Coefficient α estimates of internal reliability were .90 for FSE, .87 for OSE, and .75 for PSE. A test-retest reliability study with a third sample of 91 subjects showed subscale reliabilities of .85 for FSE, .90 for OSE, and .87 for PSE. Patients in these studies were largely female, with a mean age of 63 to 65 years and average education of 14 years (Lorig et al., 1989).

Outcome data show that levels of pain and depression at 4 months declined significantly from baseline, whereas perceived SE for pain and for other symptoms rose significantly from baseline levels for the experimental group that received the ASMC, but not for the control group. Mean baseline scores for the experimental group were FSE, 73.27; OSE, 55.62; and PSE, 52.04 (Lorig et al., 1989).

In a small ($N = 15$, experimental; $N = 15$, control), related study using efficacy-enhancing methods (individual goals, specific instructions and practice, self-relaxation with guided imagery, contracting, modeling, and reinterpretation of physiological symptoms), even greater gains in perceived SE and larger correlations with health outcomes in pain, disability, and functioning were found. Experimental patients learned psychological pain-management strategies including relaxation with guided imagery, attention refocusing, vivid imagery, dissociation, relabeling and self-encouragement; strategies were tailored for use during specific painful activities, such as climbing stairs, carrying groceries, and mopping floors. Control patients received copies of *The Arthritis Helpbook* (as did experimental patients) containing much relevant information for managing arthritis; this group achieved little or no change in SE or health outcomes. Mean subscale scores for the treatment group were PSE: 52.67, pretest; 63.40, posttest; FSE: 56.2, pretest; 64.27, posttest; and OSE: 52.53, pretest; 66.86, posttest. Mean subscale scores for the control group were PSE: 54.33, pretest; FSE: 63.64, pretest; 57.44, posttest; and OSE: 55.7, pretest; 58.33, posttest (O'Leary, Shoor, Lorig, & Holman, 1988). These findings suggest building strong efficacy-enhancing methods into programs of education for patients with arthritis and shows Arthritis Self-Efficacy Scale sensitivity to intervention (see Table 17.1).

Other studies provide further evidence supporting validity of the Arthritis SE Scale. In patients with rheumatoid arthritis, those who reported higher SE exhibited fewer pain behaviors measured by pain behavior ratings. Although the effects were small, this relationship held true for all three subscales. Mean scores for FSE were 54.5; for PSE, 51.6; and for OSE, 59.3 (Buescher et al., 1991).

The Arthritis Self-Efficacy Scale is also available in other languages. A Swedish version of the scale was tested for validity by Lomi and Nordholm (1992). Scores on the three subscales were correlated with indicators of present pain status, with scores on the Multidimensional Health Locus of Control Scales, and for FSE negatively with disease duration, all in the direction predicted by self-efficacy theory. The scales also discriminated between a group of patients with chronic pain and the rheumatology group, evidence of discriminant validity. Internal consistency was .82 to .91 and test-retest reliability .81 to .91 for the various subscales. The scale has also been translated into Spanish with preliminary psychometric testing to assess whether it is understood and easily administered to Spanish-speaking groups of varied national origin and living in different regions of the United States. The translated scale and results of validity and reliability studies on it may be found in Gonzalez, Stewart, Ritter, and Lorig (1995). The Spanish version of the scales showed an internal consistency α of .92, a test-retest reliability of .69, and item-to-scale correlations ranging from .65 to .83.

The scales have also been used to test the effects of instructions for home exercise for persons with RA, with a finding of improved OSE, increased capacity in most functional tasks, and increased joint activity among other findings (Stenstrom, 1994).

In patients with fibromyalgia, when scores on the Arthritis Self-Efficacy Scale were high, patients exhibited fewer pain behaviors, although the amount of variance in pain behavior accounted for by SE ranged from only 10% to 14% (Buckelew et al., 1994). In an intervention study of 86 patients with fibromyalgia, those who received education or education plus physical training showed significantly higher scores than did those in the control group (Burckhardt, Mannerkorpi, Hedenberg, & Bjelle, 1994).

CRITIQUE AND SUMMARY

There has been more study of these scales than of most other instruments in this book. Findings from validity studies support hypotheses that there is an association between perceived SE and both present and future health status related to arthritis, that SE can be changed by educational interventions, and growth in SE is associated with improvement in health status, consistent with construct validity of the instrument. It will also be important to test other interventions to see what has maximum effect on SE to compare instrument results with those that measure related psychological states, such as general coping skills and others as well as testing the instrument with other populations (Lorig et al., 1989).

SE is an important variable clinically. For example, Beckham, Burker, Rice, and Talton (1995) found that patient SE expectations regarding RA symptoms explained a significant proportion of variance in measures of caregiver burden and optimism. These results suggest the importance of assessing patient psychological status in evaluating caregiver responses.

REFERENCES

Beckham, J. C., Burker, E. J., Rice, J. R., & Talton, S. L. (1995). Patient predictors of caregiver burden, optimism, and pessimism in rheumatoid arthritis. *Behavioral Medicine, 20,* 171–178.

Buckalew, S. P., Parker, J. C., Keefe, F. J., Deuser, W. E., Crews, T. M., Conway, R., Kay, D. R., & Hewett, J. E. (1994). Self-efficacy and pain behavior among subjects with fibromyalgia. *Pain, 59,* 377–384.

Buescher, K. L., Johnson, J. A., Parker, J. C., Smarr, K. L., Buckelew, S. P., Anderson, S. K., & Walker, S. E. (1991). Relationship of self-efficacy to pain behavior. *Journal of Rheumatology, 18,* 968–972.

Burckhardt, C. S., Mannerkorpi, K., Hedenberg, L., & Bjelle, A. (1994). A randomized, controlled clinical trial of education and physician training for women with fibromyalgia. *Journal of Rheumatology, 21,* 714–720.

Gonzalez, V. M., Stewart, A., Ritter, P. L., & Lorig, K. (1995). Translation and validation of arthritis outcome measures into Spanish. *Arthritis and Rheumatism, 38,* 1429–1446.

Lomi, C., & Nordholm, L. A. (1992). Validation of a Swedish version of the Arthritis Self-Efficacy Scale. *Scandinavian Journal of Rheumatology, 21,* 231–237.

Lorig, K., Chastain, R. L., Ung, E., Shoor, S., & Holman, H. R. (1989). Development and evaluation of a scale to measure perceived self-efficacy in people with arthritis. *Arthritis and Rheumatism, 32,* 27–34.

O'Leary, A., Shoor, S., Lorig, K., & Holman, H. R. (1988). A cognitive-behavioral treatment for rheumatoid arthritis. *Health Psychology, 7,* 527–544.

Stenstrom, C. H. (1994). Home exercises in rheumatoid arthritis functional class II: Goal setting versus pain attention. *Journal of Rheumatology, 21,* 627–634.

ARTHRITIS SELF-EFFICACY SCALE*

Self-efficacy pain subscale

In the following questions, we'd like to know how your arthritis pain affects you. For each of the following questions, please circle the number which corresponds to your certainty that you can *now* perform the following tasks.

1. How certain are you that you can decrease your pain *quite a bit*?
2. How certain are you that you can continue most of your daily activities?
3. How certain are you that you can keep arthritis pain from interfering with your sleep?
4. How certain are you that you can make a *small-to-moderate* reduction in your arthritis pain by using methods other than taking extra medication?
5. How certain are you that you can make a *large* reduction in your arthritis pain by using methods other than taking extra medication?

Self-efficacy function subscale

We would like to know how confident you are in performing certain daily activities. For each of the following questions, please circle the number which corresponds to your certainty that you can perform the tasks as of *now*, *without* assistive devices or help from another person. Please consider what you *routinely* can do, not what would require a single extraordinary effort.

AS OF NOW, HOW CERTAIN ARE YOU THAT YOU CAN:

1. Walk 100 feet on flat ground in 20 seconds?
2. Walk 10 steps downstairs in 7 seconds?
3. Get out of an armless chair quickly, without using your hands for support?
4. Button and unbutton 3 medium-size buttons in a row in 12 seconds?
5. Cut 2 bite-size pieces of meat with a knife and fork in 8 seconds?
6. Turn an outdoor faucet all the way on and all the way off?
7. Scratch your upper back with both your right and left hands?
8. Get in and out of the passenger side of a car without assistance from another person and without physical aids?
9. Put on a long-sleeve front-opening shirt or blouse (without buttoning) in 8 seconds?

Self-efficacy other symptoms subscale

In the following questions, we'd like to know how you feel about your ability to control your arthritis. For each of the following questions, please circle the number which corresponds to the certainty that you can *now* perform the following activities or tasks.

1. *How certain* are you that you can control your fatigue?
2. *How certain* are you that you can regulate your activity so as to be active without aggravating your arthritis?
3. *How certain* are you that you can do something to help yourself feel better if you are feeling blue?
4. As compared with other people with arthritis like yours, *how certain* are you that you can manage arthritis pain during your daily activities?

5. *How certain* are you that you can manage your arthritis symptoms so that you can do the things you enjoy doing?
6. *How certain* are you that you can deal with the frustration of arthritis?

*Each question is followed by the scale:

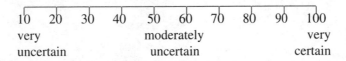

| 10 | 20 | 30 | 40 | 50 | 60 | 70 | 80 | 90 | 100 |

| very
uncertain | moderately
uncertain | very
certain |

Each subscale is scored separately, by taking the mean of the subscale items. If one-fourth or less of the data are missing, the score is a mean of the completed data. If more than one-fourth of the data are missing, no score is calculated. (The authors invite others to use the scale and would appreciate being informed of study results.)

From Lorig, K., Chastain, R. L., Ung, E., Shoor, S., & Holman, H. R. (1989). Development and evaluation of a scale to measure perceived self-efficacy in people with arthritis. *Arthritis and Rheumatism, 32*, 37–44. Copyright, American College of Rheumatology. Used with permission.

D

Asthma

18

Asthma Autonomy Preference Scale

Developed by Peter G. Gibson, Phillipa I. Talbot, Ruth C. Toneguzzi, and The Population Medicine Group 91C

INSTRUMENT DESCRIPTION, ADMINISTRATION, AND SCORING GUIDELINES

Management guidelines emphasize increased autonomy for persons with asthma, through patient education and written patient-initiated action plans. These are meant to facilitate the early detection and treatment of an exacerbation and to minimize the risk of hospitalization and death. The extent to which patients wish to be well-informed participants in the management of their illness is largely unknown. Studies of other illnesses have shown that although most patients actively sought information about their condition, few preferred to have the major role in decision making (Gibson, Talbot, Toneguzzi, & The Population Medicine Group, 1995).

The Asthma Autonomy Preference Scale (AAPS) examines preferences of patients for information about their condition and for decision making in asthma exacerbations of varying severity. The instrument takes about 10 minutes to administer. Strongest preferences in favor of decision making or information seeking by the patient are assigned scores of 5, with the weakest score 1. Overall preference is determined by adding the scores in the respective scales. Final scores were linearized to range from 1 to 100 and for each scale to a range of 0 to 10, with the lowest scores corresponding to a preference for the physician to take complete control, midrange indicating equally shared responsibility, and the highest scores for the patient to take complete control of decision making (Gibson et al., 1995).

PSYCHOMETRIC PROPERTIES

This tool was adapted to asthma using the published guidelines for management of this disease, from the Autonomy Preference Index (API) (Ende, Kazis, Ash, & Moskowitz, 1989). Items for the original index were developed from a Delphi study of clinical medical sociologists and

165

ethicists. It was tested in a study of 312 patients from a hospital-based primary care clinic. Factor analysis supported a scale on information seeking and one on decision making. Test-retest reliability for the scales was .83 and .84, and Cronbach's α for each was .82. Responses to a global item about amount of control of patient and physician correlated significantly with decision-making scores on the API, supporting concurrent validity. Scores on the decision-making scale administered to persons with diabetes adept on self-care and home monitoring were significantly higher than were scores from the general population, supporting convergent validity. Studies using the API found that although patients wanted information, their preferences for decision making were frequently weak, especially as they were asked to consider increasingly severe illnesses (Ende et al., 1989).

The AAPS consists of two scales: information-seeking preferences (8 items) and decision-making preferences (18 items). Authors of the AAPS indicated that its structure had been previously validated, based on the work done on the API. It was administered to 85 adults purchasing albuterol inhalers for asthma from community pharmacies as well as to 38 persons recently hospitalized for acute, severe asthma. Both groups indicated high preferences for information seeking (mean values over 90 out of a possible of 100), with preferences for decision making significantly lower (mean of 51 and 52, respectively). Scores on items related to the scenarios may be found in Gibson et al. (1995).

Although, on average, preferences for participation declined even further with severe exacerbation of asthma, one-third of participants indicated they still would prefer equal or greater participation in decision making under these circumstances. Quality of life in asthma was not associated with patient preference for autonomy. It is important to note that results were similar to those found with the API (Gibson et al., 1995).

CRITIQUE AND SUMMARY

The AAPS describes patient attitudes rather than the specific behaviors of patients with asthma. Although the expected results of these attitudes—namely, failure to initiate self-management in asthma exacerbations—have been documented to occur in several settings, no evidence of predictive validity could be located either for the AAPS or for the API. The number of subjects involved in studies of the AAPS is limited. In addition, no estimates of reliability and validity (apart from those that exist for API) could be located.

Two implications for patient care flow from the findings to date. First, many of the patients tested so far do not conform to the model of strong patient decision-making autonomy assumed in guidelines for asthma self-management, in that only a minority have action plans to use for management of deteriorating asthma. Studies of asthma death and severe asthma exacerbations frequently indicate delay in using medication or seeking help as potentially reversible factors in asthma death. Programs designed to improve self-management can be shown to decrease morbidity as well as decrease health care costs. Why does this occur? Do physicians not provide management plans (Gibson et al., 1995)? Do patient education programs focus solely on information about the disease and not provide explicit skill building to the point of mastery, in how to manage exacerbations? Will adequate patient programs shift the decision-making autonomy preference? If, after adequate education, patients are still resistant to strong decision-making roles, perhaps a different system of caregiving must be constructed.

Second and not surprising, because patients differ in their preferences for decision-making autonomy, it would be useful to know up front who prefers strong or weak decision-making responsibility. Particularly, if these preference tools show predictive validity with actual self-management behaviors, it would be possible to identify individuals who need backup systems to deal with serious exacerbations of their illness.

REFERENCES

Ende, J., Kazis, L., Ash, A., & Moskowitz, M. A. (1989). Measuring patients' desire for autonomy. *Journal of General Internal Medicine, 4,* 23–30.

Gibson, P. G., Talbot, P. I., Toneguzzi, R. C., & The Population Medicine Group (1995). Self-management, autonomy, and quality of life in asthma. *Chest, 107,* 1003–1008.

THE ASTHMA AUTONOMY PREFERENCE INDEX

I.   Decision-making preference scale.

    A.   General items for decision-making preferences. Scored using 5-point Likert scale, with scores ranging from "strongly agree" to "strongly disagree."

        1. The important medical decisions about your asthma should be made by your physician, not you.

        2. You should go along with your physician's advice even if you disagree with it.

        3. When hospitalized for asthma, you should not be making decisions about your own care.

        4. You should feel free to make decisions about everyday problems with your asthma.

        5. If you were sick, as your asthma became worse you would want your physician to take greater control.

        6. You should decide how frequently you need a check-up for your asthma.

    B.   Scenarios. Subjects respond to each item on a 5-point scale. Choices are "you alone," "mostly you," "the doctor and you equally," "mostly the doctor," "the doctor alone."

Stable Asthma:
Suppose you have visited your physician for a routine check-up of your asthma and to obtain prescriptions for your asthma medicines. Who should make the following decisions?

        7. When the next visit to check your asthma should be.

        8. Whether you should buy a peak flowmeter and use this to monitor your asthma.

        9. Whether you should be seen by a specialist.

    10. What action you should take if your asthma gets worse.

Mild Exacerbations:
For the last 4 days you have been feeling more wheezy and breathless than usual, and you have found it increasingly difficult to get on with your everyday activities. Last night you were awakened twice because of asthma and you found it difficult to get back to sleep. Today you wake earlier than usual and are feeling very wheezy and breathless. Who should make the following decisions?

    11. Whether you should be seen by the physician.

    12. Whether you should take more albuterol (Ventolin, Respolin) terbutaline (Bricanyl)/fenoterol (Berotec).

    13. Whether you should increase your preventive asthma inhalers (beclomethasone [Becotide, Becloforte], cromolyn [Intal], budesonide [Pulmicort]).

    14. Whether you should take prednisone or cortisone tablets.

Severe Asthma in Hospital:
Suppose you had an attack of severe asthma that was not relieved by your inhaler, frightening you enough so that you went to the hospital emergency (casualty) department. In the emergency department, physicians treat your asthma and you are taken up to the intensive care unit. Who should make the following decisions?

    15. How often the nurses should wake you up to check your temperature and blood pressure.

    16. Whether you may have visitors aside from your immediate family.

17. When you are able to be discharged.
18. Whether the nurses should wake you from sleep to give you the nebulizer.

II. Information-seeking preference scale.

A. Items for information-seeking preferences. Responses presented as a 5-point Likert scale with choices ranging from "strongly agree" to "strongly disagree."

19. As you become sicker, you should be told more and more about your asthma.
20. You should understand what is happening inside your body as a result of asthma.
21. Even if the news is bad, you should be well informed about your asthma.
22. Your physician should explain the purpose of your laboratory tests.
23. You should be given information about your asthma only when you ask.
24. It is important for you to know all the side effects of your asthma medication.
25. Information about asthma is as important as treatment.
26. When there is more than one method to treat asthma, you should be told about each one.

From Gibson, P. G., Talbot, P. I., Toneguzzi, R. C., and The Population Medicine Group. (1995). Self-management, autonomy, and quality of life in asthma. *Chest, 107,* 1003–1008.

19

Asthma Opinion Survey

Developed by James M. Richards, Jr., Jeffrey J. Dolce, Richard A. Windsor, William C. Bailey, C. Michael Brooks, and Seng-jaw Soong

INSTRUMENT DESCRIPTION, ADMINISTRATION, AND SCORING GUIDELINES

Poor self-management appears to contribute significantly to unnecessary morbidity and perhaps mortality in adults with asthma. The Asthma Opinion Survey (AOS) was designed to measure attitudes relevant to self-management in adult outpatients. Prior research has confirmed that psychological characteristics are related to effectiveness of asthma self-management. In addition to a similar tool focused on inpatient treatment, development of the AOS was guided by the Health Belief Model and by the PRECEDE diagnostic model for patient education. Thus, it includes items designed to tap predisposing (knowledge, attitudes, beliefs, and values); enabling (skills in self-management); and reinforcing factors (effects of self-management on symptoms and social support) (Richards et al., 1989).

PSYCHOMETRIC PROPERTIES

Items fall into 11 clusters: general vulnerability, specific vulnerability, attitudes toward patient knowledge, recognition of airway obstruction, accessibility of health care, panic-fear, belief in treatment efficacy, staff-patient relationships, sense of control, personal impact, and social impact (Richards et al., 1989). Because the reliability levels of these clusters vary from .48 to .87, it is suggested that future research with the AOS should rely mainly on the three factor scores: vulnerability ($\alpha = .87$), perceived quality of care ($\alpha = .76$), and recognition and control ($\alpha = .71$).

The AOS has been tested with one group of 132 adults receiving outpatient treatment in a teaching hospital in Birmingham. The full range of age and severity and duration of asthma was present in this group, and it closely reflected racial characteristics in the Birmingham, Alabama, community. AOS scores correlated with the Asthma Symptoms Checklist in ways supporting construct validity. Higher scores on the Vulnerability factor were associated with use of the more intense forms of health care, and higher scores on the Recognition and Control factor were associated with use of an emergency room. No scores could be located in published sources.

CRITIQUE AND SUMMARY

Evidence is needed both with respect to the extent to which scores on the AOS predict self-management behaviors and outcomes, and with respect to whether or not scores on the survey change in response to interventions (Richards et al., 1991). In addition, the instrument needs to be tested with more subjects in other sites because the way in which care is delivered clearly will affect responses on some items.

REFERENCE

Richards, J. M., Jr., Dolce, J. J., Windsor, R. A., Bailey, W. C., Brooks, C. M., & Soong, S. (1989). Patient characteristics relevant to effective self-management: Scales for assessing attitudes of adults toward asthma. *Journal of Asthma, 26,* 99–108.

ASTHMA OPINION SURVEY

NAME: _____ DATE: _____

Instructions: We want to learn more about your opinions concerning your asthma and the quality of care you currently are receiving from the clinic, hospital, physician, etc., where you go for asthma treatment. Please draw a circle around the number beside each of the following statements to indicate the extent to which you agree or disagree with it.

		Strongly Disagree				Strongly Agree
1.	I have asthma attacks quite often.	1	2	3	4	5
2.	People with asthma do better if they learn a lot about their disease.	1	2	3	4	5
3.	I can tell when I'm about to have an asthma attack from how I feel inside.	1	2	3	4	5
4.	When I get short of breath, I often get too upset to do much about it.	1	2	3	4	5
5.	Patients here would get a lot better treatment for their asthma somewhere else.	1	2	3	4	5
6.	I know some things to do that will help when I get short of breath.	1	2	3	4	5
7.	I would be more successful if I didn't have so many breathing problems.	1	2	3	4	5
8.	I always have to wait a long time here before I get to see the doctor.	1	2	3	4	5
9.	I generally know if I'm about to have a breathing problem.	1	2	3	4	5
10.	My asthma interferes with my social life quite a bit.	1	2	3	4	5
11.	Patients have very little to say about what happens to them here.	1	2	3	4	5
12.	When I get short of breath, I can tell if it's going to get worse from how I feel inside.	1	2	3	4	5
13.	I often worry about getting a serious disease such as cancer or a heart attack.	1	2	3	4	5
14.	The doctors, nurses, and other staff here are quite nice to patients.	1	2	3	4	5

		Strongly Disagree				Strongly Agree
15.	If an asthma attack starts to get worse, I know some things that will help me if I do them.	1	2	3	4	5
16.	Because I have asthma, I am always going to have some breathing problems.	1	2	3	4	5
17.	The doctors here are too busy to give enough time to their asthma patients.	1	2	3	4	5
18.	I usually can feel it when my chest begins to get tight from asthma.	1	2	3	4	5

Scoring instructions. The current version has been reduced to 18 items. Subjects respond in terms of a 5-point scale ranging from 1 to 5. Scores are computed for three factors by summing the items that loaded on that factor in the study reported in the *Journal of Asthma* article. The factors and the items that should be included are listed below. The scoring for some items is reversed in computing the total score on the factor. These items are identified by an asterisk (*).

Factor A—Vulnerability
Items 1, 4, 7, 10, 13, 16

Factor B—Perceived Quality of Care
Items 2, 5*, 8*, 11*, 14, 17*

Factor C—Recognition and Control
Items 3, 6, 9, 12, 15, 18

This scale was developed at the Lung Health Center, University of Alabama at Birmingham, with research funding from the Division of Lung Diseases, National Heart, Lung, and Blood Institute Grant HL 31481-02 to William C. Bailey, MD.

20

Children with Asthma: Parent Knowledge, Attitude, Self-Efficacy, and Management Behavior Survey

Developed by Ilse Mesters, R. Meertens, H. Crebolder, and G. Parcel

INSTRUMENT DESCRIPTION, ADMINISTRATION, AND SCORING GUIDELINES

Most children with asthma experience symptoms before they reach 5 years of age and account for a considerable number of hospitalizations resulting from the disease. Erroneous beliefs and attitudes held by parents were found using questionnaires and focus groups, and presumably affected their ability to care for their children. For example, preventive medication was considered ineffective because children still suffered from asthma symptoms. Parents were disappointed when the amount of medications was increased despite all their efforts and were afraid of addiction, not understanding that doses were likely to increase because of fast growth in children. Some thought that symptoms should not be suppressed but allowed to come out so that the child could get used to them and grow out of asthma. Some parents delayed the use of medicines as long as possible and tried several alternative treatments (Mesters, Pieterse, & Meertens, 1991).

Parents wanted objective indicators of the child's physical well-being and criteria by which to monitor the progress of an asthma episode, especially important because their child was too young to express verbally how and what he or she felt. The focus groups revealed that parents' knowledge appeared to be insufficient and incoherent, especially about medication, signs preceding attack and preventive activities. Parents also appeared to have an inadequate understanding about how to apply the information they received and a lack of confidence in their ability to do so. Warning signs of an asthma attack were not considered as cues to action when the symptoms were mild to moderate.

This needs assessment led to development of the surveys reviewed here. Questionnaires are available in both Dutch and English. Item scores are summed. An educational protocol consisting of 16 modules has also been developed and tested (Mesters, Meertens, Crebolder, & Parcel, 1993).

PSYCHOMETRIC PROPERTIES

The questionnaire was pretested with 10 mothers of young children with asthma, for readability and uniform interpretation. The knowledge questionnaire was constructed to test an understanding of basic concepts about the nature of asthma and general management procedures and had an α of .81. The attitude survey was based, in part, on an earlier instrument and showed an α of .59. The self-efficacy survey (SE) focused on prevention, treatment and monitoring of asthma symptoms and showed an α of .93. The management behavior survey inquired about the extent to which self-management activities were performed and showed an α of .92 (Mesters et al., 1993).

Parents participating in the education program had significantly more knowledge (mean score pretest, 38.64; posttest, 58.96); a more favorable attitude toward asthma (mean score pretest, 26.12; posttest, 35.83); and a higher SE score. Also, they reported performing self-management behaviors more frequently than they had before the program. A similar study but a randomized trial found mean posttest scores for the treatment group ($N = 31$) of 56.74 for knowledge, 34.66 for attitudes, .94 for SE, and 3.13 for self-management, all higher than scores of the control group ($N = 32$). Changes were sustained at 1 year. The treatment group was found to have decreased its emergency and nonemergency use of the physician's office and to have a reduction in reported asthma severity. Gain in knowledge was the best predictor of gain in (reported) self-management behavior, followed by gain in SE. This finding is congruent with social learning theory, which suggests that behavioral capability (which includes knowledge of what to do and how to do it) and SE mediate behavior. α levels for all scales were above .80 except for the attitude scale, which was .33 (Mesters, Meertens, Kok, & Parcel, 1994). Thus, the tools were sensitive to an appropriate intervention.

CRITIQUE AND SUMMARY

Development and testing of these tools has occurred in The Netherlands, with small and nonrandom numbers of more highly educated parents. Although results of the needs assessment provide some assurance of content validity, structured description of the domains of knowledge attitudes and self-efficacy tasks were not found, nor were other studies of validity. Reliability of the attitude scale is problematic.

Goals of asthma self-management programs are increased adherence to prescribed medication, increased ability and confidence in managing asthma attacks, and decreased anxiety and disruptions of daily life. Although the educational program for which these instruments were developed was targeted at the parents of preschool children, they may be usable with parents of older children.

REFERENCES

Mesters, I., Meertens, R., Crebolder, H., & Parcel, G. (1993). Development of a health education program for parents of preschool children with asthma. *Health Education Research, 8,* 53–68.

Mesters, I., Meertens, R., Kok, G., & Parcel, G. S. (1994). Effectiveness of a multidisciplinary education protocol in children with asthma (0–4 years) in primary health care. *Journal of Asthma, 31,* 347–359.

Mesters, I., Pieterse, M., & Meertens, R. (1991). Pediatric asthma, a qualitative and quantitative approach to needs assessment. *Patient Education and Counseling, 17,* 23–34.

PARENT KNOWLEDGE QUESTIONNAIRE

Categories: true or false for each item

A.   Most children who have asthma:
1.   need to be dressed more warmly than children without asthma
2.   have both physical and psychological problems
③.   can normally take part in any activity requiring some physical exercise
4.   cannot go on a holiday

B.   When a child has asthma:
5.   the heart sometimes doesn't work right
6.   the lungs sometimes do not work right
⑦.   the air tubes in the lungs are very sensitive to certain things
8.   something is wrong with the child's blood

C.   Asthma attacks can be caused by:
⑨.   different things in different people
10.   spicy foods like hot peppers and lots of salt
⑪.   things you are allergic to like dust, pollen, animals
⑫.   virus infections like flu
⑬.   irritants (paint, fumes, perfume, smoke, pollution)
⑭.   emotions (laughing too hard, getting upset)
15.   drinking too much liquid
⑯.   temperature difference
⑰.   bacterial infections
⑱.   physical exercise like running

D.   Preventing asthma symptoms:
19.   is never possible
⑳.   might be possible by removing those things that cause symptoms
㉑.   might be possible by staying away from those things that cause symptoms
㉒.   may be helped by performing warming-up exercises before physical exercise
23.   is something only a child's doctor can do anything about
㉔.   may be helped by taking preventive medication

E.   Children with asthma:
㉕.   have less chance of getting symptoms when they are in good physical condition
26.   can be cured with medication
㉗.   have a greater chance of keeping symptoms when the severity is worse
㉘.   will remain sensitive

F.   When asthmatic children have an attack or asthma symptoms:
㉙.   they have most trouble getting air out of the lungs
㉚.   they have shortness of breath
31.   the air tubes inside their lungs become wider
32.   the muscles in the air tubes are paralyzed
㉝.   the air passages in the lungs become filled with mucus
㉞.   the tissue of the air tubes gets swollen
㉟.   the muscles in the air tubes go into spasm and tighten

G.   Some asthma medication:
㊱.   can be used to prevent an attack or symptoms
37.   causes addiction

⑭. can be used to remedy an attack or symptoms
39. requires increasing dosages
40. causes damaging side effects even in low doses

H.   Children with allergic asthma:
⑱. react differently than other people do to the same substance
⑲. respond especially with their airways
43. only react immediately after contact with triggers
⑴. have a genetic tendency toward allergy
⑵. symptoms are triggered by the release of substances in the body after contact with a trigger

I.   If children with asthma are starting to have an asthma attack:
46. there is no way one can tell an attack is going to happen
⑷. they might notice a tight feeling in their chest before the wheezing starts
⑸. one could give medicine before the wheezing starts
49. one should give medicine only after the wheezing starts
⑺. the degree to which expiration is prolonged might indicate the severity of the attack
51. they breathe very slowly taking long breaths
⑼. sucking in the skin of the chest might indicate the severity of the attack (retractions)
⑽. using a peakflow meter might indicate the severity of the attack

J.   When the child has a moderate attack/symptoms:
54. the parent can do nothing to try and stop the attack
55. the parent must rush to the hospital before doing anything else
⒀. the parent can give medicine to stop the wheezing
⒁. it is important the child rests and tries to relax
58. the parent should try not to pay any attention to the wheezing and hope that it will go away
⒃. the child should drink lots of liquids
⒄. the parent should call the doctor if breathing does not get better shortly after taking medicine
61. always wait at least a day before calling the doctor to give medicine time to work

K.   Children with hyperreactive airways:
⒆. react sooner and longer to a substance than other people
⒇. might get out of breath during and after exercise
⒈. can trigger an attack by yelling
⒉. have more symptoms in the early morning due to the low levels of hormones in the blood

L.   Adapting the environment focuses on:
⒊. making the home as dustproof as possible
67. increasing the humidity in the home
⒌. improving ventilation in the home
⒍. removing material the child is allergic to

M.   When using:
70. a dry-powder inhaler, the powder needs to be inhaled by taking a slow and deep breath
⒏. an aerosol, the child needs to inhale the spray the moment the spray is released
⒐. a peakflow meter, the cursor needs to be moved with a single puff of breath
⒑. inhalers, the child needs to hold his/her breath for a few seconds after inhalation

True answers are circled; others are false.

ASTHMA ATTITUDE SURVEY

Categories: strongly agree (1), agree a little (2), uncertain (3), disagree a little (4), strongly disagree (5)

1. My observations of my child's asthma symptoms are important in helping to get the asthma under control
2. Missing a dose of medication won't hurt
3. Asthma is a problem, even when my child has no symptoms
4. I consider it important to do things that can prevent my child from getting asthma symptoms
5. My child is like most other kids, except that he/she has asthma
6. I don't believe it is necessary to adapt my home because of my child's asthma
7. It is important to take asthma medicines on time
8. Early detection of asthma symptoms is important for getting them under control
9. Every asthma attack needs to be treated with medication
10. I think it is important to find out which triggers cause symptoms in my child
11. I have little control over my child's asthma symptoms
12. Eating properly and/or healthy food can help my child's asthma
13. Taking asthma medication during longer periods of time isn't good for children
14. People with asthma can be successful
15. When taking medicine the advantages outweigh the disadvantages
16. The more I know about asthma the better I can help my child
17. I don't believe that medicines really help to make symptoms go away
18. Children with asthma should be disciplined pretty much like other children
19. It is important to keep my child away from triggers
20. Asthma attacks generally do not happen just like that
21. It is important to let my child get used to triggers
22. I consider it important to be able to help my child when she/he has an attack
23. It is no use asking other people to take account of the fact that my child has asthma
24. The fact that asthma symptoms can disappear during puberty is no reason not to treat asthma

Scoring for the following items is reversed: 2, 3, 6, 11, 13, 17, 21, 23

PARENT SELF-EFFICACY SURVEY

Categories: very well (1), quite well (2), uncertain (3), rather poorly (4), very poorly (5), not applicable (6)

1. Imagine giving your child medicines: HOW well can you determine the dosage?
2. Imagine your child having a mild or moderate attack: HOW well can you treat this attack?
3. Imagine your child having a severe attack: HOW well can you treat this attack?
4. Imagine your child having asthma symptoms: HOW well can you estimate the moment to start giving medicines?
5. Imagine your child having a mild or moderate attack: HOW well can you estimate the severity of the attack?
6. Imagine your child having a mild or moderate attack: HOW well can you estimate the severity from wheezing?

7. Imagine your child having a mild or moderate attack: HOW well can you estimate the severity from retractions?
8. Imagine your child having a mild or moderate attack: HOW well can you estimate the severity from your child's breathing frequency?
9. Imagine your child having a mild or moderate attack: HOW well can you estimate the severity from the relative duration of breathing in and out?
10. Imagine your child having a severe attack: HOW well can you estimate the severity of the attack?
11. Imagine your child having a severe attack: HOW well can you estimate the severity from wheezing?
12. Imagine your child having a severe attack: HOW well can you estimate the severity from retractions?
13. Imagine your child having a severe attack: HOW well can you estimate the severity from your child's breathing frequency?
14. Imagine your child having a severe attack: HOW well can you estimate the severity from the relative duration of breathing in and out?
15. HOW well can you avoid asthma symptoms?
16. Imagine the symptoms of your child become worse: HOW well can you make the right choice of medicines?
17. Imagine the symptoms of your child become less severe: HOW well can you make the right choice of medicines?
18. Imagine your child having asthma symptoms: HOW well can you judge whether the medication works?
19. HOW well can you indicate what triggers cause asthma problems in your child?
20. HOW well can you decide when to call in the help from others (primary or clinical physician)?

HOW well can you cope with triggers inside the home such as:

21. dust/housemites?
22. animal dander?
23. molds?
24. pollen from trees, grasses, and weeds?
25. change in temperature?
26. dampness?
27. cigarette/cigar smoke?
28. smells of detergents, paint, spray, or glue?

HOW well can you cope with triggers outside the home such as:

29. fog, rain, humidity?
30. air pollution?
31. HOW well can you influence your child's physical resistance?
32. HOW well can you relax your child during an attack (distracting attention away from attack)?

MANAGEMENT BEHAVIOR SURVEY

Categories: never (1), seldom (2), sometimes (3), often (4), always (5), not applicable (6)

To what extent do you take the following actions to avoid asthma symptoms in your child?

1. Give medication
2. Avoid allergic triggers outside the home

3. Avoid allergic triggers inside the home
4. Avoid chemicals (like smoke, perfumes)
5. Avoid foods my child is sensitive to
6. Ventilate the home correctly
7. Decrease the degree of humidity in the home
8. Dustproof the home
9. Pay attention to composition of furniture and textiles
10. Stimulate physical activity of my child

To what extent do you take the following actions to treat asthma symptoms in your child?

11. Give medication
12. Give liquids
13. Relax the child
14. Remove triggers
15. Let the child rest

To what extent do you take the following actions to estimate the severity of an attack?

16. Control breathing frequency
17. Control the duration of breathing in and breathing out
18. Control presence of wheezing
19. Inspect the skin around the chest
20. Use peakflow meter

STATE-ANXIETY QUESTIONNAIRE

Categories: not at all, a little, much, very much

When my child has an asthma attack:

1. I feel calm
2. I am tense
3. I feel at ease
4. I feel certain
5. I feel nervous
6. I am indecisive
7. I am relaxed
8. I am worried

From Mesters, I., Meertens, R., Crebolder, H., & Parcel, G. Development of health education program for parents of pre-school children with asthma, Table A1. *Health Education Research, 16*(1), 53–68. Reprinted with permission.

E

Pregnancy, Childbirth, and Parenting

21

Pregnancy Anxiety Scale

Developed by Jeffrey S. Levin

INSTRUMENT DESCRIPTION, ADMINISTRATION, AND SCORING GUIDELINES

Many studies have identified an association of higher anxiety and deleterious pregnancy outcomes. The Pregnancy Anxiety Scale (PAS) is a 10-item scale of maternal anxiety during pregnancy. It is intended to be useful as a diagnostic tool related to the pregnancy experience, more useful than general anxiety inventories would be. Its authors see it as useful in research. It is not yet known if it has specific clinical applications with cutoff points that would indicate a need for further assessment and intervention. The 10 items are scored 0 = no, 1 = yes, and summed (Levin, 1991).

PSYCHOMETRIC PROPERTIES

The 13-item PAS was tested on 266 postpartum mothers, largely African-American and Hispanic and showed reliability of .63. Factor analysis shows three factors: anxiety about being pregnant (items 1 to 3), anxiety about childbirth (items 4 to 7), and anxiety about hospitalization (items 8 to 10). Based on these measurement characteristics, three items were removed, leaving 10. A full and detailed description of the psychometric analysis may be found in Levin (1991).

SUMMARY AND CRITIQUE

The scale's latent structure has not yet been confirmed separately with African-American and Hispanic mothers, or with other groups like Anglo Whites.

It is reasonable to expect education to be one means of lowering excess anxiety, through teaching anxiety reduction strategies or changing misconceptions that produce anxiety. The

PAS requires additional developmental work including exploration of the use of expanded response categories and its structure after prospective use during pregnancy (Levin, 1991).

REFERENCE

Levin, J. S. (1991). The factor structure of the Pregnancy Anxiety Scale. *Journal of Health and Social Behavior, 21,* 368–381.

PREGNANCY ANXIETY

Anxiety about Being Pregnant   Yes   No

   Did any one frighten you about having a baby?
   Did you read anything that frightened you about having a
   baby?
   Did you fear that you would fall and hurt your baby?

Anxiety about Childbirth

   Were you afraid the pain of childbirth would be bad?
   Did you ask for pain medicine before childbirth?
   Did you have any fear about being torn or cut when the
   baby was born?
   Were you afraid your baby would not be normal?

Anxiety about Hospitalization

   Were you afraid you would be alone in the hospital?
   Were you worried that the doctors might not be friendly?
   Were you worried that the nurses might not be friendly?

From Levin, J. S. (1991) The Factor Structure of the Pregnancy Anxiety Scale. *Journal of Health and Social Behavior,* *32* (Dec.), 368–381. Reprinted Table 1, ''Pregnancy Anxiety Indicators by Dimensions'' with permission.

22

Childbirth Expectations Questionnaire

Developed by Annette Gupton

INSTRUMENT DESCRIPTION, ADMINISTRATION, AND SCORING GUIDELINES

Maternal childbirth expectations play an important role in determining a woman's response to her childbirth experience. A growing body of literature indicates that the degree of congruence between these expectations and the reality of actual experience has an important impact on perception of the severity of labor pain; on the subsequent evaluation of both the self and the childbirth experience including feelings of failure, grief, and loss; and on the mother-baby relationship. Yet relatively little is known about the nature of women's childbirth expectations and what influences their development. The series of studies describing development of the Childbirth Expectations Questionnaire (CEQ) is based in Janis's stress response theory that anticipatory thought processes preceding a stressful event play a major role in determining how an individual will cope during the actual event and in the succeeding period (Beaton & Gupton, 1990).

Women come to childbirth education classes already having developed expectations for their childbirth experience. Part of the educational process is to explore these expectations and promote realistic ones, especially important for women with high-risk (HR) pregnancies. Developing a birth plan should enable women to set goals for their birth experience that covers a range of circumstances and makes allowances for change. Women in Beaton and Gupton's study (1990) held high expectations of the ability of their husband/coach to help them through the experience. The education of partners is also important, as is negotiation between the couple of realistic expectations.

The CEQ consists of 35 items with four subscales confirmed by factor analysis: ability to cope with pain (items 4, 5, 12, 15, 16, 18, 21, 22, 25, 29, and 35); role of the nurse (items 2, 3, 6 to 8, 23, 26, and 28); role of the partner/coach (items 1, 9, 11, 17, 27, 31, and 34); and amount of medical intervention (items 10, 13, 14, 19, 20, 24, 30, 32, and 33). Items are scored 1 to 5 and total scores can range from 35 to 175, with high scores representing more positive expectations for the childbirth experience. Because subscales have unequal numbers of items, percentile scores are computed and allow comparison among subscales (Heaman, Beaton, Gupton, & Sloan, 1992).

PSYCHOMETRIC PROPERTIES

Steps in development of the CEQ are well documented. In-depth interviews with 11 urban Canadian women in their third trimester of pregnancy provided background for conceptualization and development of the subscales and items. The women had developed detailed expectations of the childbirth experience including the roles of support persons and health personnel. A panel of experts in maternal-infant nursing reviewed the items for relevance and clarity and sorted them into five content areas to a level of 75% agreement (Beaton & Gupton, 1990). At least three drafts were tested on a total of 400 women in a Canadian city, and items that did not correlate well or that appeared redundant were deleted. Cronbach's α for the final version total score was .82, .84 for the pain/coping subscale, .80 for the nursing support subscale, .72 for the partner/coach subscale, and .65 for the intervention subscale. A measure of test-retest reliability was .67 (Gupton, Beaton, Sloan, & Bramadat, 1991).

A study of a convenience sample of 75 HR and 77 low risk (LR) nulliparas found that anxiety was negatively related to childbirth expectations, whereas childbirth preparation was positively related to expectations. Scores were total: 122, HR; 127, LR; coping with pain subscale: 32, HR; 34, LR; support from partner/coach subscale: 29, HR; 29, LR; nursing support subscale: 32, HR; 32, LR; and intervention subscale: 28, HR; 31, LR. HR pregnant women had significantly less positive expectations for their childbirth experience than did LR pregnant women; the CEQ discriminated between the two groups. HR women expected to have more pain/more difficulty coping with pain and more medical intervention than did LR pregnant women (Heaman et al., 1992).

CRITIQUE AND SUMMARY

The CEQ or development of a birth plan might be used to explore a couple's birth expectations, and to identify those that might be unrealistic. This is a time to clarify misconceptions about interventions and purpose, decrease high anxiety, and to negotiate the role of the partner. The CEQ offers a structured way to access expectations for specific aspects of labor, as opposed to the global questions sometimes asked, and thus allows more focused interventions. Further work is needed to establish validity by comparison with other instruments and the ability of the CEQ to further discriminate among different populations of pregnant women (Gupton et al., 1991).

The population on which the CEQ has been developed (largely White, married, well educated, urban, middle-class primiparas, with a mean age in the late 20s, attending private childbirth education classes), means that its generalizability to other populations is unknown. For some groups, questions related to support by a partner/coach might not be relevant. CEQ sensitivity to instruction should be established as should longitudinal study to see whether expectations change over time. This information would assist childbirth educators in developing teaching strategies to prepare women for the realities of the childbirth experience (Gupton et al., 1991).

REFERENCES

Beaton, J., & Gupton, A. (1990). Childbirth expectations: A qualitative analysis. *Midwifery, 6*, 133–139.

Gupton, A., Beaton, U., Sloan, J., & Bramadat, I. (1991). The development of a scale to measure childbirth expectations. *The Canadian Journal of Nursing Research, 23*, 35–47.

Heaman, M., Beaton, J., Gupton, A., & Sloan, J. (1992). A comparison of childbirth expectations in high-risk and low-risk pregnant women. *Clinical Nursing Research, 1*, 252–265.

CHILDBIRTH EXPECTATIONS QUESTIONNAIRE

This questionnaire is designed to describe women's expectations regarding their impending labor and delivery experience. Your opinions along with those of other pregnant women will be used to learn more about women and childbirth.

This questionnaire contains a number of statements, each of which says something different about your labor and delivery expectations. While no one can know for sure what will happen to them in labor, we are interested in knowing what you anticipate or expect the childbirth experience will be like for you. We are asking for your "best guess" about what will happen to you in labor. For each statement, decide how you agree or disagree with the view expressed. Think about the statement. Beside each statement you will find five words used to describe your expectation. There are no right or wrong answers. People differ in their views. Your response is a matter of your personal opinion. The information you give will be completely confidential.

Thank you very much for your time and your help. Below is an example which may help you in completing the questionnaire.

EXAMPLE	Strongly Disagree	Disagree	Neutral	Agree	Strongly Agree
A. I am looking forward with great joy to the birth of my baby	❑	❑	❑	❑	☑
B. I need to know more about childbirth than I possibly could	❑	❑	☑	❑	❑

The answer to Example A, "Strongly Agree" indicates that you are quite certain that you are looking forward to the birth of your baby with great joy.

The answer to Example B, "Neutral" indicates that you cannot quite decide whether to agree or disagree with this statement.

PLEASE BE SURE TO MARK EVERY STATEMENT AND WORD(S) WHICH COMES CLOSEST TO YOUR OPINION.

With regard to my labor and delivery experience, I expect that ...

		Strongly Disagree	Disagree	Neutral	Agree	Strongly Agree
1.	My partner/coach will be happy and excited	❏	❏	❏	❏	❏
2.	The nurses will be kind to me	❏	❏	❏	❏	❏
3.	I will avoid seeking help from the nurses	❏	❏	❏	❏	❏
4.	I will be immobilized by the pain of labor	❏	❏	❏	❏	❏
5.	I will be able to cope with labor	❏	❏	❏	❏	❏
6.	I will feel reassured by the nurses' presence	❏	❏	❏	❏	❏
7.	The nurses will spend little time with me	❏	❏	❏	❏	❏
8.	My plans for birth will be ignored by the nurse	❏	❏	❏	❏	❏
9.	My partner/coach will feel quite helpless	❏	❏	❏	❏	❏
10.	I will be required to have routine procedures even if I don't want them	❏	❏	❏	❏	❏
11.	I will ask my partner/coach for help	❏	❏	❏	❏	❏
12.	I will worry about the severity of labor pain	❏	❏	❏	❏	❏
13.	There is little chance that I will end up having a cesarean section	❏	❏	❏	❏	❏
14.	Lots of medical equipment and machinery will be used	❏	❏	❏	❏	❏
15.	I will be afraid of panicking	❏	❏	❏	❏	❏
16.	I will experience discomfort but not unbearable pain	❏	❏	❏	❏	❏
17.	I will feel comforted by the presence of my partner/coach	❏	❏	❏	❏	❏
18.	I will feel intense pain	❏	❏	❏	❏	❏
19.	I will have a childbirth free of medical intervention	❏	❏	❏	❏	❏
20.	I will want to have fetal monitoring	❏	❏	❏	❏	❏

		Strongly Disagree	Disagree	Neutral	Agree	Strongly Agree
21.	I will be afraid of being a coward	❒	❒	❒	❒	❒
22.	I will be able to relax during labor	❒	❒	❒	❒	❒
23.	The nurses will offer me encouragement	❒	❒	❒	❒	❒
24.	Forceps will be used	❒	❒	❒	❒	❒
25.	The pain of labor will be agonizing	❒	❒	❒	❒	❒
26.	I will receive personal attention from the nurses	❒	❒	❒	❒	❒
27.	My partner/coach will tell me what is going on	❒	❒	❒	❒	❒
28.	The nurse will allow me to be an active participant in decision making	❒	❒	❒	❒	❒
29.	I will be scared when I think about the pain of labor	❒	❒	❒	❒	❒
30.	I will refuse to have any procedures I consider unnecessary	❒	❒	❒	❒	❒
31.	My opinion or that of my partner/coach will be sought for all major medical decisions	❒	❒	❒	❒	❒
32.	I will use anesthetics and/or pain killing drugs	❒	❒	❒	❒	❒
33.	The doctor will make most of the decisions	❒	❒	❒	❒	❒
34.	I will avoid telling my partner/coach what I am feeling	❒	❒	❒	❒	❒
35.	I will be embarrassed by my behaviour	❒	❒	❒	❒	❒

Please note the following items are reverse scored: 3, 4, 7, 8 to 10, 12, 14, 15, 18, 20, 21, 24, 25, 29, and 32 to 35.

23

Labour Agentry Scale: A Measure of a Woman's Sense of Control Over the Childbirth Experience

Developed by Ellen Hodnett

INSTRUMENT DESCRIPTION, ADMINISTRATION, AND SCORING GUIDELINES

The Labour Agentry Scale (LAS) measures perceived control during childbirth, that is, a woman's sense of mastery over internal and environmental forces. This control has been linked to improved learning and functioning on various tasks, and decreased need for analgesia and anesthesia during childbirth; and to be a key component of birth satisfaction (Hodnett & Abel, 1986). The LAS has been translated into and validated in French, Spanish, Swedish, Danish, and Hebrew. It can be used to measure either expectations or experiences of control, depending on timing of administration (antepartum or postpartum). Scores are obtained from summing item scores, with a possible range from 29 to 203. Low scores indicate low expectancies of experiences of control over oneself and one's environment during labor; high scores indicate high expectancies/experiences. The LAS takes 10 minutes to complete.

PSYCHOMETRIC PROPERTIES

Most subjects asked open-ended questions about what contributed to a positive birth experience indicated that aspects of personal control were important to them during labor. In psychometric

---

Please note that the British spelling has been retained in the "Labour Agentry Scale" but the English spelling has been used in the text.

and field studies, α reliability coefficients for the LAS have ranged from .91 to .98 (Hodnett & Abel, 1986). Subjects who experienced the highest levels of control over self and environment during labor by ambulating, foregoing analgesia and anesthesia, and having spontaneous births had the highest LAS scores, evidence supporting concurrent validity. There was also a significant inverse relationship between usage of pharmacological pain-relief measures and LAS scores, a significant positive relationship between levels of perceived human support during childbirth and LAS scores. Experienced control was distinct from but related to maternal childbirth satisfaction. Antepartum mean scores ranged from 156.5 to 162.38, with postpartum scores 152.19 to 156.89. LAS scores remained stable at 2 weeks, 1 month, and 3 months postpartum. Factor analysis and dual scaling yielded evidence of a unifactorial scale (Hodnett & Simmons-Tropea, 1987).

In one study (Hodnett & Abel, 1986), the 80 women with home births had a significantly higher mean (174.7; SD = 24.43) LAS score than did the 80 with hospital births (mean score = 150.9; SD = 25.38). Multigravidas had significantly higher mean LAS scores than did primigravidas. Such findings are congruent with perceived environmental control. Hodnett and Osborn (1989) found greater increases in LAS scores and significantly less analgesia and anesthesia when continuous support (emotional, informational, physical, and advocacy) from montrices was provided during labor than under conditions of usual nursing care. Thus, the LAS showed sensitivity to intervention.

CRITIQUE AND SUMMARY

Approximately 800 patients have been tested with the LAS. Despite this strength, the LAS has primarily been tested on patients who were middle-class, married, prenatally educated, White women in one Canadian medical center who experienced normal pregnancies and were accompanied by husband or partner during labor with vaginal deliveries delivering normal newborns. In part, the authors meant to contribute to the body of knowledge supporting management of normal childbirth, which is the norm for 85% of North American women. Other populations should be studied. Both scores and dimensions of control may be different for other groups (Hodnett & Simmons-Tropea, 1987).

Expected control has been inversely related to prenatal anxiety; education can decrease this problem. One of the key elements of professional care during labor is information and instruction. Thus, the LAS would seem to be a useful tool for patient assessment and tailoring of interventions and for research on the influence of expectations in both physiological and psychological outcomes of pregnancy and birth. LAS has also been used in studies addressing environmental conditions for birth and support during labor (Hodnett & Simmons-Tropea, 1987).

REFERENCES

Hodnett, E. D., & Abel, S. M. (1986). Person-environment interaction as a determinant of labor length variables. *Health Care for Women International, 7,* 341–356.

Hodnett, E. D., & Osborn, R. W. (1989). Effect of continuous intrapartum professional support on childbirth outcomes. *Research in Nursing and Health, 12,* 289–297.

Hodnett, E. D., & Simmons-Tropea, D. A. (1987). The Labour Agentry Scale: Psychometric properties of an instrument measuring control during childbirth. *Research in Nursing and Health, 10,* 301–310.

YOUR FEELINGS DURING LABOUR

On the following pages there are 29 statements, each describing a feeling some women have had during labour. Just as no two women are exactly alike, no two women have exactly the same experiences during labour. Please try to recall your labour as vividly as you can, and think about the feelings you experienced. Of course, you probably had many different feelings, but try to remember what it was generally like for you during this time.

For each statement, place an "X" in the space that most closely describes what labour was like for you. There are no "right" or "wrong" answers.

Thank you very much for taking the time to do this.

1.   I felt confident

Almost Always_____ : _____ : _____ : _____ : _____ : _____ : _____Rarely

    7   6   5   4   3   2   1

2.   I felt defeated

Almost Always_____ : _____ : _____ : _____ : _____ : _____ : _____Rarely

    1   2   3   4   5   6   7

3.   I felt important

Almost Always_____ : _____ : _____ : _____ : _____ : _____ : _____Rarely

    7   6   5   4   3   2   1

4.   I felt tense

Almost Always_____ : _____ : _____ : _____ : _____ : _____ : _____Rarely

    1   2   3   4   5   6   7

5.   I had a sense of understanding what was happening

Almost Always_____ : _____ : _____ : _____ : _____ : _____ : _____Rarely

    7   6   5   4   3   2   1

6.   I felt insecure

Almost Always_____ : _____ : _____ : _____ : _____ : _____ : _____Rarely

    1   2   3   4   5   6   7

7.   I felt relaxed

Almost Always_____ : _____ : _____ : _____ : _____ : _____ : _____Rarely

    7   6   5   4   3   2   1

8. I felt competent

Almost Always_____ : _____ : _____ : _____ : _____ : _____ : _____Rarely

       7   6   5   4   3   2   1

9. Someone or something else was in charge of my labour

Almost Always_____ : _____ : _____ : _____ : _____ : _____ : _____Rarely

       1   2   3   4   5   6   7

10. I felt inadequate

Almost Always_____ : _____ : _____ : _____ : _____ : _____ : _____Rarely

       1   2   3   4   5   6   7

11. I experienced a sense of distress

Almost Always_____ : _____ : _____ : _____ : _____ : _____ : _____Rarely

       1   2   3   4   5   6   7

12. Everything seemed unclear and unreal

Almost Always_____ : _____ : _____ : _____ : _____ : _____ : _____Rarely

       1   2   3   4   5   6   7

13. I was completely aware of everything that was happening

Almost Always_____ : _____ : _____ : _____ : _____ : _____ : _____Rarely

       7   6   5   4   3   2   1

14. I felt panicked

Almost Always_____ : _____ : _____ : _____ : _____ : _____ : _____Rarely

       1   2   3   4   5   6   7

15. I felt like I was falling to pieces

Almost Always_____ : _____ : _____ : _____ : _____ : _____ : _____Rarely

       1   2   3   4   5   6   7

16. I had a feeling of constriction and of being confined

Almost Always_____ : _____ : _____ : _____ : _____ : _____ : _____Rarely

       1   2   3   4   5   6   7

17.   I was in control

Almost Always_____ : _____ : _____ : _____ : _____ : _____ : _____Rarely

7   6   5   4   3   2   1

18.   I experienced a sense of being with others who care

Almost Always_____ : _____ : _____ : _____ : _____ : _____ : _____Rarely

7   6   5   4   3   2   1

19.   Everything made sense

Almost Always_____ : _____ : _____ : _____ : _____ : _____ : _____Rarely

7   6   5   4   3   2   1

20.   I felt like I was dying

Almost Always_____ : _____ : _____ : _____ : _____ : _____ : _____Rarely

1   2   3   4   5   6   7

21.   I felt I was doing everything I should have been doing

Almost Always_____ : _____ : _____ : _____ : _____ : _____ : _____Rarely

7   6   5   4   3   2   1

22.   I felt helpless

Almost Always_____ : _____ : _____ : _____ : _____ : _____ : _____Rarely

1   2   3   4   5   6   7

23.   Everything seemed peaceful and calm

Almost Always_____ : _____ : _____ : _____ : _____ : _____ : _____Rarely

7   6   5   4   3   2   1

24.   I experienced a sense of success

Almost Always_____ : _____ : _____ : _____ : _____ : _____ : _____Rarely

7   6   5   4   3   2   1

25.   I felt powerless

Almost Always_____ : _____ : _____ : _____ : _____ : _____ : _____Rarely

1   2   3   4   5   6   7

26. I experienced a sense of failure

Almost Always_____ : _____ : _____ : _____ : _____ : _____ : _____Rarely

          1   2   3   4   5   6   7

27. I was accepting what was happening

Almost Always_____ : _____ : _____ : _____ : _____ : _____ : _____Rarely

          7   6   5   4   3   2   1

28. I felt capable

Almost Always_____ : _____ : _____ : _____ : _____ : _____ : _____Rarely

          7   6   5   4   3   2   1

29. I felt bad about my behaviour during labour

Almost Always_____ : _____ : _____ : _____ : _____ : _____ : _____Rarely

          1   2   3   4   5   6   7

24

Childbirth Self-Efficacy Inventory

Developed by Nancy K. Lowe

INSTRUMENT DESCRIPTION, ADMINISTRATION, AND SCORING GUIDELINES

Self-efficacy (SE) involves an individual's evaluation of her capabilities to cope with stressful situations and perform required behaviors, certainly of concern during labor. Perceptions of self-efficacy developed before an event predict whether an individual will even try to cope with the situation and how long the effort will be sustained.

Confidence in the ability to cope with labor can be considered a motivational or conceptual factor affecting a woman's interpretation of painful labor stimuli. The importance of confidence to the perception of pain during labor is supported by data from clinical studies, which indicate that more than one half of the variance in early labor pain and about one third of the variance in active labor pain may be explained by the single variable of maternal confidence in the ability to cope. Women who express greater confidence in their ability to cope with labor report having less pain during labor. Those with the highest levels of SE will anticipate being able to execute coping behaviors during the most stressful times of labor including absence of a significant other, complications of labor, and concerns for fetal well-being. Confidence can be significantly increased by childbirth education including observation of others performing successfully during labor (Lowe, 1991).

The Childbirth Self-Efficacy Inventory (CBSEI) measures both outcome expectancies (belief that a given behavior will lead to a given outcome) and self-efficacy expectancies (conviction that one can successfully perform required behaviors in a given situation) for coping with an approaching childbirth. An individual may believe that a certain behavior could help someone cope with the potentially aversive event but feel incapable of personally performing the behavior in the particular situation (Lowe, 1993).

Reading level of the scale has been measured at grades 7 or 8. Scale scores are the sum of responses (1 to 10) to each item. In each part, the first half of the items measures outcome expectation and the second half of the items self-efficacy expectations. Thus, active labor outcome and self-efficacy scores may range from 15 to 150, whereas the parallel second-stage scores have a potential range of 16 to 160 each. Total CBSEI outcome and self-efficacy expectancy scores are the sum of the corresponding scores from active and second stage labor and may range from 31 to 310 (Lowe, 1993).

PSYCHOMETRIC PROPERTIES

Fifty-six items were generated for the CBSEI through content analysis of postpartum interviews with 23 primiparous and 25 multiparous women who had experienced the uncomplicated vaginal birth of a normal term infant within the preceding 48 hours. The interview guide elicited each subject's perceptions of the specific behaviors she used to cope with labor, the adequacy of her individual strategies, and the perceived deficiencies in her ability to cope. Fifty percent of the sample had attended childbirth preparation classes. Rating of the items by an expert panel of university professors and nurse specialists in the care of childbearing women, or self-efficacy theory and removal of redundancies reduced the item pool to 20 items.

Pilot data from 96 healthy pregnant women led to further revision including separation of items into two phases of labor: when contractions are 5 or fewer minutes apart (active labor), and when pushing the baby out to give birth; change of the response scale; and addition of outcome expectancy scales. The CBSEI was then administered to 351 women attending community-based childbirth classes in the third trimester of pregnancy. The range of scores indicated that the CBSEI was sensitive to various levels of outcome and self-efficacy expectancies for childbirth and in differentiating outcome from self-efficacy expectancies (Lowe, 1993).

Internal consistency estimates ranged from .86 to .95, and item-total correlations were greater than .30 for all items on each scale. Correlations of test-retest scores over a 2-week period ranged from .46 to .76. Validity of the CBSEI was supported by significant positive correlations with measures of generalized self-efficacy, self-esteem, and internal locus of control, and significant negative correlations with external health locus of control and learned helplessness. Validity was also supported by significantly higher self-efficacy scores for multiparous compared with nulliparous pregnant women. Factor analysis suggested that each CBSEI scale is unidimensional. Mean scores were 128 for outcome expectancy during active labor, 103 for SE during active labor, 130 for outcome expectancy during birth, 107 for SE during birth, 258 total outcome expectancy score, and 210 total SE score (Lowe, 1993).

SUMMARY AND CRITIQUE

An obvious direction for research is to investigate the effectiveness of particular strategies used in childbirth preparation to enhance women's confidence in coping with labor. It is important to understand how to tailor this education to individual variations in personality and skills that a woman may bring to her pregnancy experience including previous experience with childbirth, or stressful and painful medical events. Most of the participants on whom the instrument has been tested were White, married, highly educated, nulliparous, and recruited from childbirth education classes. The instrument must be tested in more diverse demographic samples and in women unexposed to childbirth education. In addition, prospective study using the CBSEI during pregnancy and outcome measures during labor and birth will provide additional evidence for its validity. Because outcome expectancies are not conceptually well developed in the SE theory literature, their distinctiveness from SE in relation to coping with experiences, such as childbirth, should be further studied (Lowe, 1991).

The CBSEI was developed through a well-planned and conceptualized series of studies.

REFERENCES

Lowe, N. K. (1991). Maternal confidence in coping with labor: A self-efficacy concept. *JOGN Nursing, 20,* 457–463.

Lowe, N. K. (1993). Maternal confidence for labor: Development of the Childbirth Self-Efficacy Inventory. *Research in Nursing and Health, 16,* 141–149.

CHILDBIRTH SELF-EFFICACY INVENTORY (CBSEI)

CBSEI: Part I (Labor)

Think about how you imagine labor will be and feel when you are having contractions 5 minutes apart or less. For each of the following behaviors, indicate how helpful you feel the behavior could be in helping you cope with this part of labor by circling a number between 1, *not at all helpful*, and 10, *very helpful*.

		Not at All Helpful									Very Helpful
1.	Relax my body.	1	2	3	4	5	6	7	8	9	10
2.	Get ready for each contraction.	1	2	3	4	5	6	7	8	9	10
3.	Use breathing during labor contractions.	1	2	3	4	5	6	7	8	9	10
4.	Keep myself in control.	1	2	3	4	5	6	7	8	9	10
5.	Think about relaxing.	1	2	3	4	5	6	7	8	9	10
6.	Concentrate on an object in the room to distract myself.	1	2	3	4	5	6	7	8	9	10
7.	Keep myself calm.	1	2	3	4	5	6	7	8	9	10
8.	Concentrate on thinking about the baby.	1	2	3	4	5	6	7	8	9	10
9.	Stay on top of each contraction.	1	2	3	4	5	6	7	8	9	10
10.	Think positively.	1	2	3	4	5	6	7	8	9	10
11.	Not think about the pain.	1	2	3	4	5	6	7	8	9	10
12.	Tell myself that I can do it.	1	2	3	4	5	6	7	8	9	10
13.	Think about others in my family.	1	2	3	4	5	6	7	8	9	10
14.	Concentrate on getting through one contraction at a time.	1	2	3	4	5	6	7	8	9	10
15.	Listen to encouragement from the person helping me.	1	2	3	4	5	6	7	8	9	10

Part I Continued

Continue to think about how you imagine labor will be and feel when you are having contractions 5 minutes apart or less. For each behavior, indicate how certain you are of your ability to use the behavior to help you cope with this part of labor by circling a number between 1, *not at all sure*, and 10, *completely sure*.

		Not at All Sure									Completely Sure
16.	Relax my body.	1	2	3	4	5	6	7	8	9	10
17.	Get ready for each contraction.	1	2	3	4	5	6	7	8	9	10
18.	Use breathing during labor contractions.	1	2	3	4	5	6	7	8	9	10
19.	Keep myself in control.	1	2	3	4	5	6	7	8	9	10
20.	Think about relaxing.	1	2	3	4	5	6	7	8	9	10
21.	Concentrate on an object in the room to distract myself.	1	2	3	4	5	6	7	8	9	10
22.	Keep myself calm.	1	2	3	4	5	6	7	8	9	10
23.	Concentrate on thinking about the baby.	1	2	3	4	5	6	7	8	9	10
24.	Stay on top of each contraction.	1	2	3	4	5	6	7	8	9	10
25.	Think positively.	1	2	3	4	5	6	7	8	9	10
26.	Not think about the pain.	1	2	3	4	5	6	7	8	9	10
27.	Tell myself that I can do it.	1	2	3	4	5	6	7	8	9	10
28.	Think about others in my family.	1	2	3	4	5	6	7	8	9	10
29.	Concentrate on getting through one contraction at a time.	1	2	3	4	5	6	7	8	9	10
30.	Listen to encouragement from the person helping me.	1	2	3	4	5	6	7	8	9	10

CBSEI: Part II (Birth)

Think about how you imagine labor will be and feel when you are pushing your baby out to give birth. For each of the following behaviors, indicate how helpful you feel the behavior could be in helping you cope with this part of labor by circling a number between 1, *not at all helpful*, and 10, *very helpful*.

		Not at All Helpful									Very Helpful
31.	Relax my body.	1	2	3	4	5	6	7	8	9	10
32.	Get ready for each contraction.	1	2	3	4	5	6	7	8	9	10
33.	Use breathing during labor contractions.	1	2	3	4	5	6	7	8	9	10
34.	Keep myself in control.	1	2	3	4	5	6	7	8	9	10
35.	Think about relaxing.	1	2	3	4	5	6	7	8	9	10
36.	Concentrate on an object in the room to distract myself.	1	2	3	4	5	6	7	8	9	10
37.	Keep myself calm.	1	2	3	4	5	6	7	8	9	10
38.	Concentrate on thinking about the baby.	1	2	3	4	5	6	7	8	9	10
39.	Stay on top of each contraction.	1	2	3	4	5	6	7	8	9	10
40.	Think positively.	1	2	3	4	5	6	7	8	9	10
41.	Not think about the pain.	1	2	3	4	5	6	7	8	9	10
42.	Tell myself that I can do it.	1	2	3	4	5	6	7	8	9	10
43.	Think about others in my family.	1	2	3	4	5	6	7	8	9	10
44.	Concentrate on getting through one contraction at a time.	1	2	3	4	5	6	7	8	9	10
45.	Focus on the person helping me in labor.	1	2	3	4	5	6	7	8	9	10
46.	Listen to encouragement from the person helping me.	1	2	3	4	5	6	7	8	9	10

Part II Continued

Continue to think about how you imagine labor will be and feel when you are pushing your baby out to give birth. For each behavior, indicate how certain you are of your ability to use the behavior to help you cope with this part of labor by circling a number between 1, *not at all sure*, and 10, *completely sure*.

		Not at All Sure									Completely Sure
47.	Relax my body.	1	2	3	4	5	6	7	8	9	10
48.	Get ready for each contraction.	1	2	3	4	5	6	7	8	9	10
49.	Use breathing during labor contractions.	1	2	3	4	5	6	7	8	9	10
50.	Keep myself in control.	1	2	3	4	5	6	7	8	9	10
51.	Think about relaxing.	1	2	3	4	5	6	7	8	9	10
52.	Concentrate on an object in the room to distract myself.	1	2	3	4	5	6	7	8	9	10
53.	Keep myself calm.	1	2	3	4	5	6	7	8	9	10
54.	Concentrate on thinking about the baby.	1	2	3	4	5	6	7	8	9	10
55.	Stay on top of each contraction.	1	2	3	4	5	6	7	8	9	10
56.	Think positively.	1	2	3	4	5	6	7	8	9	10
57.	Not think about the pain.	1	2	3	4	5	6	7	8	9	10
58.	Tell myself that I can do it.	1	2	3	4	5	6	7	8	9	10
59.	Think about others in my family.	1	2	3	4	5	6	7	8	9	10
60.	Concentrate on getting through one contraction at a time.	1	2	3	4	5	6	7	8	9	10
61.	Focus on the person helping me in labor.	1	2	3	4	5	6	7	8	9	10
62.	Listen to encouragement from the person helping me.	1	2	3	4	5	6	7	8	9	10

Scoring Instructions. The CBSEI is a self-report measure of outcome expectancy and self-efficacy expectancy for labor and birth. In the framework of self-efficacy theory (Bandura, 1982), *outcome expectancy* for labor and birth is defined as the belief that a given behavior will enhance coping with labor, while *self-efficacy expectancy* is a personal conviction that one can successfully perform specific behaviors during labor. This distinction is important because a woman may believe that a certain behavior could help a woman cope with labor, but feel incapable of personally performing the behavior during her own labor.

Part I of the CBSEI measures outcome expectancy and self-efficacy expectancy for active labor, while Part II measures the same constructs for second stage or birth. Scale scores are computed by summing the item responses as follows:

Outcome Expectancy Active Labor (Outcome-AL) : items 1 through 15

Self-Efficacy Expectancy Active Labor (Efficacy-AL) : items 16 through 30

Outcome Expectancy Second Stage (Outcome-SS) : items 31 through 46

Self-Efficacy Expectancy Second Stage (Efficacy-SS) : items 47 through 62

A Total Childbirth Outcome Expectancy Score (Outcome-Total) is computed by summing the Outcome-AL and Outcome-SS scale scores. A Total Self-Efficacy Expectancy Score (Efficacy-Total) is computed by summing the Efficacy-AL and Efficacy-SS scale scores.

25

Maternal Self-Efficacy Scale

Developed by Douglas M. Teti and Donna M. Gelfand

INSTRUMENT DESCRIPTION, ADMINISTRATION, AND SCORING GUIDELINES

Self-efficacy (SE) is a core construct that mediates relations between knowledge and behavior. For example, an individual may have the knowledge needed to console a distressed infant but may be unable to do so because of self-doubt. The measure yields one score by adding up the individual scores on all 10 items (Teti & Gelfand, 1991).

PSYCHOMETRIC PROPERTIES

The Maternal Self-Efficacy Scale was developed by Teti and Gelfand (1991) as part of a study of maternal depression, infant difficulty, and maternal competence. The authors propose that the influence of maternal depression, social-marital supports, and perceptions of infant temperament, all of which have been found to be related to less sensitive and punitive behavior toward infants, are mediated by feelings of efficacy in the maternal role. Those with low SE may be expected to handle their babies more indecisively, insensitively, and awkwardly because they lack the problem-solving skills or the persistence required to establish sensitive interactions with their children.

Domains of infant care, such as soothing the baby; understanding what the baby wants; getting the baby to understand the mother's wishes; maintaining joint attention and interaction with the baby; amusing the baby; knowing what the baby enjoys; disengaging from the baby; and performing daily routine tasks, such as feeding, changing, and bathing, are included in the scale. Cronbach's α was .79 based on a pilot sample of 29 mothers and .86 for a study of 48 clinically depressed and in therapy, and 38 nondepressed mothers. Evidence of concurrent validity may be seen in the strong relationship to scores on the Parenting Stress Index Sense of Competence Scale and in a measure of maternal competence and SE (Teti & Gelfand, 1991).

Teti and Gelfand's (1991) study findings support the premise that maternal self-efficacy is a central mediator of relations between mothers' competence with their infants and factors, such as maternal perceptions of infant difficulty, maternal depression, and social-marital supports. These relationships do make sense in terms of self-efficacy theory in that a difficult, irritable baby may be expected to reduce feelings of efficacy as a mother, and self-efficacy would be sensitive to social persuasion and modeling influences provided by significant others. No sample scores on the Maternal Self-Efficacy Scale could be located in published sources.

The Maternal Self-Efficacy Scale was adapted to the developmental age of toddlers in a study by LaRoche, Turner, & Kalick (1995) of toddlers' behavioral difficulties, mothers' depression, mothers' self-efficacy, and mothers' social support among 26 low income Latina mothers. It is unclear whether this revised tool is sufficiently altered to make its measurement characteristics noncumulative with the original Maternal Self-Efficacy Scale.

CRITIQUE AND SUMMARY

The population most thoroughly studied was nearly 100% White and nearly two thirds of the Mormon religion in addition to including mothers who had been diagnosed as depressed and were in therapy (Teti & Gelfand, 1991). In addition, the tool seems to underrepresent important domains of infant care, such as a wide variety of physical skills.

Teti and Gelfand (1991) suggest longitudinal investigation of the possible impact of maternal self-efficacy on developmental outcomes in infants and young children, the temporal stability of maternal self-efficacy including its sensitivity to maternal depression, child behavior and maternal competence. A study of the sensitivity of the scale to intervention could not be located. Although standard intervention elements to improve SE are well known, they may be tailored for those in particular situations. For example, because it is believed that depression predisposes individuals to low SE and poor performance because of selective activation of memories of failure experiences, the intervention should address this (Teti & Gelfand, 1991).

REFERENCES

LaRoche, M. J., Turner, C., & Kalick, S. M. (1995). Latina mothers and their toddlers' behavioral difficulties. *Hispanic Journal of Behavioral Sciences, 17,* 375–384.

Teti, D. M., & Gelfand, D. M. (1991). Behavioral competence among mothers of infants in the first year: The mediational role of maternal self-efficacy. *Child Development, 62,* 918–929.

MATERNAL EFFICACY QUESTIONNAIRE

We want to ask you some questions about *yourself and your baby*. We are trying to get a general idea of how you usually handle different situations with your baby. We realize that no one is always effective or always ineffective. We all do better in some situations than in others. So we would like to have you think about some situations that all mothers encounter.

1. When your baby is upset, fussy, or crying, how good are you at soothing him or her?

1	2	3	4
not good at all	not good enough	good enough	very good

2. How good are you at understanding what your baby wants or needs? For example, do you know when your baby needs to be changed or wants to be fed?

1	2	3	4
I do not understand my baby	I understand my baby some of the time	I understand my baby most of the time	I understand my baby all of the time

3. How good are you at making your baby understand what you want him/her to do? For example, if you want your baby to eat dinner or play quietly, how good are you at making him or her do that?

1	2	3	4
not good at all	not good enough	good enough	very good

4. How good are you at getting your baby to pay attention to you? For example, when you want your baby to look at you, how good are you at making him or her do it?

1	2	3	4
not good at all	not good enough	good enough	very good

5. How good are you at getting your baby to have fun with you? For example, how good are you at getting your baby to smile and laugh with you?

1	2	3	4
not good at all	not good enough	good enough	very good

6. How good are you at knowing what activities your baby will enjoy? For example, how good are you at knowing what games and toys your baby will like to play with?

1	2	3	4
not good at all	not good enough	good enough	very good

7. How good are you at keeping your baby occupied when you need to do housework? For example, how good are you at finding things for the baby when you need to do the dishes?

1	2	3	4
not good	not good	good enough	very good

at all   enough

8. How good do you feel you are at feeding, changing, and bathing your baby?

1	2	3	4
not good at all	not good enough	good enough	very good

9. How good are you at getting your baby to show off for visitors? For example, how good are you at making your baby smile or laugh for people who visit?

1	2	3	4
not good at all	not good enough	good enough	very good

10. In general, how good a mother do you feel you are?

1	2	3	4
not good at all	not good enough	good enough	very good

From Teti, D. M., & Gelfand, D. M. (1991). Behavioral competence among mothers of infants in the first year: The mediational role of maternal self-efficacy. *Child Development, 62,* 918–929.

26

Diabetes in Pregnancy Knowledge Screen

Developed by Anthony Spirito, Laurie Ruggerio, Andrea Bond, Lee Rotondo, and Donald R. Coustan

INSTRUMENT DESCRIPTION, ADMINISTRATION, AND SCORING GUIDELINES

For the person with diabetes to provide self-care on a day-to-day basis, an adequate understanding of the disease and the daily requirements for managing it are necessary but not sufficient. One high-risk group, pregnant women with diabetes, has been overlooked in the development of instruments to measure knowledge of diabetes and its management. Yet pregnant women are frequently open to learning because they are motivated to protect not only their own health but that of their babies. These measures have been developed to assess the baseline knowledge of the pregnant woman with diabetes or to assess the outcome of an educational intervention (Spirito, Ruggiero, Bond, Rotondo, & Coustan, 1990).

There are three versions of the Diabetes in Pregnancy Knowledge Screen (DPKS): one for women who have diabetes before becoming pregnant (overt diabetes [OD]), a second for women who develop gestational diabetes during their pregnancy and are diet controlled (GD), and a third for women who develop gestational diabetes and are placed on insulin plus diet (GDI). Eight items are common among all three forms, and varied items are common among two of the tests. Readability is 9th to 10th grade for the GD form and 7th to 8th for the OD form.

Many items have several applicable answers. They are scored 0 (incorrect), 1 (partially correct), or 2 (completely correct). Because of variation in number of items across different versions of the DPKS, scores are reported as percentage of items correct for each of the forms (Spirito et al., 1990).

PSYCHOMETRIC PROPERTIES

Participants in the study were 58 women with OD and 67 with GD, recruited from the Diabetes in Pregnancy Program at the Women and Infants Hospital of Rhode Island. Twelve to 16% of the groups were minorities. Items were developed by psychologists, nurse educators, and an obstetrician, to cover the specific teaching tasks recommended for diabetes educators working with pregnant women. These tasks include diet; blood glucose testing; insulin administration; and reactions, exercise, and sick day management. The items were revised several times on the basis of pilot testing (Spirito et al., 1990).

Internal consistency correlation coefficients ranged from .62 to .78 (Cronbach's α) and test-retest reliability from .75 to .80. All individual item-total scores exceeded correlation coefficient .2.

Woman with OD had higher mean scores on the eight items they had in common (mean = 80.2) than did women with GD (mean = 59.3) at the baseline assessment. Those who had been diagnosed longer obtained higher scores (mean = 78) than did those who had been diagnosed a shorter time (mean = 70.7). This finding provided evidence of discriminant validity because the former group had been coping with diabetes for some time. There was not a significant difference in mean scores between women who had GDI (62.8) and those with GD (55.5), even though previous research has shown the former group had more diabetes knowledge. There was partial support for the hypothesis that scores would improve at retesting because of the informal education gained by taking part in the clinic program, although the improvement could be due to practice effects of repeated testing (Spirito et al., 1990).

A subsequent study (Spirito et al., 1993) included 27 women with OD and 45 with GD, with 85% White and 85% married, from the same Rhode Island Hospital program. It found a positive though modest relationship of scores on the DPKS and self-reported measures of dietary compliance and management of insulin reactions, congruent with other studies.

CRITIQUE AND SUMMARY

It is worth noting that the average woman with GD got about 50% of the items on the DPKS correct, suggesting rudimentary knowledge of diabetes. Although refinement of item wording and scale content is to continue, its authors believe that the DPKS provides a way to pinpoint a patient's specific educational deficits quickly. Authors made a conscious decision to keep the scale brief even though this likely limits its internal consistency reliability (Spirito et al., 1990).

More specific description and justification of the knowledge domains for which items were written and selected would be helpful, as would inclusion of patient judgments about important content. Investigation of DPKS's sensitivity to a program of instruction is necessary, preferably in a study with a control group.

REFERENCES

Spirito, A., Ruggiero, L., Bond, A., Rotondo, L., & Coustan, D. R. (1990). Screening measure to assess knowledge of diabetes in pregnancy. *Diabetes Care, 13,* 712–718.

Spirito, A., Ruggiero, L., Duckworth, M., Low, K. G., Coustan, D. R., McGarvey, S. T., & Khoury, M. R. (1993). The relationship of diabetes knowledge to regimen compliance and metabolic control during pregnancy. *Psychology and Health, 8,* 345–354.

DIABETES IN PREGNANCY KNOWLEDGE SCREEN
FOR OVERT DIABETES

Instructions: Below are questions about diabetes during pregnancy. Answering these questions will help us determine your current knowledge about diabetes during pregnancy and enable us to provide the best care possible during your pregnancy. Many questions have more than one answer; therefore, circle "I don't know" rather than guessing. By answering to the best of your knowledge, we will be able to counsel you most effectively about diabetes during your pregnancy.

1. Which of the following feelings may result from a reaction? (Circle all that might happen, not just those that have happened to you)

   (A). Difficulty thinking
   (B). Blurred vision
   (C). Nervousness or shaky
   (D). Numbness
   (E). Sweating
   F. I don't know   2, 1, 0

2. What should you do if you have a reaction? (Circle all that apply)

   A. Walk it off
   (B). Sit down and rest
   (C). Eat crackers or cheese
   (D). Drink milk
   E. I don't know   2, 1, 0

3. Glycosylated hemoglobin levels are drawn about once per month during pregnancy. Why are these levels taken?

   (A). They measure previous blood sugar control
   B. They measure the amount of iron in your blood
   C. They measure how helpful your diet is in controlling your blood sugar
   D. I don't know   .   1, 0

4. When planning vigorous exercise (e.g., swimming, playing tennis), what changes should you make in your daily diabetes routine? (Circle all that apply)

   (A). Decrease insulin
   (B). Carefully time when to do your exercising
   (C). Increase amount of carbohydrates (e.g., bread, fruits) you eat
   (D). Increase the amount of protein (e.g., meat, cheese) you eat
   E. I don't know   2, 1, 0

5. On days when you are sick, what steps should you take to control your diabetes?

   (A). Increase the amount of water or other fluids
   B. Stop your insulin
   (C). Call your doctor (primary answer)
   D. I don't know   2, 1, 0
   If answer C or A & C = 2 points.
   If answer A = 1 point.

6. The normal range for blood sugar during pregnancy is:

    A.   40–150 mg/dl
    (B). 60–120 mg/dl
    C.   100–200 mg/dl
    D.   I don't know   1, 0

7. A specific meal plan has been devised for you by the dietitian. Which of the following statements about your meal plan are *correct*? (Circle all that apply)

    (A). You should eat everything on your meal plan
    B.   You can reduce the amount of food you eat if you're not hungry
    (C). You should control the amount of food you eat all the time
    D.   You can eat your meals any time during the day as long as you eat everything on your plan
    E.   I don't know   2, 1, 0

8. Bedtime snacks are an important part of your meal plan because they help you avoid having reactions overnight. (Circle one)

    True or False   1, 0

9. Margarine is mainly:

    A.   Protein
    B.   Carbohydrate
    (C). Fat
    D.   Mineral and vitamin
    E.   I don't know   1, 0

10. Rice is mainly:

    A.   Protein
    (B). Carbohydrate
    C.   Fat
    D.   Mineral and vitamin
    E.   I don't know   1, 0

11. If you don't feel like having the egg on your diet for breakfast, you can: (Circle two)

    A.   Have extra toast
    (B). Substitute one small chop
    (C). Have an ounce of cheese instead
    D.   Skip the egg, and don't eat anything else
    E.   I don't know   2, 1, 0

12. If you have problems controlling your blood sugar during pregnancy, what are some of the possible effects on your baby after birth? (Circle all that apply)

    (A). Could be born with low blood sugar (hypoglycemia)
    (B). Could be a large baby, making delivery more difficult
    (C). Could have breathing problems after birth
    D.   I don't know   2, 1, 0

13.   What does glucagon do?

      Ⓐ.   It helps the liver release more sugar into the blood.
      B.   It makes the liver stop releasing sugar into the blood.
      C.   It helps the pancreas release more insulin
      D.   It stops the pancreas from releasing insulin
      E.   I don't know   1, 0

14.   After using glucagon, it's most important to:

      A.   Drink plenty of fluids
      B.   Get plenty of rest
      Ⓒ.   Eat a meal so your blood sugar doesn't drop
      D.   None of the above
      E.   I don't know   1, 0

Scoring instructions. 2 = totally correct; 1 = partially correct; 0 = wrong, don't know.
Total possible score = 21 points for form for women with overt diabetes.

FOR GESTATIONAL DIABETES

Diabetes in Pregnancy Knowledge Test

Instructions: Below are a number of questions about diabetes during pregnancy. Answering these questions will help us determine your current knowledge about diabetes during pregnancy and enable us to provide the best care possible during your pregnancy. Please note that a number of questions have more than one answer and you should circle all correct answers. If you do not know the answer to a question, please circle "I don't know" rather than guessing. By answering to the best of your knowledge, we will be able to counsel you most effectively about diabetes during your pregnancy.

1. Blood sugar is tested during clinic visits in order to: (Circle all that apply)

    A.   Make sure your diet is working well
    B.   To see if you need another glucose tolerance test
    C.   To see if you need insulin to control your blood sugar
    D.   To see if you are gaining too much weight
    E.   I don't know   2, 1, 0

2. Gestational diabetes can be a risk factor for developing diabetes later on. After your delivery you should: (Circle all that apply)

    A.   Have regular tests for diabetes
    B.   Keep on your gestational diabetic diet
    C.   Check your blood sugar at home
    D.   Avoid being overweight
    E.   I don't know   2, 1, 0

3. If you become pregnant in the future, it's *not* likely you will develop gestational diabetes during that pregnancy. (Circle one)

    True or False   1, 0

4. When planning vigorous exercise (e.g., swimming, playing tennis, etc.), what changes should you make in your daily diabetes routine? (Circle all that apply)

    A.   Decrease amount of water or other fluids
    B.   Carefully time when to do your exercising
    C.   Increase amount of carbohydrates (e.g., bread, fruits) you eat
    D.   Increase amount of protein (e.g., meat, cheese) you eat
    E.   I don't know   2, 1, 0

5.   On days when you are sick, what steps should you take to control your diabetes?

    Ⓐ.   Increase amount of water or other fluids you drink
    B.   Increase amount of fruit you eat
    Ⓒ.   Call your doctor
    D.   I don't know   2, 1, 0
    If answer C or A & C = 2 points.
    If answer A = 1 point.

6.   The normal range for blood glucose during pregnancy is:

    A.   40–150 mgm/DL
    Ⓑ.   60–120 mgm/DL
    C.   100–200 mgm/DL
    D.   I don't know   0, 1

7.   A specific meal plan has been devised for you by the dietitian. Which of the following statements about your meal plan are *correct*? (Circle all that apply)

    Ⓐ.   You should eat everything on your meal plan
    B.   You can reduce the amount of food you eat if you're not hungry
    Ⓒ.   You should control the amount of food you eat all the time
    D.   You can eat your meals any time during the day as long as you eat everything on your plan
    E.   I don't know   2, 1, 0

8.   Margarine is mainly:

    A.   Protein
    B.   Carbohydrate
    Ⓒ.   Fat
    D.   Mineral and vitamin
    E.   I don't know   1, 0

9.   Rice is mainly:

    A.   Protein
    Ⓑ.   Carbohydrate
    C.   Fat
    D.   Mineral and vitamin
    E.   I don't know   1, 0

10.   If you don't feel like having the egg on your diet for breakfast, you can: (Circle two)

    A.   Have extra toast
    Ⓑ.   Substitute one small chop
    Ⓒ.   Have an ounce of cheese instead
    D.   Skip the egg, and don't eat anything else
    E.   I don't know   1, 0

11. If you have problems controlling your blood sugar during pregnancy, what are some of the possible effects on your baby after birth? (Circle all that apply)

   Ⓐ. Could be born with low blood sugar (hypoglycemia)
   Ⓑ. Could be a large baby, making delivery more difficult
   Ⓒ. Could have breathing problems after birth
   D. I don't know   2, 1, 0

12. Another name for gestational diabetes is: (Circle all that apply)

   Ⓐ. Pregnancy-related diabetes
   Ⓑ. Glucose intolerance during pregnancy
   C. Insulin-dependent diabetes during pregnancy
   D. Type I diabetes during pregnancy
   E. I don't know   2, 1, 0

13. Why does gestational diabetes occur in some pregnant women?

   A. Too much sugar in the diet early in pregnancy
   B. The baby's insulin doesn't work well enough
   Ⓒ. The pregnant woman's natural insulin from the pancreas doesn't work as well as usual
   D. I don't know   1, 0

14. The majority of women with gestational diabetes have blood sugar problems one month after the birth of their child. (Circle one)

   True or (False)   1, 0

Scoring instructions. 2 = totally correct; 1 = partially correct; 0 = wrong, don't know.
Total possible score for persons with gestational diabetes = 22.

FOR GESTATIONAL DIABETICS ON INSULIN

Diabetes in Pregnancy Knowledge Test

Instructions: Below are a number of questions about diabetes during pregnancy. Answering these questions will help us determine your current knowledge about diabetes during pregnancy and enable us to provide the best care possible during your pregnancy. Please note that a number of questions have more than one answer and you should circle all correct answers. If you do not know the answer to a question, please circle "I don't know" rather than guessing. By answering to the best of your knowledge, we will be able to counsel you most effectively about diabetes during your pregnancy.

1. Blood sugar is tested during clinic visits in order to: (Circle all that apply)

    (A). Make sure your diet is working well
    B.   To see if you need another glucose tolerance test
    (C). To see if you need insulin to control your blood sugar
    D.   To see if you are gaining too much weight
    E.   I don't know   2, 1, 0

2. Gestational diabetes can be a risk factor for developing diabetes later on. After your delivery you should: (Circle all that apply)

    (A). Have regular tests for diabetes
    B.   Keep on your gestational diabetic diet
    C.   Check your blood sugar at home
    (D). Avoid being overweight
    E.   I don't know   2, 1, 0

3. If you become pregnant in the future, it's *not* likely you will develop gestational diabetes during that pregnancy. (Circle one)

    True or (False)   1, 0

4. When planning vigorous exercise (e.g., swimming, playing tennis, etc.), what changes should you make in your daily diabetes routine? (Circle all that apply)

    A.   Decrease amount of water or other fluids
    (B). Carefully time when to do your exercising
    (C). Increase amount of carbohydrates (e.g., bread, fruits) you eat
    (D). Increase amount of protein (e.g., meat, cheese) you eat
    E.   I don't know   2, 1, 0

5. On days when you are sick, what steps should you take to control your diabetes?

    Ⓐ.   Increase amount of water or other fluids you drink
    B.   Increase amount of fruit you eat
    Ⓒ.   Call your doctor
    D.   I don't know   2, 1, 0
    If answer C or A & C = 2 points.
    If answer A = 1 point.

6. The normal range for blood glucose during pregnancy is:

    A.   40–150 mgm/DL
    Ⓑ.   60–120 mgm/DL
    C.   100–200 mgm/DL
    D.   I don't know   0, 1

7. A specific meal plan has been devised for you by the dietitian. Which of the following statements about your meal plan are *correct*? (Circle all that apply)

    Ⓐ.   You should eat everything on your meal plan
    B.   You can reduce the amount of food you eat if you're not hungry
    Ⓒ.   You should control the amount of food you eat all the time
    D.   You can eat your meals any time during the day as long as you eat everything on your plan
    E.   I don't know   2, 1, 0

8. Margarine is mainly:

    A.   Protein
    B.   Carbohydrate
    Ⓒ.   Fat
    D.   Mineral and vitamin
    E.   I don't know   1, 0

9. Rice is mainly:

    A.   Protein
    Ⓑ.   Carbohydrate
    C.   Fat
    D.   Mineral and vitamin
    E.   I don't know   1, 0

10. If you don't feel like having the egg on your diet for breakfast, you can: (Circle two)

    A.   Have extra toast
    Ⓑ.   Substitute one small chop
    Ⓒ.   Have an ounce of cheese instead
    D.   Skip the egg, and don't eat anything else
    E.   I don't know   1, 0

11. If you have problems controlling your blood sugar during pregnancy, what are some of the possible effects on your baby after birth? (Circle all that apply)

    Ⓐ.   Could be born with low blood sugar (hypoglycemia)
    Ⓑ.   Could be a large baby, making delivery more difficult

Ⓒ.   Could have breathing problems after birth
D.   I don't know   2, 1, 0

12.   Another name for gestational diabetes is: (Circle all that apply)

Ⓐ.   Pregnancy-related diabetes
Ⓑ.   Glucose intolerance during pregnancy
C.   Insulin-dependent diabetes during pregnancy
D.   Type I diabetes during pregnancy
E.   I don't know   2, 1, 0

13.   Why does gestational diabetes occur in some pregnant women?

A.   Too much sugar in the diet early in pregnancy
B.   The baby's insulin doesn't work well enough
Ⓒ.   The pregnant woman's natural insulin from the pancreas doesn't work as well as usual
D.   I don't know   1, 0

14.   The majority of women with gestational diabetes have blood sugar problems one month after the birth of their child. (Circle one)

True or Ⓕalse   1, 0

15.   Which of the following feelings may result from a reaction? (Circle all that might happen, not just those that have happened to you)

Ⓐ.   Difficulty thinking
Ⓑ.   Blurred vision
Ⓒ.   Nervousness or shaky
Ⓓ.   Numbness
Ⓔ.   Sweating
F.   I don't know   2, 1, 0

16.   What should you do if you have a reaction? (Circle all that apply)

A.   Walk it off
Ⓑ.   Sit down and rest
Ⓒ.   Eat crackers or cheese
Ⓓ.   Drink milk
E.   I don't know   2, 1, 0

17.   Bedtime snacks are an important part of your meal plan because they help you avoid having reactions overnight. (Circle one)

Ⓣrue or False   1, 0

18.   You should decrease your insulin before vigorous exercise. (Circle one)

Ⓣrue or False   1, 0

Questions 15 to 18 are for women with gestational diabetes on insulin.
Scoring instructions. 2 = totally correct; 1 = partially correct; 0 = wrong, or don't know.
Total possible score = 28 points for questions 1 to 18 for women with gestational diabetes on insulin.

27

Knowledge of Maternal Phenylketonuria Test

Developed by Shoshana Shiloh, Paula St. James, and Susan Waisbren

INSTRUMENT DESCRIPTION, ADMINISTRATION, AND SCORING GUIDELINES

Routine newborn screening for phenylketonuria (PKU), which identifies affected infants early enough for dietary treatment to be effective, has essentially eliminated mental retardation as a consequence of PKU in developed parts of the world. Many early treated girls with PKU are now reaching childbearing age. These women are at high risk for bearing children who have mental retardation microcephaly, congenital heart disease, and low birthweight as a consequence of the maternal disorder, which can occur regardless of whether the child does or does not have PKU. Dietary treatment during pregnancy offers at least partial protection to the developing fetus if initiated before conception. Because most young women with PKU returned to a normal diet during middle childhood, prevention of the effects of maternal PKU requires reinstitution of the difficult low-phenylalanine diet, along with careful planning of pregnancies so that the diet begins before conception (Shiloh, St. James, & Waisbren, 1990). The results of some tracking efforts indicate that women with PKU usually seek treatment after they are pregnant rather than before (Waisbren, Shiloh, St. James, & Levy, 1991).

Educational and counseling programs aimed at this problem have been conducted at several centers including Children's Hospital in Boston. In this program, group meetings include a review of PKU and definition of the maternal PKU syndrome and risk figures, and planning about reproductive health care. The Knowledge of Maternal PKU instrument was developed to assess patients' knowledge and identify misconceptions, and to evaluate and compare educational programs. One point for each correct score is summed for a total score, with a potential range of 0 to 10. The test is written at less than a 6th-grade reading level and can usually be completed in 5 minutes. Knowledge is reasonably presumed to be necessary but insufficient for the implicit goal of adherence to the regimen described previously (Shiloh, St. James, & Waisbren, 1990).

PSYCHOMETRIC PROPERTIES

Development and initial testing of the instrument was accomplished with 49 young hyperphenyla-lanimemic female patients in New England, with a mean education of 12 years. The test was developed to cover content areas of risk of maternal PKU, pregnancy planning, and dietary treatment. Initial questions from an earlier version that were answered correctly by all who took the test were excluded, and unclear questions were rephrased. Cronbach's α was .62, affected by the length of test, which restricts the validity upper limit. As evidence of validity, the authors show a moderate but statistically significant (.40) correlation with IQ scores. In addition, scores on the instrument were significantly different between patients who participated in educational sessions and those who did not. Mean test score was 7.1, with a standard deviation of 2.11. Scores for individual items may be found in Shiloh et al. (1990).

Other studies that have compared behaviors of young women with PKU, those with diabetes (who also have childbearing risks and needs for medical intervention prior and during pregnancy) and a comparison group, showed that knowledge of maternal PKU was not significantly related to frequency of contraceptive use (Waisbren et al., 1991; Waisbren, Hamilton, St. James, Shiloh, & Levy, 1995). A comparison study with Israeli women with PKU found that although the American group was more knowledgeable about both contraception and maternal PKU, it also had more unplanned pregnancies (Shiloh, Waisbren, Cohen, St. James, & Levy, 1993).

CRITIQUE AND SUMMARY

The Knowledge of Maternal PKU Test is one of a battery of tests being used to study this clinical problem including tests of knowledge about family planning; social support for family planning; and attitudes and beliefs about contraception, sex, and childbearing (Waisbren et al., 1991). From a theoretical viewpoint, it is unlikely that a test of this kind will by itself show a strong relationship to contraceptive use. Intervention programs aimed at conscious reproductive planning would likely be peer oriented and include social support in facing issues of sexuality and contraception (Waisbren et al., 1995). More explicit domain validation would be helpful to establish that the domains and items contained in the test represent those most likely to be important to what should be an explicit goal of informed patient decision making. This goal is more justifiable than is compliance with a medical regimen.

REFERENCES

Shiloh, S., St. James, P., & Waisbren, S. (1990). The development of a patient knowledge test on maternal phenylketonuria. *Patient Education and Counseling, 16,* 139–146.

Shiloh, S., Waisbren, S. E., Cohen, B. E., St. James, P., & Levy, H. L. (1993). Cross-cultural perspectives on coping with the risks of maternal phenylketonuria. *Psychology and Health, 8,* 435–446.

Waisbren, S. E., Hamilton, B. D., St. James, P. J., Shiloh, S., & Levy, H. L. (1995). Psychosocial factors in maternal phenylketonuria: Women's adherence to medical recommendations. *American Journal of Public Health, 85,* 1636—1641.

Waisbren, S. E., Shiloh, S., St. James, P., & Levy, H. L. (1991). Psychosocial factors in maternal phenylketonuria: Prevention of unplanned pregnancies. *American Journal of Public Health, 81,* 299–304.

KNOWLEDGE OF MATERNAL PKU (R)

Please circle the best answer.

1.   PKU is _____.

    A.   a blood disease
    Ⓑ.   an enzyme deficiency
    C.   a kidney disorder
    D.   a protein deficiency
    E.   an iron deficiency

2.   Mental retardation in babies born to mothers with PKU is most likely caused by _____.

    A.   an enzyme deficiency in the baby
    B.   PKU in the baby
    Ⓒ.   high blood phenylalanine in the mother during pregnancy
    D.   the father carrying a gene for PKU
    E.   too little protein in the mother's diet during pregnancy

3.   The best known treatment for maternal PKU to prevent damage to the baby is _____.

    A.   following a well-balanced diet
    B.   following a vegetarian diet
    C.   following a high-protein diet during pregnancy
    D.   following a low-phenylalanine diet after a positive pregnancy test
    Ⓔ.   following a low-phenylalanine diet before conception and throughout pregnancy

4.   In addition to mental retardation, other problems that have been seen in babies born to mothers with PKU include _____.

    A.   low birth weight
    B.   heart problems
    C.   small head size
    Ⓓ.   all of the above
    E.   none of the above

5.   Twenty mg/dl is considered a high blood phenylalanine level. On a low phenylalanine diet during pregnancy, blood phenylalanine levels should be controlled to what level?

    A.   less than 1 mg/dl
    Ⓑ.   2–6 mg/dl
    C.   6–8 mg/dl
    D.   10–15 mg/dl
    E.   16–20 mg/dl

6.   Which of the following snacks has the least amount of phenylalanine?

    A.   chocolate chip cookies
    Ⓑ.   apple
    C.   hamburger

D.   potato chips
E.   bagel with jelly

7.   Children born to mothers with PKU _____.

A.   never have PKU
B.   have a 1 in 1,000 chance of having PKU
C.   have a 1 in 100 chance of having PKU if the father carries the gene for PKU
Ⓓ.   have a 50–50 chance of having PKU if the father carries the gene for PKU
E.   will always have PKU

8.   The problems that have been seen in babies born from untreated pregnancies in mothers with PKU _____.

A.   are entirely reversible
B.   can all be corrected with surgery
C.   can be corrected by treating the baby with a low phenylalanine diet
Ⓓ.   generally result in the child having mental retardation, learning difficulties, birth defects, and the need for special services
E.   go away as the child grows older

9.   After a child is born to a mother with PKU it is important _____.
A.   to place the child on a high-protein diet
Ⓑ.   to perform newborn screening for PKU with special care and consideration so that if the child has PKU, he or she can begin dietary treatment
C.   to hold off on newborn screening for PKU for a month since the baby has had enough stress
D.   for the mother to be on a high-protein diet
E.   to immediately place the child on a low-protein diet

10.   The best advice to give a young woman with PKU who thinks she might be pregnant is to _____.

A.   wait and see if it's true
B.   wait but stop eating meat in the meantime
C.   wait but start birth control
Ⓓ.   immediately contact the PKU Clinic for guidance
E.   contact her friends for guidance

The score is the total number of correct responses (circled). Range of scores is 0 to 10.

Reprinted from Shiloh, S., St. James, P., & Waisbren, W. *The Development of a Patient Knowledge Test on Maternal Phenylketonuria,* Volume 16, 1990, pp. 139–146. With kind permission to reproduce Appendix I: Knowledge of Maternal PKU® from Elsevier Science Ireland Ltd, Bay 15K, Shannon Industrial Estate, Co. Clare, Ireland.

28

Parent Expectations Survey

Developed by Susan McClennan Reece

INSTRUMENT DESCRIPTION, ADMINISTRATION, AND SCORING GUIDELINES

Reece (1992) describes preliminary development of the Parent Expectations Survey (PES) to measure self-efficacy in early parenting. Self-efficacy (SE) in parenting is defined as the confidence a new mother has in her ability to meet the demands and responsibilities of parenthood. For the new mother, perceptions of SE in parenting stem from her own past experiences in caring for infants; her observations of other new mothers viewed as similar to herself; encouragement from others; and environmental feedback, such as that received from the baby or family. With these sources of information, the mother develops her own judgments as to whether she is capable of carrying out a certain level of performance in the care of her infant. Clinical usefulness of the PES is believed to be in identification of those women at risk for increased stress in the role of new parent because of a low level of SE (Reece, 1992).

The PES takes about 10 minutes to complete and is scored by summing individual items and dividing by the total number of items (20) to determine the mean PES score (Reece, 1992).

PSYCHOMETRIC PROPERTIES

Items were generated from the literature and clinical experience of the author and colleagues. Seven nurse and other experts in the field of SE and instrument development judged content validity. Appropriateness of the items for measuring tasks of mothering were validated by requesting feedback on the scale from four pediatric/family nurse practitioners.

The PES was then completed by 82 first-time mothers between the ages of 35 and 42 years. Most were college educated and had attended graduate school and were recruited from childbirth education programs; 45% had a cesarean section (Reece, 1992). PES scores at 1 and 3 months postpartum showed moderate correlations with the Self-Evaluation subscale of the "What Being the Parent of a Baby is Like" questionnaire (.40 to .75). Self-efficacy at 1 month ($r = .28$) and at 3 months ($r = .40$) postpartum was associated with greater maternal confidence in parenting 1 year after delivery. PES scores at 3 months postpartum had a negative association ($r = -.28$)

with perceived stress at 1 year. These results imply that women with higher self-efficacy early in the transition to parenthood have increased confidence in parenting and less stress 1 year after delivery. All of these results are supportive of validity.

The α coefficient for the PES administered at 1 month postpartum was .91 and at 3 months .86. Because of the theoretical expectation that self-efficacy in parenting would change over time, test-retest reliability was not calculated (Reece, 1992). Scores on the PES from as yet unpublished research were: mean = 7.83 and SD = 1.08 for mothers in the last trimester; mean = 7.63 and SD = .97 for fathers in the last trimester; mean = 8.77 and SD = .71 for mothers 4 months after delivery; and mean = 8.06 and SD = 1.01 for fathers 4 months after delivery (S. M. Reece, personal communication, 1996).

CRITIQUE AND SUMMARY

The PES is in preliminary stages of development and has been tested with only a group of mothers with a limited range of demographic characteristics. Correspondence with the author indicates that the PES is undergoing active revision to include interactive behaviors of the parent and infant, and affective tasks of early parenthood. PES might be used by clinicians during the perinatal period to ascertain a mother's early perceptions of self-efficacy in parenting. For those found to be low, a number of self-efficacy developing interventions could reasonably be expected to be effective including use of parenting support groups, verbal persuasion, and others (Reece, 1992). Content validity for the PES might be checked with parents as well as with practitioners. Additional studies of validity will be necessary.

REFERENCE

Reece, S. M. (1992). The Parent Expectations Survey. *Clinical Nursing Research, 1,* 336–346.

PRENATAL PARENTAL EXPECTATIONS SURVEY

The following statements describe what some parents-to-be believe about their abilities to take care of their infants. After reading each statement, please circle which number that *you* feel most closely describes how you feel about *yourself* in relation to parenting. Because these are statements about beliefs, there are no right or wrong answers. Please answer each of the 25 questions below.

1. I will be able to manage the feeding of my baby.

Cannot Do				Moderately Certain Can Do					Certain Can Do	
0	1	2	3	4	5	6	7	8	9	10

2. I will be able to manage the responsibility of my baby.

Cannot Do				Moderately Certain Can Do					Certain Can Do	
0	1	2	3	4	5	6	7	8	9	10

3. I will always be able to tell when my baby is hungry.

Cannot Do				Moderately Certain Can Do					Certain Can Do	
0	1	2	3	4	5	6	7	8	9	10

4. I will be able to deal effectively with the baby when h/she cries for "no reason."

Cannot Do				Moderately Certain Can Do					Certain Can Do	
0	1	2	3	4	5	6	7	8	9	10

5. I will be able to tell when my baby is sick.

Cannot Do				Moderately Certain Can Do					Certain Can Do	
0	1	2	3	4	5	6	7	8	9	10

6. I will be able to tell when to add different food items to my baby's diet.

Cannot Do				Moderately Certain Can Do					Certain Can Do	
0	1	2	3	4	5	6	7	8	9	10

7. I will be able to manage my household as well as before, meanwhile caring for the baby.

Cannot Do				Moderately Certain Can Do					Certain Can Do	
0	1	2	3	4	5	6	7	8	9	10

8. When I think the baby is sick, I will be able to take his/her temperature accurately.

Cannot Do				Moderately Certain Can Do					Certain Can Do	
0	1	2	3	4	5	6	7	8	9	10

9. I will be able to give my baby a bath without him/her getting cold or upset.

Cannot Do				Moderately Certain Can Do					Certain Can Do	
0	1	2	3	4	5	6	7	8	9	10

10. I will work out my concerns about working or not working once the baby arrives.

Cannot Do   Moderately Certain Can Do   Certain Can Do
0   1   2   3   4   5   6   7   8   9   10

11. I will be able to keep my baby from crying.

Cannot Do   Moderately Certain Can Do   Certain Can Do
0   1   2   3   4   5   6   7   8   9   10

12. I will be able to maintain my relationship with my partner during this next year.

Cannot Do   Moderately Certain Can Do   Certain Can Do
0   1   2   3   4   5   6   7   8   9   10

13. I will be able to meet all the demands placed on me once the baby is here.

Cannot Do   Moderately Certain Can Do   Certain Can Do
0   1   2   3   4   5   6   7   8   9   10

14. I will easily be able to get the baby and myself out for a doctor appointment.

Cannot Do   Moderately Certain Can Do   Certain Can Do
0   1   2   3   4   5   6   7   8   9   10

15. I have good judgment in deciding how to care for the baby.

Cannot Do   Moderately Certain Can Do   Certain Can Do
0   1   2   3   4   5   6   7   8   9   10

16. I can make the right decisions for my baby.

Cannot Do   Moderately Certain Can Do   Certain Can Do
0   1   2   3   4   5   6   7   8   9   10

17. I will be able to get the baby on a good nighttime routine.

Cannot Do   Moderately Certain Can Do   Certain Can Do
0   1   2   3   4   5   6   7   8   9   10

18. I will be able to give the baby the attention h/she needs.

Cannot Do   Moderately Certain Can Do   Certain Can Do
0   1   2   3   4   5   6   7   8   9   10

19. I will be able to hire a babysitter when I need one.

Cannot Do   Moderately Certain Can Do   Certain Can Do
0   1   2   3   4   5   6   7   8   9   10

20. I will be able to tell what my baby likes and dislikes.

Cannot Do   Moderately Certain Can Do   Certain Can Do
0   1   2   3   4   5   6   7   8   9   10

21. I will be able to sense my baby's moods.

Cannot Do   Moderately Certain Can Do   Certain Can Do
0   1   2   3   4   5   6   7   8   9   10

22. I will be able to show my love for my baby.

Cannot Do				Moderately Certain Can Do					Certain Can Do	
0	1	2	3	4	5	6	7	8	9	10

23. I will be able to calm my baby when h/she is upset.

Cannot Do				Moderately Certain Can Do					Certain Can Do	
0	1	2	3	4	5	6	7	8	9	10

24. I will be able to support my baby during stressful times such as at the doctor's office.

Cannot Do				Moderately Certain Can Do					Certain Can Do	
0	1	2	3	4	5	6	7	8	9	10

25. I will be able to stimulate my baby by playing with him/her.

Cannot Do				Moderately Certain Can Do					Certain Can Do	
0	1	2	3	4	5	6	7	8	9	10

POSTPARTUM PARENTAL EXPECTATIONS SURVEY

The following statements describe what some new parents believe about their abilities to take care of their infants. After reading each statement, please circle which number that *you* feel most closely describes how you feel about *yourself* in relation to parenting. Because these are statements about beliefs, there are no right or wrong answers. Please answer each of the 25 questions below.

1. I can manage the feeding of my baby.

Cannot Do   Moderately Certain Can Do   Certain Can Do
0   1   2   3   4   5   6   7   8   9   10

2. I can manage the responsibility of my baby.

Cannot Do   Moderately Certain Can Do   Certain Can Do
0   1   2   3   4   5   6   7   8   9   10

3. I can tell when my baby is hungry.

Cannot Do   Moderately Certain Can Do   Certain Can Do
0   1   2   3   4   5   6   7   8   9   10

4. I can deal effectively with the baby when h/she cries for "no reason."

Cannot Do   Moderately Certain Can Do   Certain Can Do
0   1   2   3   4   5   6   7   8   9   10

5. I can tell when my baby is sick.

Cannot Do   Moderately Certain Can Do   Certain Can Do
0   1   2   3   4   5   6   7   8   9   10

6. I can tell when to add different food items to my baby's diet.

Cannot Do   Moderately Certain Can Do   Certain Can Do
0   1   2   3   4   5   6   7   8   9   10

7. I can manage my household as well as before, meanwhile caring for the baby.

Cannot Do   Moderately Certain Can Do   Certain Can Do
0   1   2   3   4   5   6   7   8   9   10

8. When I think the baby is sick, I can take his/her temperature accurately.

Cannot Do   Moderately Certain Can Do   Certain Can Do
0   1   2   3   4   5   6   7   8   9   10

9. I can give my baby a bath without him/her getting cold or upset.

Cannot Do   Moderately Certain Can Do   Certain Can Do
0   1   2   3   4   5   6   7   8   9   10

10. I can work out my concerns about working or not working once the baby arrives.

Cannot Do				Moderately Certain Can Do					Certain Can Do	
0	1	2	3	4	5	6	7	8	9	10

11. I can keep my baby from crying.

Cannot Do				Moderately Certain Can Do					Certain Can Do	
0	1	2	3	4	5	6	7	8	9	10

12. I can maintain my relationship with my partner during this next year.

Cannot Do				Moderately Certain Can Do					Certain Can Do	
0	1	2	3	4	5	6	7	8	9	10

13. I can meet all the demands placed on me now that the baby is here.

Cannot Do				Moderately Certain Can Do					Certain Can Do	
0	1	2	3	4	5	6	7	8	9	10

14. I can easily get the baby and myself out for a doctor's visit.

Cannot Do				Moderately Certain Can Do					Certain Can Do	
0	1	2	3	4	5	6	7	8	9	10

15. I have good judgment in deciding how to care for the baby.

Cannot Do				Moderately Certain Can Do					Certain Can Do	
0	1	2	3	4	5	6	7	8	9	10

16. I can make the right decisions for my baby.

Cannot Do				Moderately Certain Can Do					Certain Can Do	
0	1	2	3	4	5	6	7	8	9	10

17. I can get the baby on a good nighttime routine.

Cannot Do				Moderately Certain Can Do					Certain Can Do	
0	1	2	3	4	5	6	7	8	9	10

18. I can give the baby the attention h/she needs.

Cannot Do				Moderately Certain Can Do					Certain Can Do	
0	1	2	3	4	5	6	7	8	9	10

19. I can hire a babysitter when I need one.

Cannot Do				Moderately Certain Can Do					Certain Can Do	
0	1	2	3	4	5	6	7	8	9	10

20. I can tell what my baby likes and dislikes.

Cannot Do				Moderately Certain Can Do					Certain Can Do	
0	1	2	3	4	5	6	7	8	9	10

21. I can sense my baby's moods.

Cannot Do				Moderately Certain Can Do					Certain Can Do	
0	1	2	3	4	5	6	7	8	9	10

22. I can show my love for my baby.

Cannot Do   Moderately Certain Can Do   Certain Can Do
0   1   2   3   4   5   6   7   8   9   10

23. I can calm my baby when h/she is upset.

Cannot Do   Moderately Certain Can Do   Certain Can Do
0   1   2   3   4   5   6   7   8   9   10

24. I can support my baby during stressful times such as at the doctor's office.

Cannot Do   Moderately Certain Can Do   Certain Can Do
0   1   2   3   4   5   6   7   8   9   10

25. I can stimulate my baby by playing with him/her.

Cannot Do   Moderately Certain Can Do   Certain Can Do
0   1   2   3   4   5   6   7   8   9   10

From Reece, M. (1992). The Parent Expectations Survey. *Clinical Nursing Research, 1,* 336–346. Copyright, Sage Publications. Reprinted by permission.

29

Infant Care Survey

Developed by Robin D. Froman and Steven V. Owen

INSTRUMENT DESCRIPTION, ADMINISTRATION, AND SCORING GUIDELINES

The Infant Care Survey (ICS) was developed to assess mothers' self-efficacy in caring for babies under 1 year of age. Social learning theory forms the framework for this work, with self-efficacy defined as a person's belief that he can successfully accomplish some particular behavior. A new mother may understand a behavior, but not attempt it because she has little confidence in her ability or expects failure. Responses on the ICS from A (very little confidence = 1) to E (quite a lot of confidence = 5) are summed into an average total score, with ranges from 1 to 5 (Froman & Owen, 1989).

PSYCHOMETRIC PROPERTIES

An initial pool of 48 statements that represent usual and important infant care behaviors was written and reviewed by nursing faculty members, visiting nurses, and hospital-based maternity nurses to assess relevance of each task to infant care, adequacy of domain sampling, and readability of the items. Items were grouped into those requiring knowledge or skill to foster feelings of efficacy and partitioned into content subgroups of health, diet, and safety behaviors. Data were collected in hospital regular and high-risk obstetrical units, home visits to new mothers, clinical nursing sites, and college classrooms among White, Hispanic, and Black groups, to provide response variation ($N = 142$) (Froman & Owen, 1989).

α internal consistency estimate for the total scale was .98, and for the subgroups of knowledge and skill items .94 and .96, respectively. Factor analysis showed a single major construct: infant care self-efficacy with modest empirical support for the groupings of items into logical subdomains. Construct validity was supported by findings that would be predicted by self-efficacy theory—behaviors commonly performed successfully or observed showed the highest means, such as holding a baby (average score = 4.46), changing diapers (average score = 4.40), and those behaviors difficult to master the lowest, such as relieving gas pains (average score = 2.82) or treating diarrhea (average score = 2.92). The fact that being female, and age and number of children was predictive of ICS scores also is congruent with self-efficacy theory because these groups have more opportunity to perform infant care successfully (Froman & Owen, 1989).

A second study of a convenience sample of 200 new mothers and the nurses caring for them addressed not only variables related to mothers' sense of infant care self-efficacy as indicated by scores on the ICS but also differences between the mothers' reports and nurses' ratings of mothers' skill at those tasks. Factor analysis and measure of internal consistency were consistent with the first study as was the relationship with number of children and age. Other more specific relationships between demographic variables and self-efficacy for various parenting tasks measured in the ICS may be found in Froman and Owen (1990).

Trends between health of the child and self-efficacy ratings suggested that mothers of special care neonates do not share the same sense of confidence for infant care activities that mothers of healthy infants enjoy. The implication of this finding is that extra time and special effort should be spent to build these mothers' self-confidence even beyond demonstration of adequate skill in the care of these infants. In this sample, there is little evidence that nurses' estimates of mothers' proficiency explain perceptions beyond established demographic factors. This means that nurses should not base decisions about how much teaching mothers need on demonstrated skill alone (Froman & Owen, 1990).

CRITIQUE AND SUMMARY

ICS incorporates both knowledge and confidence in the ability to perform a task, both of which are necessary for real-world performance. Teaching should focus on including the multiple ways in which self-efficacy can be developed (actual successful experience, modeling, and persuasion). Because providing such potent learning experiences may require special effort in most health care settings, the ICS can be used to evaluate how well current teaching efforts are doing to yield high self-efficacy.

The predictive worth of ICS needs to be documented (Froman & Owen, 1989), and further study is needed to show whether specific efficacy-building attempts by nurses are associated with changes in maternal self-beliefs (Froman & Owen, 1990). In response to the first study, Barnard (1989) suggests addition of a new domain called Communication Skills: talking to your baby, expressing love and affection, sensing the baby's moods, helping the baby modulate state, communicating security to the baby, recognizing distress cues, and responding contingently to the baby—an important part of social and emotional infant care. She also notes that future samples should include parents of preterm infants, adolescent mothers, and adoptive parents. The second study does address health of the infant.

Although mean self-ratings were found to be high, there was also wide variation in efficacy perceptions among mothers and across tasks. Routine use of the ICS before discharge may help to identify those mothers who seem skilled but suffer from low-efficacy expectations and offer diagnostic advice to help individualize maternity education. It may also be used to assess those at risk and those needing to be drawn into the health care system (Froman & Owen, 1990). The ICS has apparently not been used to study parenting self-efficacy of fathers.

REFERENCES

Barnard, K. (1989). Response to "Infant care self-efficacy." *Scholarly Inquiry for Nursing Practice: An International Journal, 3,* 213–215.

Froman, R. D., & Owen, S. V. (1989). Infant care self-efficacy. *Scholarly Inquiry for Nursing Practice: An International Journal, 3,* 199–211.

Froman, R. D., & Owen, S. V. (1990). Mothers' and nurses' perceptions of infant care skills. *Research in Nursing and Health, 13,* 247–253.

INFANT CARE SURVEY

Directions: Your responses are confidential and will help us to improve our services. There are no right or wrong answers.

How much confidence do you have about doing each of the behaviors listed below?

A   B   C   D   E
very   quite
little   ← —— —— —— —— —— —— —— —— —— —— —— —— →   a lot
                                    CONFIDENCE

Health Knowledge

1. Knowing immunization schedules.
2. Knowing schedule for physical exam.
3. Recognizing signs of an ear infection.
4. Identifying diaper rash.
5. Knowing when to get help from the clinic, emergency room, or doctor.
6. Recognizing teething.
7. Knowing regular breathing sounds of babies.
8. Recognizing congestion.
9. Recognizing an allergic response.
10. Recognizing croup.
11. Knowing expected weight gain patterns for an infant.
12. Recognizing constipation.
13. Recognizing diarrhea.
14. Recognizing gas pains.
15. Knowing normal growth and development patterns.

Diet Knowledge

16. Knowing how much to feed your baby.
17. Selecting the best formula.
18. Selecting baby foods.
19. Planning a balanced diet for your baby.
20. Knowing how to use a baby bottle.

Safety Knowledge

21. Identifying safety hazards in the house.
22. Choosing safe baby toys.
23. Choosing safe baby furniture.
24. Choosing safe baby clothes.
25. Knowing which medications are dangerous.
26. Knowing safe positions for a baby after feeding.
27. Knowing what articles are safe to leave with your baby in the crib or baby seat.

Health Skills

28. Treating diaper rash.
29. Burping your baby.
30. Weighing your baby.
31. Taking your baby's temperature.

A	B	C	D	E
very				quite

← —— —— —— —— —— —— —— —— —— —— →

CONFIDENCE

little   a lot

32. Changing a diaper.
33. Relieving pain from teething.
34. Relieving congestion.
35. Giving your baby a liquid medication.
36. Relieving croup.
37. Treating constipation.
38. Treating diarrhea.
39. Relieving gas pains.
40. Establishing a sensible sleeping schedule.
41. Soothing your crying baby.

Diet Skills

42. Breast or bottle feeding your baby (whichever way your baby is fed).
43. Spoon feeding your baby.
44. Preparing baby food.
45. Introducing new food into baby's diet.
46. Establishing a sensible feeding schedule.

Safety Skills

47. Holding your baby.
48. Demonstrating a tonic neck reflex.
49. Bathing your baby.
50. Using a car seat.
51. Walking while holding your baby.
52. Playing with your baby.

Note: Item 48 was not included in the original scale; it is now being studied as a possible lie item.
Copyright © 1985 by R. D. Froman and S. V. Owen.

From Froman, R. D., & Owen, S. V. (1989). Infant care self-efficacy. *Scholarly Inquiry for Nursing Practice, 3,* 199–215.

30

How I Deal with Problems Regarding Care of My Baby Questionnaire

Developed by Karen F. Pridham and Audrey S. Chang

INSTRUMENT DESCRIPTION, ADMINISTRATION, AND SCORING GUIDELINES

The way in which parents of new infants view their problem-solving competence is clinically important and likely to influence their adaptation to parenting, how stressful they perceive the experience to be, and how they cope with it. Experience in caring for a new infant requires continuing accommodation to the infant's developing biological processes and rhythms, and may affect perceptions of competence (Pridham & Chang, 1991).

This is a self-report instrument assessing parents' sense of their skills in problem-solving phases: scanning (noticing things about the baby that are likely to be important and do so soon enough); formulating (how well figure out what is one or why it is happening); appraising (figuring out whether or not should do something different or take action regarding baby); planning (planning or thinking through how to deal with a concern); implementing solutions (carrying out plans to deal with a concern); and evaluating (thinking through how well have dealt with the concern) (Pridham & Chang, 1991).

Items 1 and 11 to 15 are descriptive and included to provide a context of the parent's problem solving (PPS). Scores for items 2 to 10 are summed. An earlier version of the PPS has separate scales assessing perceived problem-solving competence with feeding and the baby's physical condition (Pridham & Chang, 1991).

PSYCHOMETRIC PROPERTIES

An early study of 49 mothers showed α coefficients of .85 for each of two administrations of the PPS at 30 and 90 days postpartum. Convergent validity was supported by significant correlations between primary care physicians' and nurse practitioners' ratings of mothers' problem-solving skills at 30 days ($r = .52$) and of mothers' and nurses' ratings at 90 days ($r = .34$).Construct validity of the PPS received support from the predicted finding that a mother's assessment of need for her personal action concerning infant care issues influences her perception of her problem-solving competence (Pridham, Chang, & Hansen, 1987). At 2 and 4 months, mean scores for perceived competence ranged from 5.9 to 6.9, with PPS scores increasing as the infants grew older. This may mean that the items were measuring a similar construct, or mothers perceived themselves as being relatively competent in all problem-solving phases (Pridham & Chang, 1991).

CRITIQUE AND SUMMARY

PPS authors believe that early assessment of mothers' perceptions of their competence in processes used in solving infant care issues should help to identify those at risk for parenting difficulties and to specify required clinician support and assess its effectiveness. The tool has primarily been used with well-educated mothers, not with fathers or those with lesser education. All mothers had sufficient resources to use health care services for themselves and their infant regularly. The correspondence between competence in performance and perceived competence in solving infant care issues is not expected to be perfect (Pridham & Chang, 1991).

These authors have also developed a method of examining parent problem-solving skill for child care problems, with particular interest in the quality and quantity of solutions generated. Assistive solutions involve parents' clarifying for their children what is expected of them, supplying reasons for parental action, anticipating with and informing the child what will be encountered and what may be the consequences of the child's behavior, and guiding him or her through a problem-solving process. Coercive solutions have none of these characteristics. Although problem-solving processes can be developed by clinicians, it is not clear how well parental responses to the simulated problems in the instrument correspond with actual problem solving (Pridham, Denney, Pascoe, Chiu, & Creasey, 1995).

REFERENCES

Pridham, K. F., & Chang, A. S. (1991). Mothers' perceptions of problem-solving competence for infant care. *Western Journal of Nursing Research, 13,* 164–180.

Pridham, K. F., Chang, A. S., & Hansen, M. F. (1987). Mothers' problem-solving skill and use of help with infant-related issues: The role of importance and need for action. *Research in Nursing and Health, 10,* 163–175.

Pridham, K., Denney, N., Pasco, J., Chiu, Y-M, & Creasey, D. (1995). Mothers' solutions to childrearing problems: Conditions and processes. *Journal of Marriage and the Family, 57,* 785–799.

HOW I DEAL WITH PROBLEMS REGARDING CARE OF MY BABY

For each question, please indicate how things are for you by circling the number that best describes your need for help.

For example: 1____2____3____④____5____6____7____8____9

1. A. *How things are going* in relation to *care of my new baby.*

    1____2____3____4____5____6____7____8____9
    Not well at all   Very well

   B. *How things are going* in relation to care *of my older child/children.*

    1____2____3____4____5____6____7____8____9
    Not well at all   Very well

    _____ Not applicable.

2. *Skill in solving problems* concerning baby care.

    1____2____3____4____5____6____7____8____9
    Unskilled   Very skilled

3. Extent to which I get involved in *thinking about and dealing with things having to do with baby care.*

    1____2____3____4____5____6____7____8____9
    Not at all   To a great extent

4. My accuracy in *being right about what is going on* in regard to the things about the baby that I notice.

    1____2____3____4____5____6____7____8____9
    Not at all accurate   Very accurate

5. A. Extent to which I *notice things about the baby* that are likely to be important.

    1____2____3____4____5____6____7____8____9
    Never notice things that are important   Always notice things that are important

   B. Extent to which I *notice things about the baby* that are likely to be important *soon enough.*

    1____2____3____4____5____6____7____8____9
    Never notice things   Always notice things
    that are likely to   that are likely to
    be important *soon enough*   be important *soon enough*

6. How well I *figure out what things are like or why something is happening*.

1_____2_____3_____4_____5_____6_____7_____8_____9
Not well at all   Very well

7. How well I *make decisions* as to *whether or not I should do something* regarding the baby or his/her care.

1_____2_____3_____4_____5_____6_____7_____8_____9
Not well at all   Very well

8. *How well* I plan (think through *how to deal with a concern* about baby care).

1_____2_____3_____4_____5_____6_____7_____8_____9
Not well at all   Very well

9. How *successful* I am in *carrying out my plans* to deal with concerns about care of the baby.

1_____2_____3_____4_____5_____6_____7_____8_____9
Unsuccessful   Very successful

10. How well I *think through how I have dealt with a concern* about the baby or his/her care.

1_____2_____3_____4_____5_____6_____7_____8_____9
Not well at all   Very well

11. For problems concerning your baby, how much help with *problem-solving* do you think you need?

1_____2_____3_____4_____5_____6_____7_____8_____9
None at all   A great deal

12. Sometimes there is a change in a baby's condition or behavior. For example, a baby may seem fussier than usual, or may want to eat less. When this kind of change happens for your baby:

    A. How much help do you think you need to figure out what is going on?

1_____2_____3_____4_____5_____6_____7_____8_____9
None at all   A great deal

    B. How much help do you think you need in figuring out what to do?

1_____2_____3_____4_____5_____6_____7_____8_____9
None at all   A great deal

13. On the whole, how troublesome have the problems in caring for your baby been for you?

1_____2_____3_____4_____5_____6_____7_____8_____9
Not at all troublesome   Somewhat troublesome   Greatly troublesome

14. When you need help, how good at getting the needed help are you?

1_____2_____3_____4_____5_____6_____7_____8_____9
Not good at all   Very good

15. When you take everything into consideration—your child, your adult life, etc.—how would you describe your current life situation?

   _____ 1. Things are very bad right now.

   _____ 2. Things are fairly bad right now.

   _____ 3. Things are OK—not bad and not good.

   _____ 4. Things are fairly good.

   _____ 5. Things are very good.

   _____ 6. Other (please explain): _____

Scoring instructions. Sum the scores for items 2 to 10. Items 1 and 11 to 15 are descriptive and included to provide a context of the parent's problem solving.

Copyright © Karen Pridham, University of Wisconsin–Madison.

31

Toddler Care Questionnaire

Developed by Deborah Gross and Lorraine Rocissano

INSTRUMENT DESCRIPTION, ADMINISTRATION, AND SCORING GUIDELINES

The Toddler Care Questionnaire (TCQ) is a measure of maternal confidence specifically for the developmental issues that arise in children between 12 and 36 months of age. Changing behaviors in the developing child require changing behaviors in the parent so that skills learned during the first year of life are not necessarily the most relevant skills for the second year of life. Such a measure is important because maternal confidence has been correlated with indices of maternal and child competence including mothers' self-esteem, mental health, adaptation to parenthood, and perception of infant temperament (Conrad, Gross, Fogg, & Ruchala, 1992). TCQ was designed to be used as a research measure and clinical assessment tool (Gross & Tucker, 1994).

Maternal confidence is defined as a mother's perception that she can effectively manage a variety of tasks or situations related to parenting her toddler. The theoretical framework used to guide this program of research is Bandura's theory of self-efficacy. Knowing what is typical behavior of a 2-year-old is not the same as feeling confident that you can manage your 2-year-old's behavior. The TCQ can be completed in about 5 minutes. Item responses are scored with A to E as 1 to 5; TCQ score is the sum of the items, ranging from 37 to 185, which shows greater maternal confidence. Respondents are also asked to circle those items for which they wish more information, which offers a base for working with mothers. Because completion of the tool requires 5 minutes, it is well suited for use in busy clinical settings (Gross & Rocissano, 1988).

PSYCHOMETRIC PROPERTIES

TCQ was first tested on a convenience sample of 20 and then 50 additional middle-class mothers of toddlers. TCQ has been reviewed for content validity by five experts in the fields of maternal-child nursing, child development, and psychometrics. Each item refers to a specific parenting task or situation that typically arises during toddlerhood; making the item task specific makes the tool consistent with self-efficacy theory. Multiple estimates of α reliability have ranged between .91 and .96. Test-retest reliability over a 4-week interval was .87 (Gross & Rocissano, 1988; Gross, Rocissano, & Roncali, 1989).

Multiple studies of validity have shown a negative correlation between TCQ scores and maternal depression, a negative relationship with dimensions of difficult toddler temperament, a positive relationship with other measures of maternal confidence, extent of prior childcare experience, maternal effectiveness ratings based on observations of structured mother-toddler interactions (Gross, Conrad, Fogg, Willis, & Garvey, 1993) and with maternal knowledge of child development and parenting, as would be predicted by self-efficacy theory. Lack of difference in TCQ scores between mothers of a first- versus second-born child could not be supported by SE theory. The combined effects of maternal knowledge and confidence were related to quality of mother-toddler interactions, congruent with SE theory. Mean TCQ scores in this study were 155.5 (SD = 16.5). The TCQ has not been significantly related to scores on the Marlow-Crowne Social Desirability Scale (Conrad et al., 1992).

A study of 70 mothers of toddlers who had been full term and 62 whose toddlers had been preterm showed no difference in their TCQ scores except if the mother reported the preterm child had cerebral palsy, which would present many novel, unpredictable, and stressful experiences for parents. There may be several possible reasons for the lack of difference between the groups—that these preterms were relatively healthy, the TCQ does not adequately detect the issues of concern to mothers of preterms, or these mothers may have received additional support services. Future research on this question should use multiple measures and methods (Gross, Rocissano, & Roncoli, 1989).

Gross, Conrad, Fogg, and Wothke (1994) studied 126 mothers of 1-year-olds and 126 mothers of 2-year-olds three times during a year. Data analyzed with structural equation modeling supported a model whereby (a) the more depressed the mother feels, the more likely she is to rate her toddler's temperament as difficult; (b) the more difficult the child's temperament is perceived to be, the lower the mother's estimates of her parenting self-efficacy; (c) the lower the mother's self-efficacy, the greater her depression; and (d) the more depressed the mother feels at one point in time, the more likely she is to remain depressed 6 months later. The study by Gross and Tucker (1994) compares factors that appear to influence scores on TCQ for mothers and fathers, and finds them to be different.

Gross, Fogg, and Tucker (1995) found the TCQ to be sensitive to interventions, particularly for those who completed a higher portion of the intervention and in comparison with groups who did not have the intervention. The 10-week intervention program systematically taught parents who judged their 2-year-olds as behaviorally difficult, child management techniques, such as how to play with and help their children learn; how to use praise and rewards effectively; how to set limits effectively; and how to manage misbehavior. Participants practiced problem solving using videotaped vignettes (vicarious learning), home work assignments (mastery experiences), and verbal persuasion and reinforcement in the group.

The training program led to significant increases in maternal SE, decreases in maternal stress, and improvements in the quality of mother-toddler interactions and perceived improvements in child behavior. Fathers participated less in the program. The authors suggest use of the intervention with a group of children more difficult to parent (Gross et al., 1995).

CRITIQUE AND SUMMARY

Although TCQ has been studied with ethnically diverse populations (Gross, Conrad, Fogg, Willis, & Garvey, 1993), all have been middle class and most were married, from an urban health maintenance organization population; in some samples, two thirds were college educated or beyond. The authors suggest additional longitudinal research to explore continuities and discontinuities of maternal confidence across developmental periods, and to examine the consequences for the mother-child relationship (Conrad, Gross, Fogg, & Ruchala, 1992) and experimental research to confirm the validity of the model of the longitudinal relationship found between maternal self-efficacy, depression, and difficult temperament during toddlerhood (Gross et al., 1994).

TCQ has undergone considerable testing. Seven hundred seventy parents have taken the TCQ through the seven studies cited subsequently. Its internal consistency levels are in the range adequate for clinical use as well as for research. Its most obvious use is to focus interventions with mothers who have low levels of confidence in parenting their toddlers.

REFERENCES

Conrad, B., Gross, D., Fogg, L., & Ruchala, P. (1992). Maternal confidence, knowledge, and quality of mother-toddler interactions: A preliminary study. *Infant Mental Health Journal, 13,* 353—361.

Gross, D., Conrad, B., Fogg, L., Willis, L., & Garvey, C. (1993). What does the NCATS measure? *Nursing Research, 42,* 260–265.

Gross, D., Conrad, B., Fogg, L., & Wothke, W. (1994). A longitudinal model of maternal self-efficacy, depression, and difficult temperament during toddlerhood. *Research in Nursing and Health, 17,* 207–215.

Gross, D., Fogg, L., & Tucker, S. (1995). The efficacy of parent training for promoting positive parent-toddler relationships. *Research in Nursing and Health, 18,* 489–499.

Gross, D., & Rocissano, L. (1988). Maternal confidence in toddlerhood: Its measurement for clinical practice and research. *Nurse Practitioner, 13*(3), 19–27.

Gross, D., Rocissano, L., & Roncoli, M. (1989). Maternal confidence during toddlerhood: Comparing preterm and fullterm groups. *Research in Nursing and Health, 12,* 1–9.

Gross, D., & Tucker, S. (1994). Parenting confidence during toddlerhood. *Nurse Practitioner, 19*(10), 25–34.

TODDLER CARE QUESTIONNAIRE

Dear Parents,

Please complete the items below. Your responses on the questionnaire are confidential and will help us to improve our services to parents of young children. Circle the appropriate letter to indicate how much confidence you have with the following:

A	B	C	D	E
Very ←				→ Quite
Little		CONFIDENCE		a Lot

A B C D E   1.   Knowing which toys are appropriate for your child's age.

A B C D E   2.   Knowing how to encourage your child's language development.

A B C D E   3.   Knowing about common fears children have at this time.

A B C D E   4.   Knowing what to do to help your child develop hand coordination (for example, using a spoon, stacking blocks, etc.).

A B C D E   5.   Knowing how to help your child develop body coordination (for example, walking, climbing, etc.).

A B C D E   6.   Knowing how to manage toilet training.

A B C D E   7.   Knowing how feeding patterns change between 12 and 36 months.

A B C D E   8.   Knowing which situations are likely to upset your child.

A B C D E   9.   Knowing how to make your home safe for your child.

A B C D E   10.   Knowing which situations your child is likely to enjoy.

A B C D E   11.   Predicting how your child will respond to new people and places.

A B C D E   12.   Knowing your child's daily sleep schedule.

A B C D E   13.   Knowing what foods your child will and won't eat.

A B C D E   14.   Predicting whether your child will like a new toy.

A B C D E   15.   Knowing what your child's different cries mean (for example, tiredness, hunger, pain, fear, boredom, frustration, etc.).

A B C D E   16.   Knowing how to relieve your child's distress (for example, due to being tired, hungry, in pain, frightened, bored, frustrated, etc.).

A B C D E   17.   Involving your child in activities you both enjoy.

A B C D E   18.   Knowing when your child seems to want affection from you.

A B C D E   19.   Being comfortable in showing affection to your child.

A B C D E   20.   Getting your child to smile or laugh.

A B C D E   21.   Developing your child's interest in new things.

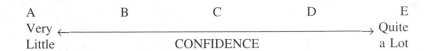

A	B	C	D	E
Very				Quite
Little		CONFIDENCE		a Lot

A B C D E 22. Knowing your child's favorite toys and games.

A B C D E 23. Knowing how to help your child play with other children.

A B C D E 24. Helping your child adjust to new situations (for example, a new babysitter, entering daycare, vacationing, etc.).

A B C D E 25. Setting limits on your child's destructive behaviors (for example, tearing books, breaking valuable items).

A B C D E 26. Setting limits on your child's behavior when it looks dangerous (for example, playing with matches, electric outlets and wires, etc.).

A B C D E 27. Knowing what types of discipline do not work with your child.

A B C D E 28. Knowing what to do when your child has a temper tantrum.

A B C D E 29. Getting your child to bed without a struggle.

A B C D E 30. Keeping a consistent bedtime hour for your child.

A B C D E 31. Knowing when rules can be "bent" or modified and when they should not be.

A B C D E 32. Getting back to "friendly terms" with your child soon after a problem behavior has ended.

A B C D E 33. Knowing whether your style of parenting will "spoil" your child.

A B C D E 34. Managing your child's aggressiveness with other children (for example, hitting, biting, or pushing).

A B C D E 35. Finding supportive services and people in your community for you and your child (for example, other parents of young children, play groups, daycare services, preschools, etc.).

A B C D E 36. Knowing how to manage non-emergency illnesses at home (for example, fever, diarrhea, minor injuries).

A B C D E 37. Managing separations from your child (for example, to go to the store, to go to work, to go out for the evening).

38. Now go back and circle the numbers of any item you would like to know more about.

Thank you.

32

Contraceptive Self-Efficacy Scale

Developed by Ruth Andrea Levinson

INSTRUMENT DESCRIPTION, ADMINISTRATION, AND SCORING GUIDELINES

Contraceptive Self-Efficacy (CSE) is not only the name of this tool but also a concept believed to be important for teenagers because their sexual activity and its consequences (including sexually transmitted disease and pregnancy) are so strongly linked to their ability to control their adult lives. CSE is defined as the strength of a teenager's conviction that she should and can exercise control within sexual and contraceptive situations to achieve contraceptive protection.

Items for the CSE Scale are constructed in a hierarchy of task difficulty related to situations with increasing levels of stress. Items were based on literature that distinguishes between successful and unsuccessful contraceptive users and on the author's teaching experience with the target population.

The behavioral situations contained in the items simulate the kinds of conditions in which teenagers have been reported not to use contraceptives. They are drawn from three bodies of research literature: family planning, developmental psychology, and social psychology. They involve obtaining contraceptives, using contraceptives with a partner, talking to a partner about contraceptive use, using contraceptives despite partner or parental disapproval, interrupting an episode of unplanned sex to talk about or use a contraceptive, and preventing episodes of unprotected intercourse. Scores on the CSE are obtained by averaging item scores, with higher numbers indicating higher CSE. Items 2, 5, 6, 8, 9, 11, 12, 14, and 15 are reverse scored. The instrument takes 10 minutes to complete (Levinson, 1986).

PSYCHOMETRIC PROPERTIES

Reliability coefficient for the CSE was .73.

The CSE has been shown to be sensitive to interventions based on self-efficacy theory, with the goal of influencing teenagers to believe that they should and could influence control in sexual and contraceptive situations and to be contraceptively protected. Interventions used role-playing situations, video-cassette episodes, and salient role models with persuasive communications. Several studies have found that an increase in SE contributed significantly to females' contraceptive use. Some adolescents were strongly resistant to instruction or consideration of the consequences of being sexually active (Heinrich, 1993; Levinson, 1984).

CSE has now been used with four diverse samples: suburban lower-middle– to middle-class teenage girls who attended a family-planning clinic in Northern California (21% Hispanic); in a French version with 9th- and 10th-grade male and female high school students in Montreal; in a predominantly White middle-class college sample in the United States; and inner-city primarily poverty to middle-class African-American (94%) teenage women in Chicago. Some of these samples were at high risk for pregnancy because of high frequency of unprotected intercourse and irregular use of contraceptives. Mean score for the college sample was 4.07, 3.79 for less effective user groups, and 4.26 for highly effective user groups. Item means for each of the four populations may be found in Levinson, Jaccard, Wan, and Beamer (1996), and serve as norms for other similar populations.

Although four factors emerged from factor analysis in most of the research, correlations between items have been relatively low, suggesting large amounts of unique variance in them. The factors are conscious acceptance of sexual activity (items 2, 5, 6, 12, 14, and 15); assumption of responsibility for sexual activity and contraception (items 1 and 13a to 13c); assertiveness in preventing sexual intercourse (items 4, 7, and 13d); and strong feelings of sexual arousal (items 3 and 8 to 11) (Heinrich, 1993; Levinson, 1986). At least two of the studies raised questions about which items belong to which factor and which factors are most highly predictive of contraceptive behavior.

CSE items have operated distinctly in the Chicago sample, where only item 3 was significantly correlated with contraceptive behavior. For the California sample, items 8, 10, 11, and 13c were the primary predictors of contraceptive use; for the Montreal group, items 3, 8, and 12 were the most relevant; for the college sample, items 2, 6, and 8 were most relevant. Although the CSE items as a totality were significant predictors of contraceptive behavior in all four samples, there were variations in their predictive power in different samples (Levinson et al., 1996).

CSE operated least powerfully in predicting contraceptive behavior in the Chicago sample, perhaps representing cultural differences in the issues impacting contraceptive behavior. The authors believe that although the total item set be used, the relationship between each item and contraceptive behavior should be analyzed separately because items may offer unique information about what issues are most salient to any given sample. Norms for each item for each sample described previously are available and may be used for comparison for like samples (Levinson et al., 1996).

CRITIQUE AND SUMMARY

Contraceptive behavior is clearly complex, and the authors are to be congratulated for testing the CSE with nearly 900 adolescents from four diverse populations to establish generalizability and to set guidelines for use of the scale (Levinson et al., 1996). Clearly, cultural assumptions are important to attaining a tool predictive of contraceptive behavior, and it must be understood that the outcome behavior will not be valued by everyone. More important, the issues embedded in the CSE Scale may not be the most relevant issues impacting these young women's sexual and contraceptive behavior. Reliability for the CSE is still low, and work remains to be done to obtain internally consistent factors. Most of the work on the CSE has been done with teenage girls and less with boys; yet the work already accomplished is impressive.

Because individuals who feel relatively contraceptively self-efficacious on some items might not feel so on others, it is useful to look at item scores. Yet to be established is some target score level that could be used to judge the efficacy of interventions. Theory would suggest that a teenager would need to feel relatively self-efficacious across several items.

REFERENCES

Heinrich, L. B. (1993). Contraceptive self-efficacy in college women. *Journal of Adolescent Health, 14,* 269–276.

Levinson, R. A. (1984). Contraceptive self-efficacy: A primary prevention strategy. *Journal of Social Work and Human Sexuality, 3,* 1–15.

Levinson, R. A. (1986). Contraceptive self-efficacy: A perspective on teenage girls' contraceptive behavior. *Journal of Sex Research, 22,* 347–369.

Levinson, R. A., Jaccard, J., Wan, C. K., & Beamer L. A. (1996). *The Contraceptive Self-Efficacy Scale: Analysis in four samples.* Unpublished manuscript.

CONTRACEPTIVE SELF-EFFICACY INSTRUMENT

The items on the following page are a list of statements. Please rate each item on a 1 to 5 scale according to how true the statement is of you. Using the scale, circle one number for each question.

> 1 = Not at all true of me
> 2 = Slightly true of me
> 3 = Somewhat true of me
> 4 = Mostly true of me
> 5 = Completely true of me

1. 1 2 3 4 5   When I am with a boyfriend, I feel that I can always be responsible for what happens sexually with him.

2. 1 2 3 4 5   Even if a boyfriend can talk about sex, I can't tell a man how I really feel about sexual things.

3. 1 2 3 4 5   When I have sex, I can enjoy it as something that I really wanted to do.

4. 1 2 3 4 5   If my boyfriend and I are getting "turned on" sexually and I don't really want to have sexual intercourse (go all the way, get down), I can easily tell him "No" and mean it.

5. 1 2 3 4 5   If my boyfriend didn't talk about the sex that was happening between us, I couldn't either.

6. 1 2 3 4 5   When I think about what having sex means, I can't have sex so easily.

7. 1 2 3 4 5   If my boyfriend and I are getting "turned on" sexually and I don't really want to have sexual intercourse (go all the way, get down), I can easily stop things so that we don't have intercourse.

8. 1 2 3 4 5   There are times when I'd be so involved sexually or emotionally that I could easily have sexual intercourse even if I weren't protected (using a form of birth control).

9. 1 2 3 4 5   Sometimes I just go along with what my date wants to do sexually because I don't think I can take the hassle of trying to say what I want.

10. 1 2 3 4 5   If there were a man (boyfriend) to whom I was very attracted physically and emotionally, I could feel comfortable telling him that I wanted to have sex with him.

11. 1 2 3 4 5   I couldn't continue to use a birth control method if I thought that my parents might find it.

12. 1 2 3 4 5   It would be hard for me to go to the drugstore and ask for foam (Encare Ovals, a diaphragm, a pill prescription, etc.) without feeling embarrassed.

13. If my boyfriend and I were getting really heavy into sex and moving towards intercourse and I wasn't protected . . .

(a) 1 2 3 4 5   I could easily ask him if he had protection (or tell him that I didn't).

(b) 1 2 3 4 5   I could excuse myself to put in a diaphragm or foam (if I used them for birth control).

(c) 1 2 3 4 5   I could tell him I was on the pill or had an IUD (if I used them for birth control).

1 = Not at all true of me
2 = Slightly true of me
3 = Somewhat true of me
4 = Mostly true of me
5 = Completely true of me

(d)   1   2   3   4   5   I could stop things before intercourse, if I couldn't bring up the subject of protection.

14.   1   2   3   4   5   There are times when I should talk to my boyfriend about using contraceptives, but I can't seem to do it in the situation.

15.   1   2   3   4   5   Sometimes I end up having sex with a boyfriend because I can't find a way to stop it.

Note: The CSE scale was previously published in "Contraceptive Self-Efficacy: A perspective on teenage girls' contraceptive behavior" by R. A. Levinson (1986). *Journal of Sex Research, 22,* 351.

F

Other Clinical Topics

33

Hussey's Medication Knowledge and Compliance Scale, and Hussey's Picture Schedule

Developed by Leslie C. Hussey

INSTRUMENT DESCRIPTION, ADMINISTRATION, AND SCORING GUIDELINES

Although one of the major factors in prolongation and increased quality of life has been the use of medications, the significant dangers associated with incorrect prescription use of multiple drugs is particularly significant in the elderly. Education that assures that these patients understand instructions for how to take the medications, correct dosage and scheduling, and reactions and interactions are important.

Low literacy will contribute to confusion in taking medications, and yet literacy skills are seldom assessed by health care providers teaching patients. If persons with low literacy are questioned, they frequently will indicate that they understand even if they do not. Hussey's Medication Knowledge and Compliance Scale (MKCS) was designed to elicit information about the patient's knowledge of and compliance with the medication regimen. Compliance was defined as the appropriate use of legal medications taken according to the physician's prescribed directions. One MKCS is used for each medication the patient is taking. The nine items are scored 1 = correct and 0 = wrong or does not know, and scores are added and averaged. An acceptable level of compliance is deemed to be 80%, based on evidence that at such a level therapeutic effects are observed. An average score of .8 or higher was graded as 1 or correct. No reported scores from the study groups were available (Hussey, 1994).

Hussey's Picture Schedule was used as part of the instruction to simplify a medication regimen for patients who have difficulty reading or following it. It appears on page 258. The lines next to the clock contained colored dots, representing each medication, with the number of dots indicating the number of tablets to be ingested. The medication bottle was coded with the same color. The Picture Schedule was enlarged to 8.5 × 14 inches and enclosed in a plastic cover so that the patient could cross out the dose after taking it, with a nonpermanent marker (Hussey, 1994).

PSYCHOMETRIC PROPERTIES

Content validity of the MKCS was established by a panel of 20 nurses who were active participants in the hospital's patient education program and pilot tested on 25 elderly patients with chronic health problems but who were not from the study population. Reliability as measured by the Kuder-Richardson formula was .85. The scale was administered to 80 patients in a geriatric outpatient clinic in a large county hospital in the southwestern United States, serving a primarily indigent population with self-reported reading skills at the 3rd- and 4th-grade reading level. Sixty-two percent were African-American. Patients receiving verbal medication instruction only or instruction with the visual medication schedule did not differ in knowledge, although those in the visual instruction group who had the lowest reported compliance scores on pretest did show increase in compliance. On posttest 3 weeks after instruction, the entire group did show changes in both knowledge and reported compliance (Hussey, 1994), supporting sensitivity of the MKCS to instruction. The Picture Schedule proved effective in increasing reported compliance for those who on pretest had the most difficulty complying with their medication regimens (Hussey, 1994).

CRITIQUE AND SUMMARY

The MKCS represents an example of a criterion-referenced standard, in that an average score of .8 was considered correct. This approach does not consider the fact that some answers to each question are more crucial for safe medication taking than are others.

Both the meaning of the term *compliance* and the term itself are now controversial because they have been used in the past to imply that patients who were not following a physician's prescription were reprehensible. The problematic assumption is that the provider is always right. In addition, self-reported compliance may not be strongly related to actual compliance (however that may be defined).

The MKCS does focus on an important group (low literacy, chronically ill, and indigent), for which there is little research, but great need for well-established tools and teaching approaches.

REFERENCE

Hussey, L. C. (1994). Minimizing effects of low literacy on medication knowledge and compliance among the elderly. *Clinical Nursing Research, 3,* 132–145.

HUSSEY'S MEDICATION KNOWLEDGE
AND COMPLIANCE SCHEDULE[a]

	Correct 1	Wrong/ Doesn't Know 0
1. What is the name of your medicine?		
2. What is this medicine for?		
3. What side effects of your medicine would you call your nurse or doctor about?		
4. When do you take your medicine?		
5. When should you take your medicine?		
6. How much of this medicine do you take?		
7. Are there any special instructions you need to follow when you take your medicine?		
8. If #7 is yes, what are they?		
9. Do you follow these special instructions when you take your medicine?		

Medication: _____

[a]This scale is used so the patient's knowledge and compliance are tested on the medications individually.

L. C. Hussey, Medication Knowledge and Compliance Scale. Used with permission.

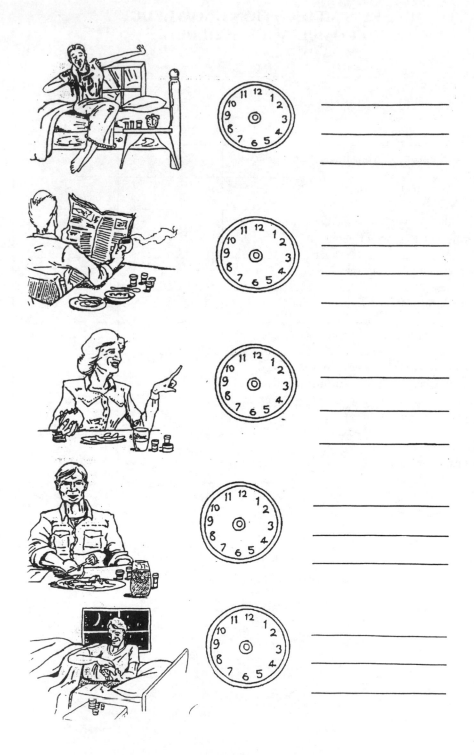

HUSSEY'S PICTURE SCHEDULE

L. C. Hussey, The Picture Schedule, Copyright, 1989. Used with permission.

34

Patient/Family Pain Questionnaires: Patient Pain Questionnaire and Family Pain Questionnaire

Developed by Betty R. Ferrell, Michelle Rhiner, and Lynne M. Rivera

INSTRUMENT DESCRIPTION, ADMINISTRATION, AND SCORING GUIDELINES

Ferrell, Ferrell, Rhiner, and Grant (1991) remind us that two of every three American families will have at least one member diagnosed with cancer. Family members become active caregivers whether or not they feel competent to do so, and home care is increasing as the site of cancer care, frequently for many years.

Researchers have consistently found pain to be a major concern of family caregivers including fear of drug addiction, respiratory depression, or drug tolerance. These fears may lead to undermedication of patients even though they are experiencing unrelieved pain. In addition, pain management has become increasingly complex, with use of multiple medications, adjunct drugs, and complex delivery systems, such as patient-controlled analgesia pumps, epidural catheters, or continuous parenteral infusions.

The Family Pain Questionnaire (FPQ) was developed to measure caregivers' knowledge of basic pain management. The Patient Pain Questionnaire (PPQ) and FPQ include the same items; nine are in the knowledge subscale, with a higher score indicating higher knowledge, and seven items in the experience scale, with lower scores indicating more positive experience. Scale and subscale scores are sums of item scores.

PSYCHOMETRIC PROPERTIES

The FPQ was modeled after tools that have been used extensively to measure knowledge and attitudes of health care professionals about pain but modified to be appropriate for patients and family using results of interviews and surveys of families and patients describing their pain experience. The PPQ and FPQ was first tested with 85 patients/families with cancer pain in a community hospital, a cancer center, and a home-based community hospice program. Seventy-seven percent were White. The FPQ received 90% to 100% acceptance for content validity by a panel of six cancer pain management experts. Test-retest reliability was .92 and Cronbach's α .81 (Ferrell, Rhiner, & Rivera, 1993).

The two subscales of knowledge and experience were defined through factor analysis. The experience subscale captures the caregivers' personal experiences, such as perceptions of the intensivity of the patient's pain, and his or her own distress regarding the patient's pain (Ferrell, Rhiner, & Rivera, 1993).

Several other studies by the authors, using these instruments, have been reported. Ferrell, Ferrell, Ahn, and Tran (1994) report a study of an educational intervention for pain management delivered during home visits to 80 patients 60 years and older and their family caregivers. Topics included assessment of pain, use of pain-rating scales, the use of pharmacological and nonpharmacological agents, and the need to relieve pain to promote overall comfort and quality of life. Mean of the knowledge subscale was 54 and the experience subscale 52 before the intervention. Areas of lowest scores for knowledge and attitudes included fear of respiratory depression (mean score = 43), pain distress (mean score = 38), and need to take low doses of medicines (mean score = 38).

Significant improvement was verified in eight of the experience subscales before and after the educational treatment, providing support for sensitivity of the instrument. Scores of 50 family caregivers of these patients on the FPQ before the educational intervention are reported in Ferrell, Grant, Chan, Ahn, and Ferrell (1995). Mean score on the knowledge subscale was 53 and on the experience subscale 39. Caregivers showed lowest knowledge about the inevitability of addiction, a perception that patients were often overmedicated, and the relationship between medication and respiratory distress. Again, 10 of the 14 items showed significant improvement after the educational intervention, as did the two subscale scores. Overall, patients showed more positive responses than did family members.

A study of the family experience of cancer pain management in children used the FPQ. Participants were families of patients in a pediatric cancer hospital and a community hospice. Scores on individual items of the FPQ may be seen in a report of that research. Again, low scores were found in knowledge of the danger (mean item score = 56), dose (mean item score = 44), and constancy of pain medications (mean item score = 56) (Ferrell, Rhiner, Shapiro, & Strause, 1994).

CRITIQUE AND SUMMARY

Ferrell, Ferrell, Ahn, and Tran (1994) believe that structured pain education should be provided to all patients with cancer who experience this symptom, just as it is expected that diabetes education will be provided to all who have diabetes. Indeed, the studies cited previously indicate that patients and family caregivers have important educational needs in areas related to routine dosing, pain assessment, addiction, and respiratory depression. They also show the effectiveness of an educational intervention (Ferrell et al., 1995), although the most optimally effective intervention has still not been adequately investigated. Meanings that might be attached to different levels of scores are not immediately clear. Studies of the predictive validity of the scores and patient/family pain management behavior would be useful.

REFERENCES

Ferrell, B. R., Ferrell, B. A., Ahn, C., & Tran, K. (1994). Pain management for elderly patients with cancer at home. *Cancer, 74,* 2139–2146.

Ferrell, B. R., Ferrell, B. A., Rhiner, M., & Grant, M. (1991). Family factors influencing cancer pain. *Post Graduate Medical Journal, 67*(Suppl. 2), S64–S69.

Ferrell, B. R., Grant, M., Chan, J., Ahn, C., & Ferrell, B. A. (1995). The impact of cancer pain education on family caregivers of elderly patients. *Oncology Nursing Forum, 22,* 1211–1218.

Ferrell, B., Rhiner, M., & Rivera, L. M. (1993). Development and evaluation of the Family Pain Questionnaire. *Journal of Psychosocial Oncology, 10*(4), 21–35.

Ferrell, B. R., Rhiner, M., Shapiro, B., & Strause, L. (1994). The family experience of cancer pain management in children. *Cancer Practice, 2,* 441–445.

The Family Pain Questionnaire (FPQ) is a 16-item ordinal scale that measures the Knowledge and Experience of a family caregiver in managing chronic cancer pain. This tool can be useful in clinical practice as well as for research. This instrument can be administered by mail or in person.

Directions: The caregiver is asked to read each question thoroughly and decide if he/she agrees with the statement or disagrees. The caregiver is then asked to circle a number to indicate the degree to which he/she agrees or disagrees with the statement according to the word anchors on each end of the scale.

The FPQ includes 9 items that measure knowledge about pain and 7 items that measure the caregivers' experience with pain. All of the items have been formatted such that 0 = the most positive outcome and 10 = the most negative outcome. We have found it most helpful to analyze the data by focusing on the subscales as well as the individual items as each item has important implications.

You are welcome to use this instrument in your research/clinical practice to gain information about caregiver knowledge and experience to formulate or evaluate pain management programs. You have permission to duplicate this tool.

This tool is used in conjunction with a version created for use by patients, the Patient Pain Questionnaire (PPQ). The FPQ tool has been tested with established reliability (test retest, internal consistency) and validity (content, construct, concurrent). A series of psychometric analyses were performed on the instrument including content validity (CVI = .90), construct validity (ANOVA, $p. < .05$), concurrent validity ($r = .60$, $p. < .05$), factor analysis and test-retest reliability ($r = .80$) established with a retest of caregivers ($N = 67$).

FAMILY PAIN QUESTIONNAIRE

Below are a number of statements about cancer pain and pain relief. Please circle a number on the line to indicate your response.

Knowledge

1. Cancer pain can be effectively relieved.

    Agree   0   1   2   3   4   5   6   7   8   9   10   Disagree

2. Pain medicines should be given only when pain is severe.

    Disagree   0   1   2   3   4   5   6   7   8   9   10   Agree

3. Most cancer patients on pain medicines will become addicted to the medicines over time.

    Disagree   0   1   2   3   4   5   6   7   8   9   10   Agree

4. It is important to give the lowest amount of medicine possible to save larger doses for later when the pain is worse.

    Disagree   0   1   2   3   4   5   6   7   8   9   10   Agree

5. It is better to give pain medications around the clock (on a schedule) rather than only when needed.

   Agree 0 1 2 3 4 5 6 7 8 9 10 Disagree

6. Treatments other than medications (such as massage, heat, relaxation) can be effective for relieving pain.

   Agree 0 1 2 3 4 5 6 7 8 9 10 Disagree

7. Pain medicines can be dangerous and can often interfere with breathing.

   Disagree 0 1 2 3 4 5 6 7 8 9 10 Agree

8. Patients are often given too much pain medicine.

   Disagree 0 1 2 3 4 5 6 7 8 9 10 Agree

9. If pain is worse, the cancer must be getting worse.

   Disagree 0 1 2 3 4 5 6 7 8 9 10 Agree

Experience

10. Over the past week, how much pain do you feel your family member has had?

    No Pain 0 1 2 3 4 5 6 7 8 9 10 A Great Deal

11. How much pain is your family member having now?

    No Pain 0 1 2 3 4 5 6 7 8 9 10 A Great Deal

12. How much pain relief is your family member currently receiving?

    A Great Deal 0 1 2 3 4 5 6 7 8 9 10 No Relief

13. How distressing do you think the pain is to your family member?

    Not At All 0 1 2 3 4 5 6 7 8 9 10 A Great Deal

14. How distressing is your family members' pain to you?

    Not At All 0 1 2 3 4 5 6 7 8 9 10 A Great Deal

15. To what extent do you feel you are able to control the patient's pain?

    A Great Deal 0 1 2 3 4 5 6 7 8 9 10 Not At All

16. What do you expect will happen with your family member's pain in the future?

    Will Get Better 0 1 2 3 4 5 6 7 8 9 10 Will Get Worse

Used with permission: Betty R. Ferrell, City of Hope National Medical Center, Duarte, California.

The Patient Pain Questionnaire (PPQ) is a sixteen item ordinal scale that measures the Knowledge and Experience of a patient in managing chronic cancer pain. This tool can be useful in clinical practice as well as for research. This instrument can be administered by mail or in person.

Directions: The patient is asked to read each question thoroughly and decide if he/she agrees with the statement or disagrees. The patient is then asked to circle a number to indicate the degree to which he/she agrees or disagrees with the statement according to the word anchors on each end of the scale.

The PPQ includes 9 items that measure knowledge about pain and 7 items that measure the patient's experience with pain. All of the items have been formatted such that 0 = the most positive outcome and 10 = the most negative outcome. We have found it most helpful to analyze the data by focusing on the subscales as well as the individual items as each item has important implications.

You are welcome to use this instrument in your research/clinical practice to gain information about caregiver knowledge and experience to formulate or evaluate pain management programs. You have permission to duplicate this tool.

This tool is used in conjunction with a version created for use by family members, the Family Pain Questionnaire (FPQ). The PPQ tool has been tested with established reliability (test retest, internal consistency) and validity (content, construct, concurrent). A series of psychometric analyses were performed on the PPQ instrument including content validity (CVI = .90), construct validity (ANOVA, p. < .05), concurrent validity (r = .60, p. < .05), factor analysis and test-retest reliability (r = .80) established with a retest of caregivers (N = 67). The PPQ was recently revised to the current form and is being used in our current research.

PATIENT PAIN QUESTIONNAIRE

Below are a number of statements about cancer pain and pain relief. Please circle a number on the line to indicate your response.

Knowledge

1. Cancer pain can be effectively relieved.

    Agree   0   1   2   3   4   5   6   7   8   9   10   Disagree

2. Pain medicines should be given only when pain is severe.

    Disagree   0   1   2   3   4   5   6   7   8   9   10   Agree

3. Most cancer patients on pain medicines will become addicted to the medicines over time.

    Disagree   0   1   2   3   4   5   6   7   8   9   10   Agree

4. It is important to give the lowest amount of medicine possible to save larger doses for later when the pain is worse.

    Disagree   0   1   2   3   4   5   6   7   8   9   10   Agree

5. It is better to give pain medications around the clock (on a schedule) rather than only when needed.

   Agree 0   1   2   3   4   5   6   7   8   9   10   Disagree

6. Treatments other than medications (such as massage, heat, relaxation) can be effective for relieving pain.

   Agree 0   1   2   3   4   5   6   7   8   9   10   Disagree

7. Pain medicines can be dangerous and can often interfere with breathing.

   Disagree 0   1   2   3   4   5   6   7   8   9   10   Agree

8. Patients are often given too much pain medicine.

   Disagree 0   1   2   3   4   5   6   7   8   9   10   Agree

9. If pain is worse, the cancer must be getting worse.

   Disagree 0   1   2   3   4   5   6   7   8   9   10   Agree

Experience

10. Over the past week, how much pain have you had?

    No Pain 0   1   2   3   4   5   6   7   8   9   10   A Great Deal

11. How much pain are you having now?

    No Pain 0   1   2   3   4   5   6   7   8   9   10   A Great Deal

12. How much pain relief are you currently receiving?

    A Great Deal 0   1   2   3   4   5   6   7   8   9   10   No Relief

13. How distressing is the pain to you?

    Not At All 0   1   2   3   4   5   6   7   8   9   10   Extremely

14. How distressing is your pain to your family members?

    Not At All 0   1   2   3   4   5   6   7   8   9   10   Extremely

15. To what extent do you feel you are able to control your pain?

    A Great Deal 0   1   2   3   4   5   6   7   8   9   10   Not At All

16. What do you expect will happen with your pain in the future?

    Pain Will Get Better 0   1   2   3   4   5   6   7   8   9   10   Will Get Worse

Used with permission: Betty R. Ferrell, City of Hope National Medical Center, Duarte, California.

35

Toronto Informational Needs Questionnaire–Breast Cancer

Developed by Susan Galloway, Jane Graydon, Dianne Harrison, Sherrol Palmer-Wickham, Stephanie Burlein-Hall, Louanne Rich-van der Bij, Pamela West, and Barbara Evans-Boyden

INSTRUMENT DESCRIPTION, ADMINISTRATION, AND SCORING GUIDELINES

The Toronto Informational Needs Questionnaire–Breast Cancer (TINQ-BC) is designed to elicit women's perceptions of their informational needs related to their experience of breast cancer. It takes women about 20 minutes to complete the questionnaire. Each item begins with the stem: "To help me with my illness it is important for me to know" and rates each item on a scale of 1 (not important) to 5 (extremely important). The questionnaire yields a total score with a minimum of 52 and a maximum of 260. Higher scores represent more importance being placed on information to help the woman deal with the illness. Individual subscales may be calculated (Galloway et al., n.d.)

PSYCHOMETRIC PROPERTIES

Items were generated from findings in the literature and 11 oncology nurse experts. Each expert independently placed each item on one subscale, yielding an interrater reliability of item assignment to category of .91. Thirty-four women, including those with and without breast cancer, lay people, and health care providers, assessed the questionnaire for clarity in the wording of items. The TINQ-BC was administered to 114 women with a recent diagnosis of breast cancer during chemotherapy ($n = 39$), radiation therapy ($n = 40$), or surgery ($n = 35$). The items applied to 90% of the women with interitem correlations between .20 and .80. The five subscales may be seen in Table 35.1. Informational needs of the women were high with mean scores over 200 and the greatest needs in the areas of diagnosis or treatment (Galloway, 1993).

There is beginning evidence of construct validity. Women newly diagnosed with breast cancer report high informational needs as measured by the TINQ-BC, and women experiencing a recurrence of breast cancer also place high importance on having information. These findings are congruent with the theoretical perspective of Lazarus and Folkman (1984) that people in threatening situations will seek information to understand what is happening, and with results of previous studies. Younger women reported a greater need for information than did older women. Scores on the TINQ-BC have shown variability in women's responses. The instrument has shown internal consistency reliabilities between .85 and .90 for the subscales and .93 for the total questionnaire (Galloway et al., n.d.).

In a second study of 20 female breast cancer patients after excisional biopsy and axillary node dissection, 20 completed TINQ-BC in the 1st week of radiation therapy, and 20 did so in the first clinic visit after completion of radiation therapy. Although all women had informational needs on all TINQ scales, treatment was the highest area of informational need, with the physical subscale being second. These findings were common with both groups and at both times in the treatment cycle. In general, patient informational needs were high (Harrison-Woermke & Graydon, 1993).

CRITIQUE AND SUMMARY

This instrument is still in early stages of development. It requires further evaluation of construct validity by factor analysis and longitudinal studies to determine how informational needs alter over time to determine the best timing and methods for delivering information (Galloway, 1993) as well as other studies of validity.

TINQ-BC can be used in needs assessment for individuals or groups of women, so that teaching interventions can be targeted. Availability of the information patients need should contribute to realistic expectations, to self-care, to a sense of control, and to trust with providers. Sensitivity of TINQ-BC to instruction and its ability to predict these important outcomes should be established including with patients who cope best by avoidance of information.

TABLE 35.1   Subscale Definitions of the TINQ-BC

Subscale	Definition and item nos.
Disease	Description of the disease, its process and prognosis. (Items: 2, 7, 10, 12, 14, 18, 37, 42, 50)
Investigative tests	Description of the rationale, process, and sensations associated with diagnostic procedures used to monitor the disease and treatments. (Items: 1, 15, 16, 19, 33, 47, 48, 51)
Treatments	Rationale and implications of methods used for disease control including how methods work, how they are done, sensations and possible side effects and actions to minimize the side effects. (Items: 3, 5, 6, 9, 13, 17, 27, 28, 29, 30, 32, 35, 40, 41, 45, 46)
Physical	Description of the preventive, restorative, and maintenance care which the body requires as a result of the disease. (Items: 4, 21, 23, 24, 31, 36, 38, 39, 43, 44, 52)
Psychosocial	Description of how to obtain assistance in dealing with feelings and social concerns arising as a result of the illness. (Items: 8, 11, 20, 22, 25, 26, 34, 49)

This tool should also be useful as one of several measures to evaluate the quality of communication in a care program for persons with breast cancer to see that most patients get the information they need and want, and to feel secure with their care. Perception of inadequate information can occur because patients cannot absorb what is being given to them or feel that no one has a sustained interest in and commitment to their care and symptoms. Sometimes it is not information that patients desire but rather intensified support of their hopes, concern for their person, and confirmation of the validity of what they think they know (Cassileth, Volckmar, & Goodman, 1980).

REFERENCES

Cassileth, B. R., Volckmar, D., & Goodman, R. L. (1980). The effect of experience on radiation therapy patients' desire for information. *International Journal Radiation Oncology Biophysics, 6,* 493–496.

Galloway, S. (1993). Informational needs questionnaire for women with breast cancer. *Oncology Nursing Forum, 20,* 336.

Galloway, S., Graydon, J., Harrison, D., Palmer-Wickham, S., Evans-Boyden, B., Burlein-Hall, S., Rich-van der Bij, L., & West, P. (n.d.). *Toronto Informational Needs Questionnaire–Breast Cancer.* University of Toronto, Ontario, Canada.

Harrison-Woermke, D. E., & Graydon, J. E. (1993). Perceived informational needs of breast cancer patients receiving radiation therapy after excisional biopsy and axillary node dissection. *Cancer Nursing, 16,* 449–455.

Lazarus, R., & Folkman, S. (1984). *Stress, appraisal and coping.* New York: Springer.

TORONTO INFORMATIONAL NEEDS
QUESTIONNAIRE–BREAST CANCER

We are interested in knowing the types of information women with breast cancer need. Please read each of the following statements and circle the number that best describes how important it is for you to have this information.

1 = not important
2 = slightly important
3 = moderately important
4 = very important
5 = extremely important

It is important for me to know:

1.	How I will feel during the tests (e.g., x-ray, bone scans).	1	2	3	4	5
2.	If the breast cancer will come back.	1	2	3	4	5
3.	How to prepare for my treatment.	1	2	3	4	5
4.	When to examine my breasts.	1	2	3	4	5
5.	How I will feel after my treatment.	1	2	3	4	5
6.	Who I should call if I have questions while I am still getting treatment.	1	2	3	4	5
7.	How breast cancer acts in the body.	1	2	3	4	5
8.	If there are groups where I can talk with other people with cancer.	1	2	3	4	5
9.	If there are ways to prevent treatment side effects.	1	2	3	4	5
10.	How the illness may affect my life over the next few months.	1	2	3	4	5
11.	If there will be changes in the usual things I can do with and for my family.	1	2	3	4	5
12.	If there is cancer anywhere else in my body.	1	2	3	4	5
13.	Who I should call if I have questions after all the treatments are over.	1	2	3	4	5
14.	If it is known what causes breast cancer.	1	2	3	4	5
15.	How the tests (e.g., x-rays, bone scans) are done.	1	2	3	4	5
16.	Why they need to test my blood.	1	2	3	4	5
17.	Who to talk with if I hear about treatments other than surgery, radiation, or chemotherapy.	1	2	3	4	5
18.	How the illness may affect my life in the future.	1	2	3	4	5
19.	What the results of my blood tests mean.	1	2	3	4	5

1 = not important
2 = slightly important
3 = moderately important
4 = very important
5 = extremely important

It is important for me to know:

20.	Where my family can go if they need help dealing with my illness.	1	2	3	4	5
21.	How to care for my wound or incision.	1	2	3	4	5
22.	What to do if I become concerned about dying.	1	2	3	4	5
23.	If I can continue my usual hobbies and sports.	1	2	3	4	5
24.	If I can wear a brassiere.	1	2	3	4	5
25.	Where I can get help to deal with my feelings about my illness.	1	2	3	4	5
26.	How to talk to family/friends about my illness.	1	2	3	4	5
27.	If I have side effects, how to deal with them.	1	2	3	4	5
28.	The possible side effects of my treatment.	1	2	3	4	5
29.	What side effects I should report to the doctor/nurse.	1	2	3	4	5
30.	If I am prone to infection because of my treatment.	1	2	3	4	5
31.	How long my wound/incision will take to heal.	1	2	3	4	5
32.	How long I will be receiving treatment.	1	2	3	4	5
33.	How I will feel after the tests (e.g., x-rays, bone scans).	1	2	3	4	5
34.	Where I can get help if I have problems feeling as attractive as I did before.	1	2	3	4	5
35.	How the treatment works against the cancer.	1	2	3	4	5
36.	If there are special arm exercises to do.	1	2	3	4	5
37.	The medical name for my type of breast cancer.	1	2	3	4	5
38.	If there are any physical things I should not do.	1	2	3	4	5
39.	If I'm going to need help taking care of myself.	1	2	3	4	5
40.	How my treatment is done.	1	2	3	4	5
41.	If the treatment will alter the way that I look.	1	2	3	4	5
42.	How to tell if the cancer has come back.	1	2	3	4	5
43.	Which foods I can or cannot eat.	1	2	3	4	5
44.	If I can take a bath or shower.	1	2	3	4	5
45.	What types of treatment are available.	1	2	3	4	5
46.	Why the doctor suggested this treatment plan for me.	1	2	3	4	5

1 = not important
2 = slightly important
3 = moderately important
4 = very important
5 = extremely important

It is important for me to know:

47.	The reasons my doctor suggests certain tests (e.g., x-rays, bone scans).	1	2	3	4	5
48.	How to prepare for the tests (e.g., x-rays, bone scans).	1	2	3	4	5
49.	What to do if I feel uncomfortable in social situations.	1	2	3	4	5
50.	If my illness is hereditary.	1	2	3	4	5
51.	When to have a mammogram.	1	2	3	4	5
52.	If I can continue my usual social activities.	1	2	3	4	5

36

Colorectal Cancer Knowledge Questionnaire

Developed by Sally P. Weinrich, Martin C. Weinrich, Marlyn D. Boyd, Edna Johnson, and Marilyn Frank-Stromberg

INSTRUMENT DESCRIPTION, ADMINISTRATION, AND SCORING GUIDELINES

Colorectal cancer is the second leading cause of death in the United States; yet the survival rate for patients could be increased with screening and early detection in conjunction with appropriate management. Although not sufficient by itself to promote behavioral change, adequate levels of knowledge are prerequisite to such behavior. The possible range of scores on the questionnaire is 0 to 12, with each correct answer counting as 1 point. Responses were obtained by interview for those who had difficulty reading and writing, with each interview lasting 12 minutes (Weinrich, Weinrich, Boyd, Johnson, & Frank-Stromberg, 1992.)

PSYCHOMETRIC PROPERTIES

Only one study using the questionnaire could be located. Participants were socioeconomically disadvantaged adults with an average age of 72 years, contacted in 12 Southern congregate meal sites sponsored by the Council on Aging (Weinrich et al., 1992). A socioeconomically disadvantaged population has been shown to be least likely to participate in screening and also most likely to die from colorectal cancer, and studies have documented inadequate knowledge of cancer among this group. Half of the participants in the present study were Black and half White.

The Colorectal Cancer Knowledge Questionnaire (CCKQ) was adapted for the study population from the American Cancer Society's Colorectal Health Check Questionnaire. The CCKQ was administered before and after a program using four different educational methods to which participants were randomly assigned: peer education, educational modification to accommodate normal aging changes including increased time for learning and decrease in short-term memory, combination of these approaches, and traditional method. Pretest scores ranged from 2 to 12, with an overall mean of 8 and SD of 2.6; posttest scores administered 6 days later had a range of 1 to 12, mean of 8.7, and SD of 2.5, a significant change in scores. Cronbach's α was 0.69, with a test-retest reliability of 0.65 for a subset of 19 people from the sample.

Fewer of this sample had undergone screening for colorectal cancer than the national average, although having had screening was not significantly associated with cancer knowledge. Score on the CCKQ was a predictor of participation in fecal occult blood testing made available at the time of education.

CRITIQUE AND SUMMARY

Little information about validity of the CCKQ, including content validity, was made available. Particularly with a knowledge test, explicit definition of the domains from which items were generated and then chosen is expected. Relationship between CCKQ scores and additional target behaviors, such as diet, would also be helpful. Reliability is modest. In addition, the questionnaire has been tested with only one sociodemographically homogeneous set of participants. Because more educated persons could be anticipated to have greater knowledge of cancer, it is not clear whether ceiling effects might occur when such persons were tested with the CCKQ. This is a particular problem when testing sensitivity to teaching interventions.

REFERENCE

Weinrich, S. P., Weinrich, M. C., Boyd, M. D., Johnson, E., & Frank-Stromborg, M. (1992). Knowledge of colorectal cancer among older persons. *Cancer Nursing, 15,* 322–330.

KNOWLEDGE OF COLORECTAL CANCER QUESTIONNAIRE

Tell me if you think these questions are true, false, or don't know.

Do you think or believe that:	Yes (true)	No (false)	Don't know
1. Men get cancer of the bowel more often than women.	T	F	DK
2. Bowel cancer is always a deadly disease.	T	F	DK
3. To check for blood in your bowel movement, you need to have a bowel movement blood test.	T	F	DK
4. You think you would always have pain if you had cancer of the bowel.	T	F	DK
5. You think your chances of getting cancer of the bowel are greater if you have a family member who had cancer of the bowel.	T	F	DK
6. Blood in your bowel movement means you have cancer for sure.	T	F	DK
7. You need to check your bowel movement for blood even if your bowel habits are normal.	T	F	DK
8. You think testing bowel movements for hidden blood would be very painful.	T	F	DK
9. Almost all the people who get bowel cancer are 50 years old or older.	T	F	DK
10. Most people who get cancer of the bowel could be saved if it were found and treated at an early stage.	T	F	DK
11. A diet with a lot of roughage, like fruits, vegetables, and grains, may reduce your chances of getting cancer of the bowel.	T	F	DK
12. You should have your bowel movement tested for hidden blood every year if you are 50 years or older.	T	F	DK

Correct answers: 1, 2, 4, 6, and 8 are false; 3, 5, 7, 9, 10, 11, and 12 are true.

From Weinrich, S. P., Weinrich, M. C., Boyd, M. D., Johnson, E., & Frank-Stromberg, M. (1992). Knowledge of colorectal cancer among older persons. *Cancer Nursing, 15*(5), 322–330.

37

Cardiac Diet and Exercise Self-Efficacy Instruments: Cardiac Diet Self-Efficacy Instrument and Cardiac Exercise Self-Efficacy Instrument

Developed by Mairead L. Hickey, Steven V. Owen, and Robin D. Froman

INSTRUMENT DESCRIPTION, ADMINISTRATION, AND SCORING GUIDELINES

Inactivity and improper diet are two frequent and modifiable cardiac risk factors. These instruments measure an important predictor of behavior—an individual's perceived self-efficacy to carry out that specific behavior. The authors suggest that mean score rather than a sum be used in calculating overall scores (Hickey, Owen, & Froman, 1992).

PSYCHOMETRIC PROPERTIES

Content validity was supported by a process of domain identification, item generation, and instrument formation (Hickey et al., 1992). Conceptual definitions of cardiac diet self-efficacy and cardiac exercise self-efficacy were developed and reviewed by 10 experts in cardiac rehabilitation and self-efficacy, defined as the confidence individuals ascribe to these behaviors within a variety of contexts. Experts rated how well items that had been generated fit within each subdimension and were retained based on the judgment of their fit. Ten cardiac rehabilitation participants reviewed the scales for readability and item format. Three hundred seventy participants in outpatient cardiac rehabilitation programs and 109 marathon runners provided data, the latter to study known groups' construct validity. Based on the important influence of past experience, individuals who have been successful with a specific behavior are more confident about their future ability to perform the behavior. An additional 101 participants in cardiac rehabilitation programs provided information for study of the relationship between diet and exercise self-efficacy, and subsequent diet and exercise goal attainment (predictive validity).

Factor analysis for the Cardiac Diet Self-Efficacy Instrument (CDSEI) supported its sampling one general construct. Mean item scores ranged from 3.49 to 4.44 (where 5 = quite a lot), suggesting that these subjects were generally confident about their ability to perform the cardiac diet behaviors listed on the CDSEI. Marathon runners were more confident about their diet behaviors than were cardiac rehabilitation program participants, and significant positive relationship was found between the diet self-efficacy levels of the cardiac rehabilitation program participants and their subsequent diet goal attainment.

Factor analysis for the Cardiac Exercise Self-Efficacy Instrument (CESEI) suggested that it drew from one construct. Mean item scores of the CESEI ranged from 3.47 to 4.61; this sample was also confident about performing each of the behaviors in the CESEI. The marathon runners reported significantly higher exercise self-efficacy than did cardiac rehabilitation program participants, and participants' mean CESEI scores correlated significantly with subsequent exercise goal attainment. For both instruments, those more highly confident attained more of their diet and exercise goals than did those who were less self-confident.

Both instruments had α coefficients of .90 and test-retest reliability (3 days apart) of .86 for CDSEI and .87 for CESEI.

CRITIQUE AND SUMMARY

The findings cannot be generalized to cardiac patients who do not enter rehabilitation programs. The validity and reliability data reported support experimental use of these two instruments in cardiac rehabilitation programs. The authors suggest that future research be conducted with other samples to confirm the factor structures found to date (Hickey et al., 1992). Evidence of changes in self-efficacy from properly designed interventions would also be helpful. These instruments have been developed with a careful and well described process.

REFERENCE

Hickey, M. L., Owen, S. V., & Froman, R. D. (1992). Instrument development: Cardiac diet and exercise self-efficacy. *Nursing Research, 41*, 347–351.

SCORING INSTRUCTIONS FOR CDSEI AND CESEI

In calculating overall CDSEI and CESEI scores, we prefer calculating a mean rather than a sum. With missing data (e.g., omitted items), a sum score is incorrect; the mean considers missing data without penalizing the respondent. Also, the mean score is in the original metric of the scale, so there is a simple frame of reference for interpreting scores.

Users may wish to change the questionnaire instructions to best fit your application. For example, if you need informed consent, you might say something like ''Filling out this questionnaire is completely voluntary and confidential. There are no penalties for not participating, and you may quit at any time.''

CARDIAC EXERCISE SELF-EFFICACY INSTRUMENT

Beside each item below, please circle the number that represents how much confidence you have about performing it.

1	2	3	4	5
Very Little		Confidence		Quite a Lot

1 2 3 4 5   1. ''Warming up'' before exercise.

1 2 3 4 5   2. Exercising without getting chest pain.

1 2 3 4 5   3. Knowing when I have exercised too much and need to stop.

1 2 3 4 5   4. Exercising when it is inconvenient.

1 2 3 4 5   5. Knowing what my heart rate should be before and after exercise.

1 2 3 4 5   6. ''Cooling down'' after exercise.

1 2 3 4 5   7. Fitting exercise into a busy day.

1 2 3 4 5   8. Enduring strenuous exercise.

1 2 3 4 5   9. Knowing what exercise is healthy for me.

1 2 3 4 5   10. Knowing when I can increase my exercise level.

1 2 3 4 5   11. Enduring moderate exercise.

1 2 3 4 5   12. Taking my heart rate before and after exercise.

1 2 3 4 5   13. Resuming my pre-hospital level of activity.

1 2 3 4 5   14. Enduring light exercise.

1 2 3 4 5   15. Exercising for at least twenty minutes three times each week.

1 2 3 4 5   16. Exercising at home by myself.

CARDIAC DIET SELF-EFFICACY INSTRUMENT

Beside each item below, please circle how much confidence you have about performing it.

1	2	3	4	5

Very Little   Confidence   Quite a Lot

1 2 3 4 5   1. Reaching my ideal weight by eating healthy food.

1 2 3 4 5   2. Decreasing the amount of fat and cholesterol in my diet.

1 2 3 4 5   3. Staying on a healthy diet when I am busy or in a rush.

1 2 3 4 5   4. Staying on a healthy diet when no one at home is on it.

1 2 3 4 5   5. Staying on a healthy diet when I eat at a restaurant.

1 2 3 4 5   6. Staying on a healthy diet when I am not at home to eat.

1 2 3 4 5   7. Staying on a healthy diet on special occasions or holidays.

1 2 3 4 5   8. Knowing what foods I should eat on a healthy diet.

1 2 3 4 5   9. Cutting out unhealthy snacks during the day or evening.

1 2 3 4 5   10. Increasing the amount of fiber and vegetables in my diet.

1 2 3 4 5   11. Staying at my ideal weight once I have reached it.

1 2 3 4 5   12. Knowing how to cook healthy meals.

1 2 3 4 5   13. Preparing a healthy meal for myself when I eat alone.

1 2 3 4 5   14. Limiting the number of egg yolks I eat in a week.

1 2 3 4 5   15. Knowing what food to buy at the store.

1 2 3 4 5   16. Decreasing the amount of sugar and sweets in my diet.

38

Knowledge Inventory:
A Measure of Knowledge
of Important Factors
in Cardiac Rehabilitation

**Developed by Pamela McHugh Schuster,
Cynthia Wright, and Patricia Tomich**

INSTRUMENT DESCRIPTION, ADMINISTRATION,
AND SCORING GUIDELINES

Patients in need of cardiac rehabilitation may elect to participate in structured programs (20%) or more likely be given information on home rehabilitation programs that can be performed independently on discharge. Patients are also given reading materials and exercise instructions. It is well known that knowledge is one of the several elements necessary for successfully accomplishing self-care and lifestyle behavioral changes necessary for rehabilitation. The Knowledge Inventory was used in a study comparing the outcomes of structured and home rehabilitation programs. It assesses the patient's knowledge of heart disease, bypass surgery, diagnostic tests, exercise guidelines, smoking, nutrition, medications, and stress. Scores range from 0 to 50 with 50 indicating greatest knowledge (Schuster, Wright, & Tomich, 1995).

PSYCHOMETRIC PROPERTIES

Sixty-four patients who had coronary bypass surgery at a single Ohio medical center were studied. All but one were White. The test was reviewed for clarity, content, and face validity by 10 cardiac rehabilitation professionals (nurses and exercise physiologists) and administered to 10 rehabilitation patients to establish its clarity, adequacy, and freedom from bias. It was pilot tested on 54 hospitalized and outpatient cardiac patients before being used in the study. Internal consistency measured at .84. Findings of the study showed that males but not females in structured cardiac rehabilitation programs showed increased knowledge. Mean scores for males and females in home and in structured rehabilitation programs ranged from 28 to 39 as long as 6 months postprogram; further breakdown in scores may be found in Schuster et al. (1995). The authors describe the Knowledge Inventory as a criterion-referenced mastery test, which means that each learner should attain a certain score level to be successful.

CRITIQUE AND SUMMARY

Further details or an independent assessment of content validity are needed. Although the domains indicated are those commonly included in cardiac rehabilitation programs, it is not clear whether judges including patients explicitly concurred that the items adequately represent these domains and whether other domains are important. Testing on a larger and more diverse population of patients is necessary, as is further evidence of sensitivity of the inventory to instruction. Because adequate cardiac rehabilitation is the desired outcome goal, the ability of the inventory and other measures, such as self-efficacy and -care practices to predict rehabilitation is an essential step. It is particularly essential in selecting the criterion score on the Knowledge Inventory that should be reached with or without instruction. No such score could be located in the report of development and use of this instrument.

REFERENCE

Schuster, P. M., Wright, C., & Tomich, P. (1995). Gender differences in the outcomes of participants in home programs compared to those in structured cardiac rehabilitation programs. *Rehabilitation Nursing, 20,* 93–101.

KNOWLEDGE INVENTORY

1.   The function of the coronary arteries is to

    Ⓐ.   supply the heart muscle with blood and oxygen.
    B.   connect the heart to the lungs.
    C.   maintain an even rate of the heart.
    D.   circulate blood to the rest of the body.
    E.   Don't know

2.   Atherosclerosis is

    A.   chest pain not relieved by medication.
    B.   a clot in the coronary artery.
    Ⓒ.   a build-up of cholesterol and other materials inside the arteries.
    D.   an inflammation around the sac covering the heart.
    E.   Don't know

3.   A heart attack means the heart

    A.   has a hole in it.
    Ⓑ.   has been damaged.
    C.   has been enlarged.
    D.   stops beating.
    E.   Don't know

4.   Angina or chest pain is caused by

    A.   a muscle spasm of the chest.
    B.   a blood clot in the lungs.
    C.   leaking of blood around the heart.
    Ⓓ.   lack of oxygen to the heart muscle.
    E.   Don't know

5.   A heart attack usually begins with

    A.   nausea.
    Ⓑ.   chest discomfort.
    C.   palpitations.
    D.   dizziness.
    E.   Don't know

6.   If the incision (in your chest) from cardiac surgery is draining a yellowish, thick, foul-smelling substance you should

    A.   cover it with a clean bandage and change it every day.
    B.   wash it with soap and water and place alcohol around the edge.
    Ⓒ.   contact your physician and follow his instructions.

D.   leave it open to the air so it can heal faster.
E.   Don't know

7.   Which of the following situations will indicate the need to call your doctor

A.   weight gain of 1 1/2 pounds in one week.
B.   feeling of breathlessness when you run up the stairs.
C.   weight gain of 3–4 pounds overnight.
D.   increase of 15 beats of your resting heart rate during your exercise program.
E.   Don't know

8.   The purpose of coronary artery bypass surgery is to

A.   clean and open up the arteries in the heart.
B.   remove an artery from the leg.
C.   increase the amount of blood to the heart muscle.
D.   prevent blockages from developing in the heart's arteries.
E.   Don't know

9.   The healing of the breast bone (sternum) after cardiac surgery usually takes

A.   2 weeks.
B.   4–6 weeks.
C.   3 months.
D.   1 year.
E.   Don't know

10.   Which statement is TRUE about smoking?

A.   Cigarettes with filters and low tar are safe.
B.   Smoking decreases the heart rate.
C.   Smoking decreases the amount of oxygen to the heart.
D.   Men's hearts are more affected by smoking than women's hearts.
E.   Don't know

11.   Which statement about nicotine in cigarettes is TRUE?

A.   It is non-addictive.
B.   It lowers blood pressure.
C.   It raises heart rate.
D.   It lowers pulse rate.
E.   Don't know

12.   Once you stop smoking, how long before your risk of smoking is reduced to that of a non-smoker?

A.   1 year
B.   5 years
C.   10 years
D.   Never
E.   Don't know

13.   The amount of salt intake is directly related to INCREASED

A.   appetite.

B.   chest pain.
C.   heart rate.
Ⓓ.   water retention.
E.   Don't know

14. An increase of which food items is strongly recommended after a heart attack?

A.   Citrus fruits.
B.   Red meats.
C.   Yellow vegetables.
Ⓓ.   High fiber foods.
E.   Don't know

15. Which sandwich has the highest amount of cholesterol?

A.   A hot dog sandwich.
Ⓑ.   An egg sandwich.
C.   A sardine sandwich.
D.   A peanut butter sandwich.
E.   Don't know

16. The appropriate selection of an entree at a restaurant would be

Ⓐ.   broiled fish.
B.   fried chicken.
C.   steamed liver.
D.   a western omelet.
E.   Don't know

17. Which practice would be useful to lower blood cholesterol?

A.   Increase fiber in food.
Ⓑ.   Reduce saturated fat intake.
C.   Weight reduction.
D.   Decrease salt intake.
E.   Don't know

18. How many calories must be eliminated to loose one pound?

A.   500
B.   1,000
C.   1,500
Ⓓ.   3,500
E.   Don't know

19. The medication commonly prescribed for the relief of chest pain (angina) is

A.   lasix.
B.   lanoxin.
Ⓒ.   nitroglycerin.
D.   quinidine.
E.   Don't know

20.   If you are experiencing chest pain (angina) and have a prescription for nitroglycerine, the total number of tablets you may take before going to the hospital is

    A.   one.
    B.   two.
    C.   three.
    D.   four.
    E.   Don't know

21.   You took three nitroglycerin tablets as prescribed. The chest pain is NOT relieved. You should

    A.   go to the emergency room.
    B.   take two tablets at once and wait 20 minutes.
    C.   lay down for the rest of the day.
    D.   take an antacid.
    E.   Don't know

22.   You take a heart medication every eight hours at 8 am, 4 pm, and 12 midnight. This morning it is 10:30 am and you remember your 8 am dosage of medication. The best thing to do is

    A.   skip the 8 am dose and double the 4 pm dosage.
    B.   take half the dose at the time you remembered it and take the full dose at 4 pm and 12 midnight.
    C.   take this dose and delay the 4 pm dose about an hour and resume the normal schedule at 12 midnight.
    D.   skip the 8 am dose and just take the 4 pm and 12 midnight dose for that day.
    E.   Don't know

23.   The process of emotionally adjusting to heart disease in most people usually takes

    A.   1–6 months.
    B.   7–12 months.
    C.   2 years.
    D.   5 years.
    E.   Don't know

24.   You are in a traffic jam, and will probably be late for work. You would

    A.   find another route, and try to get there as soon as you can.
    B.   blow your horn, shout and try to get the traffic moving.
    C.   leave your car and find a ride to work.
    D.   realize that you will probably be late and practice some relaxation.
    E.   Don't know

25.   A recommended method of relaxation for the person with heart disease is to

    A.   tighten the muscle of your extremities for 15 seconds and relax them for 5 seconds.
    B.   breathe shallow and rapidly for 30 seconds.
    C.   take a deep breath and hold it for 10 seconds.
    D.   inhale slowly through your nose and exhale slowly through your mouth.
    E.   Don't know

26. Continued prolonged stress on the body may result in

    A.   reduced blood pressure.
    B.   high energy levels.
    C.   increased exercise endurance.
    Ⓓ.   high blood pressure.
    E.   Don't know

27. In order to develop and maintain fitness, what is the minimum number of days per week exercise should be done?

    A.   One.
    B.   Two.
    Ⓒ.   Three.
    D.   Four.
    E.   Don't know

28. Which of these factors is LEAST important to an exercise prescription?

    A.   Current fitness level.
    B.   Intensity and duration of exercise.
    C.   Frequency and type of exercise.
    Ⓓ.   Body composition.
    E.   Don't know

29. In general, as the intensity of exercise INCREASES

    A.   blood pressure decreases.
    B.   breathing rate decreases.
    Ⓒ.   heart rate increases.
    D.   pulse rate decreases.
    E.   Don't know

30. In order to maintain fitness, the length of each exercise session (not counting warm-up and cool-down periods)

    A.   should be 5–10 minutes each session.
    Ⓑ.   should be 15–60 minutes each session.
    C.   should be 65–70 minutes each session.
    D.   should be 75–80 minutes each session.
    E.   Don't know

31. Warm-up before exercise is important because it

    Ⓐ.   prevents injury to muscles.
    B.   extends the exercise time period.
    C.   reduces body fat.
    D.   builds muscle strength.
    E.   Don't know

32. The cool-down phase

    A.   increases blood pressure.
    Ⓑ.   decreases heart rate gradually.
    C.   increases the chance of skipped heart beats.

D.   decreases the chance of having a heart attack.
E.   Don't know

33.   What action should be taken when symptoms occur during exercise (chest discomfort, shortness of breath)?

A.   Heart rate should be kept in the heart rate range.
B.   The heart rate can be exceeded.
C.   The exercise should be gradually discontinued.
D.   Exercise can be done even if symptoms occur.
E.   Don't know

34.   All of the following symptoms indicate that the intensity of exercise should be decreased except

A.   Chest discomfort.
B.   Skipped heart beats.
C.   Flushed skin color.
D.   Shortness of breath.
E.   Don't know

35.   You have just finished your exercise program. You are beginning to cool down and your heart rate is 15 beats above your resting heart rate. You should

A.   complete your cool-down exercises and stretches and recheck your pulse.
B.   skip cool-down activities and relax the rest of the day.
C.   reduce the time of cool down to two minutes.
D.   resume your exercise program.
E.   Don't know

36.   After your exercise program it is acceptable to feel

A.   pleasantly tired.
B.   chest tightness and heaviness.
C.   your heart racing.
D.   dizzy and sweating.
E.   Don't know

37.   The temperature outside is "0" F, and there is a heavy wind. The doctor has instructed you to walk 30 minutes per day. You should

A.   cancel the walk for that day.
B.   walk only half the recommended distance.
C.   walk indoors.
D.   call the doctor for instructions.
E.   Don't know

38.   After a heart attack, sexual intercourse with your usual partner generally can be safely resumed how long after discharge from the hospital?

A.   Immediately.
B.   2–4 weeks.
C.   3 months.
D.   Never again.
E.   Don't know

39. After bypass surgery, sexual intercourse with your usual partner generally can be safely resumed how long after discharge from the hospital?

 A. Immediately.
 B. 2–4 weeks.
 C. 3 months.
 D. Never again.
 E. Don't know

40. When should the pulse rate be counted?

 A. Before and after each activity.
 B. Before and during each activity.
 C. During and after each activity.
 D. Before, during, and after each activity.
 E. Don't know

41. Which of the following is the BEST way to check the pulse during exercise?

 A. Count the pulse for 10 seconds and multiply the number by 6.
 B. Count the pulse for 60 seconds.
 C. There is no need to count the pulse because the pulse rate does not have to be checked during exercise.
 D. Count the pulse for 15 seconds and multiply the number by 4.
 E. Don't know

42. What are the three major risk factors associated with the development of coronary artery disease that can be controlled?

 A. Smoking, high blood pressure, cholesterol
 B. High blood pressure, age, stress
 C. Heredity, cholesterol, stress
 D. Obesity, diabetes, sex
 E. Don't know

43. A heart catheterization is a diagnostic test that

 A. measures the size of the heart.
 B. records the electrical activity of the heart.
 C. visualizes the blood vessels and chambers of the heart.
 D. calculates the strength of the heart.
 E. Don't know

44. An electrocardiogram (EKG) is a test that

 A. looks the same for everyone.
 B. records the electrical impulses generated by the heart.
 C. is rarely done since new tests have become available.
 D. uses sound waves to outline the chambers of the heart.
 E. Don't know

45. Which statement is true about a stress test (exercise test)?

 A. It determines the extent of blockage of the coronary arteries.
 B. It measures the size of the chest.

      C.   It provides very little information about the heart.
      Ⓓ.   It determines how much work the heart can safely do.
      E.   Don't know

Correct answer circled.

46.   What are the risk factors that you believe influenced your development of heart disease?
       Circle those that apply to you.

        don't know
        high blood pressure   lack of exercise   smoking
        high cholesterol   stress   heredity
        overweight   diabetes   age

47.   What is the highest heart rate (maximum heart rate) that you should not go above
       WHILE EXERCISING?

       _____ beats per minute

       _____ don't know

48.   What is the lowest heart rate (minimum heart rate) that you should not go below
       WHILE EXERCISING?

       _____ beats per minute

       _____ don't know

49.   What is your (average) resting heart rate?

       _____ beats per minute

       _____ don't know

50.   List your medications and what they are for.

1. example: Nitroglycerine for chest discomfort
_____

2. _____

3. _____

4. _____

5. _____

Answers are individualized, based on patient paramenters.

39

Caretaker and Adolescent Confidence in Managing Cystic Fibrosis

Developed by L. Kay Bartholomew, Guy S. Parcel, Paul R. Swank, and Danita I. Czyzewski

INSTRUMENT DESCRIPTION, ADMINISTRATION, AND SCORING GUIDELINES

Self-management refers to the behaviors that patients and family members perform to lessen the impact of a chronic illness. It is different from strict compliance to medical regimens in that it includes the complex cognitive-behavioral skills of self-monitoring, decision making, and communicating about both symptoms and treatment regimens. Behaviors required for cystic fibrosis (CF) self-management are especially complex because the health care of a child with this disease is usually intensive, even when the child is doing well, and includes chest physical therapy and respiratory therapy, diet, and medication. Enhancing self-efficacy (SE) through education may be critical to learning and performing CF home care routines because even good self-management may not be followed by noticeable improvement of physical symptoms or health status, and thus may not be reinforced over long periods (Bartholomew, Parcel, Swank, & Czyzewski, 1993). These instruments test confidence (SE) for adolescents and caretakers, in managing cystic fibrosis.

The instrument has a 6th-grade reading level. Scoring is by summing item scores, with the outcomes scores separate (Bartholomew et al., 1993). Scores were not available in published sources.

PSYCHOMETRIC PROPERTIES

Items for the instrument were sampled from 150 self-management performance objectives for CF that represented eight domains of care including aspects of medical care, coping, and communication (Bartholomew et al., 1993). Ratings by a panel of experts and a survey of CF center directors provided evidence for agreement from the practice community that the objectives were important for self-management of CF. This evidence supports content validity.

After pilot work, the instruments were administered to members of 199 families (patients and their primary caretakers) from two CF centers. Twelve of the patients were African-American. Factor analysis yielded solutions reflecting five theorized aspects of self-management for the caretaker instrument: medical judgment and communication, coping, communication, compliance, and acceptance of CF. Cronbach's αs ranged from .73 to .88. Four factors were found for the adolescent SE instrument: communication with the health care team, acceptance and coping, medical judgment and communication, and medical treatment. Moderate correlations between factors justify their use as subscales representing related yet conceptually consistent domains of SE. Test-retest reliability was not performed because SE is not expected to be a stable trait (Bartholomew et al., 1993).

Both the caretaker version and the adolescent version also include items on outcome expectations that are beliefs about the effect of self-management on the patient's disease process and quality of life. Expectations for positive outcomes from carrying out these activities should also predict self-management behaviors. Results showed that at low levels of outcome expectations, SE was not strongly related to self-management. Cronbach's α coefficients of internal consistency for these items was .84 for the caretaker instrument and .75 for the adolescent instrument.

SE contributed significantly to the prediction of self-management on the part of both caretakers and adolescents with CF, providing evidence of criterion validity (Bartholomew et al., 1993).

CRITIQUE AND SUMMARY

Content validity should also be supported by patient experts. In addition, both socioeconomic status and education were high for those in the pilot study. The authors suggest that these instruments can be used to assess educational needs of CF patient caretakers and of the adolescent patients themselves. Interventions can be targeted toward behaviors with the lowest SE scores. The instruments can also be used to monitor over time patients' and caretakers' progress toward becoming confident in their ability and to evaluate the effectiveness of educational interventions designed to increase behavioral capability and SE for CF self-management. Studies documenting the usefulness of these instruments for these purposes should be completed. Evidence that changes in SE can lead to improvements in self-management of CF would be important.

REFERENCE

Bartholomew, L. K., Parcel, G. S., Swank, P. R., & Czyzewski, D. I. (1993). Measuring self-efficacy expectations for the self-management of cystic fibrosis. *Chest, 103,* 1524–1530.

ADOLESCENT CONFIDENCE IN MANAGING CYSTIC FIBROSIS - SCALE D

We are interested in how sure you feel that you can do things to manage your cystic fibrosis. Please circle the answer that comes closest to describing how sure you feel. Your first reaction to each question should be your answer. Please answer all questions.

In general in your everyday life—How sure are you that you can do the following?	Not Sure at All	A Little Sure	Fairly Sure	Mostly Sure	Very Sure
1. Notice changes in cough, sputum, and shortness of breath that might indicate a lower respiratory infection	1	2	3	4	5
2. Tell when symptoms (for example, coughing, weight loss, and changes in sputum) mean that you have developed a lower respiratory infection	1	2	3	4	5
3. Do chest PT (clapping) the number of times a day that your doctor suggests	1	2	3	4	5
4. Perform breathing treatments (respiratory therapy) as many times a day as your doctor suggests	1	2	3	4	5
5. Watch for signs of changes in your digestion (for example, observe stools and observe for bloating)	1	2	3	4	5
6. Take enzymes when food is eaten	1	2	3	4	5
7. Notice when you are losing weight	1	2	3	4	5
8. Notice whether or not you have a good appetite and are eating enough	1	2	3	4	5
9. Take antibiotics as prescribed	1	2	3	4	5
10. Perform chest PT (clapping) the way you were shown	1	2	3	4	5
11. Tell the difference between poor digestion due to cystic fibrosis and poor digestion due to other stomach problems (such as a "stomach virus" or "flu")	1	2	3	4	5
12. Eat enough high calorie foods (get enough calories)	1	2	3	4	5
13. Correctly perform breathing treatments (for example, measuring and drawing up medication)	1	2	3	4	5
14. Take the right amount of enzymes for the amount and type of food eaten	1	2	3	4	5

In general in your everyday life—How sure are you that you can do the following?	Not Sure at All	A Little Sure	Fairly Sure	Mostly Sure	Very Sure
15. Notice changes in your appetite and weight that might indicate a lower respiratory infection	1	2	3	4	5
16. Accept cystic fibrosis as your diagnosis (acknowledge the effects that cystic fibrosis will have on your life)	1	2	3	4	5
17. Accept that cystic fibrosis may present new problems to you and your family at any time	1	2	3	4	5
18. Accept that cystic fibrosis related problems will demand that you and your family make changes and adjustments	1	2	3	4	5
19. Identify what problems in your life are causing you to be stressed	1	2	3	4	5
20. Notice signs that you are becoming too stressed or not coping with stress well	1	2	3	4	5
21. Recognize when something is going to cause a problem for you or your family	1	2	3	4	5
22. *Figure out* several ways to solve a problem	1	2	3	4	5
23. *Figure out* several ways to make yourself feel better when you have a problem or are distressed	1	2	3	4	5
24. *Try* several ways of solving different problems	1	2	3	4	5
25. *Use* several methods to make yourself feel better when you have a problem or are distressed	1	2	3	4	5
26. Judge when a problem has been solved	1	2	3	4	5
27. Continue to try and solve a problem even after your first try at solving it has been unsuccessful	1	2	3	4	5
28. Decide what you need to talk about with your doctor or nurse	1	2	3	4	5
29. Decide which doctor or nurse to talk with	1	2	3	4	5
30. Ask your doctor or nurse clear questions	1	2	3	4	5
31. Ask other questions when you do not get an answer or do not understand an answer from your doctor or nurse	1	2	3	4	5
32. Use the right words when talking about your cystic fibrosis or describing symptoms to your doctor or nurse	1	2	3	4	5
33. Notice whether or not your doctor or nurse is understanding what you are saying	1	2	3	4	5

In general in your everyday life—How sure are you that you can do the following?	Not Sure at All	A Little Sure	Fairly Sure	Mostly Sure	Very Sure
34. Identify feelings in yourself that you wish to discuss with your doctor or nurse	1	2	3	4	5
35. Judge how your doctor or nurse will react when you talk about your feelings	1	2	3	4	5
36. Let your doctor or nurse know that you have understood what you have been told	1	2	3	4	5

Outcome Expectations

We are interested in how sure you feel that the following things you do to manage your cystic fibrosis will be helpful to your well-being. Please circle the answer that comes closest to describing how sure you feel that doing these things will delay the progression of cystic fibrosis, will improve how you feel, or will improve your quality of life. Your first reaction to each question should be your answer. Please answer all questions.

Regarding your well-being—How sure are you that the following will be helpful?	Not Sure at All	A Little Sure	Fairly Sure	Mostly Sure	Very Sure
37. Making sure that your lower respiratory infections are found early and treated	1	2	3	4	5
38. Performing breathing treatments the way your doctor has prescribed	1	2	3	4	5
39. Performing chest PT (clapping) the way your doctor has prescribed	1	2	3	4	5
40. Making sure that you eat enough food (get enough calories)	1	2	3	4	5
41. Making sure that you take the right amount of enzymes to control poor digestion	1	2	3	4	5
42. Communicating well with your doctor or nurse	1	2	3	4	5
43. Coping well with any problems caused by cystic fibrosis and its management	1	2	3	4	5
44. Making sure you engage in physical activities several times a week (for example, swimming, running, or bike riding)	1	2	3	4	5

CARETAKER CONFIDENCE IN MANAGING
CYSTIC FIBROSIS - SCALE A

We are interested in how sure you feel that *you* can do things to manage your child's cystic fibrosis. Please circle the answer that comes closest to describing how sure you feel. Your first reaction to each question should be your answer. Please answer all questions.

In general in your everyday life—How sure are you that *you* can do the following?	Not Sure at All	A Little Sure	Fairly Sure	Mostly Sure	Very Sure
1. Accept that cystic fibrosis may present new problems to your family at any time	1	2	3	4	5
2. Ask other questions when you do not get an answer or do not understand an answer from your child's doctor or nurse	1	2	3	4	5
3. Do chest PT (clapping) the number of times a day that your doctor suggests	1	2	3	4	5
4. Perform breathing treatments (respiratory therapy) as many times a day as your doctor suggests	1	2	3	4	5
5. Accept that cystic fibrosis related problems will demand that you and your family make changes and adjustments	1	2	3	4	5
6. Let your child know that you have understood what he or she has told you	1	2	3	4	5
7. Talk to your child about your feelings	1	2	3	4	5
8. Judge how your child will react when you talk about your feelings	1	2	3	4	5
9. Identify feelings in yourself that you wish to discuss with your child's doctor or nurse	1	2	3	4	5
10. *Figure out* several ways to make yourself feel better when you have a problem or are distressed	1	2	3	4	5
11. Accept cystic fibrosis as your child's diagnosis (acknowledge the effects that cystic fibrosis will have on your child's life)	1	2	3	4	5
12. Decide what you need to talk about with your child's doctor or nurse	1	2	3	4	5
13. Notice changes in cough, sputum, and shortness of breath that might indicate a lower respiratory infection in your child	1	2	3	4	5

In general in your everyday life—How sure are you that *you* can do the following?	Not Sure at All	A Little Sure	Fairly Sure	Mostly Sure	Very Sure
14. Use the right words when talking about your child's cystic fibrosis or describing symptoms to your child's doctor or nurse	1	2	3	4	5
15. Judge when a problem has been solved	1	2	3	4	5
16. Correctly perform breathing treatments (for example, measuring and drawing up medication)	1	2	3	4	5
17. Notice whether or not your child's doctor or nurse is understanding what you are saying	1	2	3	4	5
18. *Use* several methods to make yourself feel better when you have a problem or are distressed	1	2	3	4	5
19. Tell when symptoms (for example, coughing, weight loss, and changes in sputum) mean that your child has developed a lower respiratory infection	1	2	3	4	5
20. Perform chest PT (clapping) the way you were shown	1	2	3	4	5
21. Notice signs that you are becoming too stressed or not coping with stress well	1	2	3	4	5

Outcome Expectations

We are interested in how sure you feel that the following things you do to manage your child's cystic fibrosis will be helpful to your child's well-being. Please circle the answer that comes closest to describing how sure you feel that doing these things will delay the progression of cystic fibrosis, will improve how your child feels, or will improve your child's quality of life. Your first reaction to each question should be your answer. Please answer all questions.

Regarding your child's well-being—How sure are you that the following will be helpful?	Not Sure at All	A Little Sure	Fairly Sure	Mostly Sure	Very Sure
22. Making sure that your child's lower respiratory infections are found early and treated	1	2	3	4	5
23. Performing breathing treatments the way your doctor has prescribed	1	2	3	4	5
24. Performing chest PT (clapping) the way your doctor has prescribed	1	2	3	4	5
25. Making sure that your child eats enough food (gets enough calories)	1	2	3	4	5

In general in your everyday life—How sure are you that *you* can do the following?	Not Sure at All	A Little Sure	Fairly Sure	Mostly Sure	Very Sure
26. Making sure that your child takes the right amount of enzymes to control poor digestion	1	2	3	4	5
27. Communicating well with your child's doctor or nurse	1	2	3	4	5
28. Coping well with any problems caused by cystic fibrosis and its management	1	2	3	4	5
29. Making sure your child engages in physical activities several times a week (for example, swimming, running, or bike riding)	1	2	3	4	5

40

Kidney Disease Questionnaire

Developed by Gerald M. Devins, Yitzchak M. Binik, Henry Mandin, P. K. Letourneau, David J. Hollomby, Paul E. Barre, and Sara Prichard

INSTRUMENT DESCRIPTION, ADMINISTRATION, AND SCORING GUIDELINES

The Kidney Disease Questionnaire (KDQ) is a measure of patient knowledge about end-stage renal disease and its treatment. The KDQ is available in a 26-item version or as two parallel 13-item tests. Parallel forms exist to facilitate retesting, for example, for the evaluation of knowledge gains subsequent to educational interventions. Readability level is grade 9. Scoring guidelines may be found in the footnote at the end of the KDQ (Devins et al., 1990).

PSYCHOMETRIC PROPERTIES

A pool of items was developed in consultation with nephrology nurses and physicians, related to domains thought to be relevant and including normal kidney function, kidney diseases, and current treatment options including maintenance hemodialysis, peritoneal dialysis, and renal transplantation. The items were administered to groups expected to differ in end-stage renal disease (ESRD)-relevant knowledge: dialysis nurses, ESRD patients, and undergraduate psychology students. Item analysis was subsequently performed to select a subset of 25 items that maximized discrimination among the groups. The test also differentiated patients thought to be well informed from those deemed not to be and reflected the fact that patients know more about their own particular treatment modalities than about others with which they are less familiar. These findings are supportive of validity. Cronbach's coefficient α for the final 26-item test was .94; for Form A, .75; and for Form B, .85. Detailed explanation of procedures followed may be found in Devins et al. (1990).

A second study of 270 patients showed that those who received an enhanced education intervention showed a significant increase in KDQ scores, whereas those who received a standard education intervention did not show an increase, with a similar effect related to starting dialysis.

These findings indicate sensitivity of the test to the enhanced educational intervention. Although the test is also available in French, limited data are available about its psychometric adequacy (Devins et al., 1990).

CRITIQUE AND SUMMARY

Patients were not involved in the definition of important domains of knowledge. Since the reading level may be difficult for patients who do not have the equivalent of a high school diploma, the authors recommend that the KDQ be administered to these patients by a health professional familiar with kidney disease. No scores on the KDQ from the tested population could be located.

The availability of parallel forms is useful for those who wish to conduct repeated assessments of illness knowledge as in evaluating the benefits of education. The full 26-item test can be used for a single testing because its reliability is somewhat higher (Devins et al., 1993).

The KDQ has also been used in a study of education provided to patients with chronic deteriorating kidney disease, before the usual time of education at initiation of renal replacement therapy. Compared with a control group receiving the usual education in the clinical setting, those receiving an enhanced educational program showed significantly higher difference scores (preeducation to posteducation). Interestingly, this group on average survived 4.6 months longer without requiring the initiation of renal replacement therapy. The potential mediating mechanisms are not known (Binik et al., 1993).

REFERENCES

Binik, Y. M., Devins, G. M., Mandin, H., Letourneau, P. K., Hollomby, D. J., Barre, P. E., & Prichard, S. (1993). Live and learn: Patient education delays the need to initiate renal replacement therapy in end-stage renal disease. *Journal of Nervous and Mental Disease, 181,* 371–376.

Devins, G. M., Binik, Y. M., Mandin, H., Letourneau, P. K., Hollomby, D. J., Barre, P. E., & Prichard, S. (1990). The Kidney Disease Questionnaire: A test for measuring patient knowledge about end-stage renal disease. *Journal of Clinical Epidemiology, 43,* 297–307.

KIDNEY DISEASE QUESTIONNAIRE—FORM A*

1. (1)   People normally have two kidneys in the body.
    (a)   True
    (b)   False
    (c)   Don't know

2. (5)   When a person has kidney disease, his kidneys must be removed from his body before he can get treatment with a dialysis machine.
    (a)   True
    (b)   False
    (c)   Don't know

3. (3)   Kidneys do many important things in the body, but they function only at night while the person is sleeping.
    (a)   True
    (b)   False
    (c)   Don't know

4. (25)   What is the term used to describe the vibration or buzzing sensation that can be felt over the vein of a shunt or fistula?
    (a)   Hypoplasia
    (b)   Lobulation
    (c)   Enervation
    (d)   Thrill or bruit
    (e)   Don't know

5. (11)   In CAPD, waste substances pass from the blood, across the peritoneal membrane and into the dialysate fluid by a process called:
    (a)   Diffusion
    (b)   Transport
    (c)   Excretion
    (d)   Chemical breakdown
    (e)   Don't know

6. (17)   In addition to removing wastes from the blood, the artificial kidney also functions to remove excess water from the blood. This water-removal process is called:
    (a)   Ultra-filtration
    (b)   Ultra-refraction
    (c)   Osmosis
    (d)   Catharsis
    (e)   Don't know

7. (9)   A patient with kidney disease can experience high blood pressure, swelling and rapid weight gain when his body becomes overloaded with:
    (a)   Protein
    (b)   Urea
    (c)   Water
    (d)   Don't know

8. (7)   Which one of these foods has a lot of potassium?
    (a)   Rice
    (b)   Ice cream

(c)   Bananas
(d)   Don't know

9. (15)   Approximately how many times a week do hemodialysis patients usually have their sessions on the kidney dialysis machine?
(a)   1
(b)   3
(c)   6
(d)   Don't know

10. (14)   A patient with chronic kidney disease may have a living relative who wants to donate a kidney to the patient for transplantation. Which one of the following items about the donor is FALSE?
(a)   The donor will have to undergo a series of medical tests before the transplant operation.
(b)   The donor runs very little risk to his own health when he donates one kidney.
(c)   The donor will need to take immunosuppressive drugs for life.
(d)   After the transplant operation the donor's remaining kidney will enlarge in size.
(e)   Don't know

11. (18)   Which one of the following items about kidney transplantation is FALSE?
(a)   Sometimes a transplanted kidney will begin to function as soon as the blood vessels are connected on the operating table.
(b)   Kidney transplants are placed in the patient's pelvis rather than in the usual kidney location.
(c)   A person who has recovered from transplant surgery and has a new well-functioning kidney will no longer need dialysis treatment.
(d)   A patient can receive a kidney from a living relative but the donor's kidney must be removed one week before the transplant for close observation.
(e)   Don't know

12. (20)   CAPD is a form of dialysis treatment which is used as an alternative to hemodialysis. One *advantage* of CAPD is that:
(a)   It allows the patient to walk about freely during the course of treatment.
(b)   It only needs to be performed once a week.
(c)   It does not involve any preparatory surgical procedure.
(d)   It makes it easier for the patient to bathe and swim.
(e)   Don't know

13. (23)   Patients with chronic kidney disease are advised to eat limited quantities of potassium-rich foods. Elevated potassium levels in the blood is dangerous because:
(a)   It can cause fluid overload.
(b)   It can raise the patient's hematocrit.
(c)   It can decrease the production of white blood cells.
(d)   It can cause the heart to beat irregularly and even stop.
(e)   Don't know

KIDNEY DISEASE QUESTIONNAIRE—FORM B[†]

1. (2)   Kidney disease is a problem that comes with old age—young people do not get this disease.
   (a)   True
   (b)   False
   (c)   Don't know

2. (4)   Most types of kidney disease last about 5 years. After this the kidneys start to work normally again.
   (a)   True
   (b)   False
   (c)   Don't know

3. (6)   Peritonitis, an infection of the abdominal cavity, is one of the major problems for patients on CAPD.
   (a)   True
   (b)   False
   (c)   Don't know

4.   Kidney transplantation is the best form of treatment for patients with kidney disease because after the transplant the patients are less likely to get infections from bacteria or virus.
   (a)   True
   (b)   False
   (c)   Don't know

5. (24)   There are about one million tiny filters in the human kidney. They are called:
   (a)   Ribosomes
   (b)   Ureters
   (c)   Glomeruli
   (d)   Organelles
   (e)   Don't know

6. (13)   In kidney failure, waste products in the blood build up to abnormal levels and this causes a condition called:
   (a)   Absorption
   (b)   Uremia
   (c)   Libido
   (d)   Adaptation
   (e)   Don't know

7. (16)   The artificial kidney is called:
   (a)   Henle's Loop
   (b)   Transferrin
   (c)   Bun
   (d)   Dialyzer
   (e)   Don't know

8. (21)   A new type of dialysis for treating kidney disease is called CAPD. Which part of the body makes this type of dialysis possible?
   (a)   Peritoneum
   (b)   Bladder

(c)   Renal pelvis
(d)   Don't know

9. (8)   Patients with kidney disease are told not to eat salty foods because salt has a lot of:
(a)   Potassium
(b)   Sodium
(c)   Calcium
(d)   Don't know

10. (10)   Immunosuppressive drugs are given to transplant patients in order to:
(a)   Prevent and treat rejection of the kidney graft.
(b)   Treat blood clotting in the new kidney.
(c)   Prevent infection of the kidney by virus or bacteria.
(d)   Raise the patient's hematocrit.
(e)   Don't know

11. (19)   Bone disease is a medical problem that could result from chronic kidney disease. It can occur because:
(a)   The diseased kidney can no longer rid the body of excess water in a normal fashion.
(b)   The diseased kidney loses its ability to keep calcium and phosphate levels in the proper range in the body.
(c)   The diseased kidney loses its ability to excrete excess potassium from the bloodstream.
(d)   The body is no longer able to use protein foods.
(e)   Don't know

12. (12)   Which medication is sometimes prescribed to control the level of potassium in the patient's body?
(a)   Riopan
(b)   Kayexalate
(c)   Amphojel
(d)   Aldomet
(e)   Don't know

13. (22)   In the regular procedure for CAPD, dialysate fluid is introduced into the patient's abdominal cavity through an implanted tube just below the navel. The dialysate fluid is then:
(a)   Left inside the abdominal cavity for several hours and then drained out.
(b)   Left inside the abdominal cavity until it is completely absorbed into the body.
(c)   Transferred into an artificial kidney through another tube.
(d)   Transferred into an artificial kidney through the same tube.
(e)   Don't know

Note. Items that comprise the 25-item version of the KDQ, described in Study 1, are indicated in parentheses.
[*]Correct responses for Form A of the KDQ are as follows: item 1 (alternative A), 2 (B), 3 (B), 4 (D), 5 (A), 6 (A), 7 (C), 8 (C), 9 (B), 10 (C), 11 (D), 12 (A), 13 (D). Individual item scores (i.e., 0 vs 1) are summed to generate a total score which can, thus, range between 0 and 13.
[*]Correct responses for Form B of the KDQ are as follows: item 1 (alternative B), 2 (B), 3 (A), 4 (B), 5 (C), 6 (B), 7 (D), 8 (A), 9 (B), 10 (A), 11 (B), 12 (B), 13 (A). Individual item scores (i.e., 0 vs 1) are summed to generate a total score which can, thus, range between 0 and 13.

From Devins, G. M., Binik, Y. M., Mandin, H., Letourneau, P. K., Hollomby, D. J., Barre, P. E., & Prichard, S. (1990). The Kidney Disease Questionnaire: A test for measuring patient knowledge about end-stage renal disease. *Journal of Clinical Epidemiology, 43,* 297–307.

41

Endoscopy Confidence Questionnaire

Developed by Suzanne M. Gattuso, Mark D. Litt, and Terence E. Fitzgerald

INSTRUMENT DESCRIPTION, ADMINISTRATION, AND SCORING GUIDELINES

High levels of anxiety related to invasive medical and dental procedures have been associated with a variety of adverse effects including negative affective responses, prolonged and more difficult recoveries, and increased need for pain medication. These findings have prompted the development of numerous preparatory interventions designed to help patients cope with invasive and stressful procedures. It has been suggested that successful coping after preparatory interventions results from changes in certain cognitive mechanisms, such as perceived self-efficacy. Self-efficacy (one's confidence in her ability to behave in a particular way) is situation specific and thus likely to be a good predictor of behavior. Self-efficacy also appears to be manipulable and applicable to clinical intervention (Gattuso, Litt, & Fitzgerald, 1992).

The Endoscopy Confidence Questionnaire (ECQ) is a nine-item scale to assess patients' estimates of confidence in their ability to engage in six specific behaviors that contribute to successful coping with endoscopy. Scale score is an average of the ratings for the items; mean scores ranged from 3.8 to 4.8 preintervention and 4.5 to 4.9 postintervention (Gattuso et al., 1992).

PSYCHOMETRIC PROPERTIES

The ECQ was used in an intervention study with 48 male patients in a Veterans Administration Hospital. Internal reliability αs for the ECQ preintervention and postintervention were .90 and .92, respectively. Changes in self-efficacy judgments predicted changes in affective distress over the same period, and this effect was most pronounced after an intervention intended to raise self-efficacy. The ECQ was sensitive to this intervention (Gattuso et al., 1992).

SUMMARY AND CRITIQUE

There is little discussion of content validity for ECQ, although some evidence of construct validity, sensitivity to instruction, and adequate reliability. Additional testing of the ECQ with a broader population will be necessary.

REFERENCE

Gattuso, S. M., Litt, M. D., & Fitzgerald, T. E. (1992). Coping with gastrointestinal endoscopy: Self-efficacy enhancement and coping style. *Journal of Consulting and Clinical Psychology, 60,* 133—139.

ENDOSCOPY CONFIDENCE QUESTIONNAIRE (ECQ)

For each of the questions below, please *circle the number* which represents the best description of your feelings *right now:*

1. How confident are you that you can swallow the tube without difficulty during the upcoming examination?

1	2	3	4	5	6	7
Not at All Confident			Somewhat Confident			Very Confident

2. How confident are you that you can keep your body still during the examination?

1	2	3	4	5	6	7
Not at All Confident			Somewhat confident			Very Confident

3. How well do you think you can relax your body during the examination?

1	2	3	4	5	6	7
Not at All			Somewhat			Completely

4. How comfortable do you think you will be during the examination?

1	2	3	4	5	6	7
Not at All Comfortable			Somewhat Comfortable			Extremely Comfortable

5. How easily do you think you will swallow the tube during the examination?

1	2	3	4	5	6	7
Not at All Easy			Somewhat Easy			Extremely Easy

6. How much medication (sedative) do you think you will need to relax during the examination?

1	2	3	4	5	6	7
A Great Deal of Medication			Some Medication			No Medication

7. How confident are you that you can complete this examination without any medication to help you relax?

1	2	3	4	5	6	7
Not at All Confident			Somewhat Confident			Extremely Confident

8. How much time do you think the examination will take?

1	2	3	4	5	6	7
More Time than Usual			About the same Time as Usual			Less Time than Usual

9. Overall, how confident are you that you will get through the examination without any difficulty?

1	2	3	4	5	6	7
Not at All Confident			Somewhat Confident			Extremely Confident

42

Osteoporosis Health Belief, Self-Efficacy, and Knowledge Tests

Developed by Katherine K. Kim, Mary Horan, Phyllis Gendler, and Minu Patel

INSTRUMENT DESCRIPTION, ADMINISTRATION, AND SCORING GUIDELINES

This set of three instruments developed to measure important aspects of osteoporosis self-care is in early stages of development.

The Osteoporosis Health Belief Scale (OHBS) is based on the Health Belief Model (HBM) and especially designed to assess beliefs related to exercise and calcium intake in the elderly. Questions have a readability level of 5th grade. The revised OHBS, included here, is scored by awarding 1 for "strongly disagree" to 5 for "strongly agree." Because there are six items in each subscale, the possible score for each ranges from 6 to 30. The instrument can be administered in 20 minutes (Kim, Horan, Gendler, & Patel, 1991).

HBM elements include susceptibility (perceived risk of developing osteoporosis); seriousness (perception of threat from having osteoporosis including to physical health, role and social status, and ability to complete desired tasks); benefits (belief in the effectiveness of specific behaviors to prevent the occurrence of the disease); barriers (beliefs about the negative components of the behaviors that would be undertaken to prevent the disease); and health motivation (general tendency for an individual to engage in health behaviors). Self-efficacy (SE) is now also part of the model, which predicts that health behaviors are more likely to occur if an individual believes in personal susceptibility to the condition; believes that having the condition would have serious consequences; recognizes the impact of health motivation, perceived barriers, and benefits; and feels self-confident (SE) in taking the specific health actions necessary to prevent osteoporosis (Kim et al., 1991).

Osteoporosis Self-Efficacy Scale (OSES) is scored by measuring distance of the patient's mark from the left anchor in millimeters; thus, the range is 0 to 100. There are two subscales. OSES Exercise includes items 1 to 6 and OSES Calcium items 7 to 12. The score for each subscale is obtained by totaling item scores and dividing by 6.

Osteoporosis Knowledge Test (OKT) also has two subscales: OKT Exercise (items 1 to 16) and OKT Calcium (items 1 to 9 and 17 to 24). Correct answers are summed (K. K. Kim, personal communication, March, 1996).

PSYCHOMETRIC PROPERTIES

OHBS was revised based on a pilot study of 16 elderly individuals. The tools were then administered to 150 individuals recruited from senior citizen centers (80% female). This group had a mean age of 74 years and were neither cognitively impaired, nor reported that they had osteoporosis. A review of the literature and input from nurses around elements of the HBM were used to generate items (Kim et al., 1991).

OHBS items form six subscales supported by factor analysis: susceptibility (items 1 to 6, α .82, test-retest .84); seriousness (items 7 to 12, α .71, test-retest .79); benefits from exercise (items 13 to 18, α .81, test-retest .63); benefits from calcium intake (items 19 to 24, α .80, test-retest .52); barriers exercise (items 25 to 30, α .82, test-retest .80); barriers calcium intake (items 31 to 36, α .74, test-retest .68); and health motivation (items 37 to 42, α .73, test-retest .67). Discriminant classification of the OHBS exercise scores correctly classified 66% of cases of self-reported low and high levels of exercise, and 69% of those with self-reported low and high calcium intake, in evaluation of concurrent validity (Kim, 1996).

OSES Exercise subscale and OSES Calcium subscale each have reliability coefficients for internal consistency of .90. Construct validity of the OSES has been evaluated by factor analysis and concurrent validity by discriminant function analysis (Kim, 1996). Details in published form could not be located.

OKT Exercise subscale internal consistency reliability coefficient was .69; OKT Calcium subscale internal consistency reliability coefficient was .72. Validity of the OKT was evaluated by factor analysis and discriminant function analysis (Kim, 1996). Details in published form could not be located.

Both the OHBS and the OSES were used in a study of stages of readiness for osteoporosis prevention in 452 women ages 35 to 45. Osteoporosis-specific beliefs showed little relationship to women's decisions to exercise. Compared with those who were not engaged in adopting exercise precautions, those who were so engaged had higher OSES scores (Blalock et al., 1996). Such a finding is consistent with self-efficacy theory and, therefore, supportive of validity. Blalock et al. (1996) also found that for both calcium and exercise as measured by the OHBS, perceived benefits were higher among currently engaged women compared with never-engaged women but with no differences between these groups on perceived barriers.

CRITIQUE AND SUMMARY

Much of the testing of these instruments may be found only in unpublished sources and, therefore, is not readily available. This includes details of validity testing for OKT and OSES and sample scores.

The focus of these instruments is preventive behavior on the part of elderly subjects within the context of the HBM. The process for establishing content was not described in detail. Self-report measures for exercise and calcium intake may themselves suffer from limitations of reliability and validity, and not constitute strong measures of concurrent validity for the OHBS. Ability of the HBM to predict health actions has been widely studied and is variable. Therefore, early findings that the OHBS was marginally related to decision to take the preventive actions may reflect limitations of the model. Nursing interventions related to osteoporosis prevention have consisted primarily of educational programs aimed at changing dietary and exercise habits, and at removing perceived barriers to these actions (Kim et al., 1991). It is, therefore, important to have evidence of these scales' sensitivity to instruction.

REFERENCES

Blalock, S. J., DeVellis, R. F., Giorgino, B., DeVellis, B. M., Gold, D. T., Dooley, M. A., Anderson, J. J. B., & Smith, S. L. (1996). Osteoporosis prevention in premenopausal women: Using a stage model approach to examine the predictors of behavior. *Health Psychology, 15*, 84–93.

Kim, K. K., Horan, M. L., Gendler, P., & Patel, M. K. (1991). Development and evaluation of the Osteoporosis Health Belief Scale. *Research in Nursing and Health, 14*, 115–163.

OSTEOPOROSIS HEALTH BELIEF SCALE

(Interviewer: Read the following instruction *slowly*)

Osteoporosis (os-teo-po-ro-sis) is a condition in which the bones become excessively thin (porous) and weak so that they are fracture prone (they break easily).

I am going to ask you some questions about your beliefs about osteoporosis. There are no right or wrong answers. Everyone has different experiences that will influence how they feel. After I read each statement, tell me if you STRONGLY DISAGREE, DISAGREE, are NEUTRAL, AGREE, or STRONGLY AGREE with the statement. I am going to show you a card with these five choices. When I read each statement, tell me which one of the five is your choice.

It is important that you answer according to your actual beliefs and not according to how you feel you should believe or how you think we want you to believe. We need the answers that best explain how *you* feel.

(Interviewer: Before administration of the scale, check whether the participant can read the five choices on the card. If the person is unable to read them, you need to read the five choices after each statement.)

Strongly Disagree 1	Disagree 2	Neutral 3	Agree 4	Strongly Agree 5		
SD	D	N	A	SA	1.	Your chances of getting osteoporosis are high.
SD	D	N	A	SA	2.	Because of your body build, you are more likely to develop osteoporosis.
SD	D	N	A	SA	3.	It is extremely likely that you will get osteoporosis.
SD	D	N	A	SA	4.	There is a good chance that you will get osteoporosis.
SD	D	N	A	SA	5.	You are more likely than the average person to get osteoporosis.
SD	D	N	A	SA	6.	Your family history makes it more likely that you get osteoporosis.
SD	D	N	A	SA	7.	The thought of having osteoporosis scares you.
SD	D	N	A	SA	8.	If you had osteoporosis you would be crippled.

Scoring Instructions. The Osteoporosis Health Belief Scale (OHBS) is scored by awarding 5 for responses of "strongly agree" to 1 for "strongly disagree" for each item. The OHBS has 7 subscores. Because there are 6 items in each subscale, the possible score for each ranges from 6 to 30.

Susceptibility	OHB01-OHB06	Barriers Exercise	OHB25-OHB30
Seriousness	OHB07-OHB12	Barriers Calcium Intake	OHB31-OHB36
Benefits Exercise	OHB13-OHB18	Health Motivation	OHB37-OHB42
Benefits Calcium Intake	OHB19-OHB24		

Strongly Disagree 1	Disagree 2	Neutral 3	Agree 4	Strongly Agree 5	
SD	D	N	A	SA	9. Your feelings about yourself would change if you got osteoporosis.
SD	D	N	A	SA	10. It would be very costly if you got osteoporosis.
SD	D	N	A	SA	11. When you think about osteoporosis you get depressed.
SD	D	N	A	SA	12. It would be very serious if you got osteoporosis.
SD	D	N	A	SA	13. Regular exercise prevents problems that would happen from osteoporosis.
SD	D	N	A	SA	14. You feel better when you exercise to prevent osteoporosis.
SD	D	N	A	SA	15. Regular exercise helps to build strong bones.
SD	D	N	A	SA	16. Exercising to prevent osteoporosis also improves the way your body looks.
SD	D	N	A	SA	17. Regular exercise cuts down the chances of broken bones.
SD	D	N	A	SA	18. You feel good about yourself when you exercise to prevent osteoporosis.

(Interviewer: Read the following instruction *slowly*)

For the following 6 questions, when I say "taking in enough calcium" it means taking enough calcium by eating calcium-rich foods and/or taking calcium supplements.

SD	D	N	A	SA	19. Taking in *enough calcium* prevents problems from osteoporosis.
SD	D	N	A	SA	20. You have lots to gain from taking in *enough calcium* to prevent osteoporosis.
SD	D	N	A	SA	21. Taking in *enough calcium* prevents painful osteoporosis.
SD	D	N	A	SA	22. You would not worry as much about osteoporosis if you took in *enough calcium*.
SD	D	N	A	SA	23. Taking in *enough calcium* cuts down on your chances of broken bones.
SD	D	N	A	SA	24. You feel good enough about yourself when you take in *enough calcium* to prevent osteoporosis.
SD	D	N	A	SA	25. You feel like you are not strong enough to exercise regularly.
SD	D	N	A	SA	26. You have no place where you can exercise.
SD	D	N	A	SA	27. Your spouse or family discourages you from exercising.

Strongly Disagree 1	Disagree 2	Neutral 3	Agree 4	Strongly Agree 5	
SD	D	N	A	SA	28. Exercising regularly would mean starting a new habit which is hard for you to do.
SD	D	N	A	SA	29. Exercising regularly makes you uncomfortable.
SD	D	N	A	SA	30. Exercising regularly upsets your every day routine.
SD	D	N	A	SA	31. Calcium-rich foods cost too much.
SD	D	N	A	SA	32. Calcium-rich foods do not agree with you.
SD	D	N	A	SA	33. You do not like calcium-rich foods.
SD	D	N	A	SA	34. Eating calcium-rich foods means changing your diet which is hard to do.
SD	D	N	A	SA	35. In order to eat more calcium-rich foods you have to give up other foods that you like.
SD	D	N	A	SA	36. Calcium-rich foods have too much cholesterol.
SD	D	N	A	SA	37. You eat a well-balanced diet.
SD	D	N	A	SA	38. You look for new information related to health.
SD	D	N	A	SA	39. Keeping healthy is very important for you.
SD	D	N	A	SA	40. You try to discover health problems early.
SD	D	N	A	SA	41. You have a regular health check-up even when you are not sick.
SD	D	N	A	SA	42. You follow recommendations to keep you healthy.

OSTEOPOROSIS S-E SCALE

We are interested in learning how confident you feel about doing the following activities. Everyone has different experiences which will make each person more or less confident in doing the following things. Thus, there are no right or wrong answers to this questionnaire. It is your opinion that is important. In this questionnaire, EXERCISE means activities such as walking, swimming, golfing, biking, aerobic dancing.

Place your "X" anywhere on the answer line that you feel best describes your confidence level.

If it were recommended that you do any of the following THIS WEEK, how confident or certain would you be that you could:

1. begin a new or different exercise program

    Not at All ———————————————————————————— Very
    Confident   Confident

2. change your exercise habits

    Not at All ———————————————————————————— Very
    Confident   Confident

3. put forth the effort required to exercise

    Not at All ———————————————————————————— Very
    Confident   Confident

4. do exercises even if they are difficult

    Not at All ———————————————————————————— Very
    Confident   Confident

5. exercise for the appropriate length of time

    Not at All ———————————————————————————— Very
    Confident   Confident

6. do the type of exercises that you are supposed to do

    Not at All ———————————————————————————— Very
    Confident   Confident

Scoring instructions. When scoring the Osteoporosis Self-Efficacy Scale (OSES), first with a ruler, measure from the left anchor on the visual analogue in millimeters to the line where the subject has marked, on each item. The line from "Not at All Confident" to "Very Confident" should measure exactly 10 cm (100 mm). The subject's score on each item should be measured to the nearest millimeter. Thus, the range for each item is 0–100. As with the OKT, the OSES has two subscales. Exercise includes OSE01-OSE06. Calcium includes OSE07-OSE12. Total the scores for the six items from each subscale. Divide each score by 6 to obtain the individual scores. The total possible for each subscale ranges from 0 to 100.

7. increase your calcium intake

    Not at All ——————————————————————————————————— Very
    Confident   Confident

8. change your diet to include more calcium-rich foods

    Not at All ——————————————————————————————————— Very
    Confident   Confident

9. eat calcium-rich foods as often as you are supposed to do

    Not at All ——————————————————————————————————— Very
    Confident   Confident

10. select appropriate foods to increase your calcium intake

    Not at All ——————————————————————————————————— Very
    Confident   Confident

11. stick to a diet which gives an adequate amount of calcium

    Not at All ——————————————————————————————————— Very
    Confident   Confident

12. obtain foods that give an adequate amount of calcium even when they are not readily available

    Not at All ——————————————————————————————————— Very
    Confident   Confident

OSTEOPOROSIS KNOWLEDGE TEST

(Interviewer: Read the following instruction *slowly*)

Osteoporosis (os-teo-po-ro-sis) is a condition in which the bones become very brittle and weak so that they break easily.
I am going to read a list of things which may or may not affect a person's chance of getting osteoporosis. After I read each one, tell me if you think the person is:

    MORE LIKELY TO GET OSTEOPOROSIS, or
    LESS LIKELY TO GET OSTEOPOROSIS, or
    IT HAS NOTHING TO DO WITH GETTING OSTEOPOROSIS.

I am going to show you a card with these 3 choices. When I read each statement, tell me which one of the 3 will be your best answer. (Test administrator. *Do not read "don't know" choice.* If the participants say "don't know," circle this option.)

	More Likely	Less Likely	Neutral	Don't Know
1. Eating a diet *low* in milk products	(ML)	LL	NT	DK
2. Being menopausal; "change of life"	(ML)	LL	NT	DK
3. Having big bones	ML	(LL)	NT	DK
4. Eating a diet high in dark green leafy vegetables	ML	(LL)	NT	DK
5. Having a mother or grandmother who has osteoporosis	(ML)	LL	NT	DK
6. Being a white woman with fair skin	(ML)	LL	NT	DK
7. Having ovaries surgically removed	(ML)	LL	NT	DK
8. Taking cortisone (steroids, e.g., Prednisone) for long time	(ML)	LL	NT	DK
9. Exercising on a regular basis	ML	(LL)	NT	DK

(Interviewer: Read the following instruction *slowly*)

For the next group of questions, you will be asked to choose one answer from several choices. Be sure to choose only one answer. If you think there is more than one answer, choose the best answer. If you are not sure, just say "I don't know."

10. Which of the following exercises is the *best way* to reduce a person's chance of getting osteoporosis?
 A. Swimming.
 Ⓑ. Walking briskly.
 C. Doing kitchen chores, such as washing dishes or cooking.
 D. Don't know

11. Which of the following exercises is the *best way* to reduce a person's chance of getting osteoporosis?
 Ⓐ. Bicycling.
 B. Yoga.
 C. Housecleaning.
 D. Don't know

12. *How many days a week* do you think a person should exercise to strengthen the bones?
 A. 1 day a week.
 B. 2 days a week.
 Ⓒ. 3 or more days a week.
 D. Don't know

13. What is the *least amount of time* a person should exercise on each occasion to strengthen the bones?
 A. Less than 15 minutes.
 Ⓑ. 20 to 30 minutes.
 C. More than 45 minutes.
 D. Don't know

14. Exercise makes bones strong, but it must be *hard enough to make breathing*:
 A. Just a little faster.
 B. So fast that talking is not possible.
 Ⓒ. *Much faster*, but talking is possible.
 D. Don't know

15. Which of the following exercises is the *best way* to reduce a person's chance of getting osteoporosis?
 Ⓐ. Jogging or running for exercise.
 B. Golfing using golf cart.
 C. Gardening.
 D. Don't know

16. Which of the following exercises is the *best way* to reduce a person's chance of getting osteoporosis?
 A. Bowling.
 B. Doing laundry.
 Ⓒ. Aerobic dancing.
 D. Don't know

(Interviewer: Read the following statement *slowly*)

Calcium is one of the nutrients our body needs to keep bones strong.

17. Which of these is a good source of calcium?
    A. Apple.
    Ⓑ. Cheese.
    C. Cucumber.
    D . Don't know

18. Which of these is a good source of calcium?
    A. Watermelon.
    B. Corn.
    Ⓒ. Canned sardines.
    D. Don't know

19. Which of these is a good source of calcium?
    A. Chicken.
    Ⓑ. Broccoli.
    C. Grapes.
    D. Don't know

20. Which of these is a good source of calcium?
    Ⓐ. Yogurt.
    B. Strawberries.
    C. Cabbage.
    D. Don't know

21. Which of these is a good source of calcium?
    Ⓐ. Ice cream.
    B. Grapefruit.
    C. Radishes.
    D. Don't know

22. Which of the following is the recommended amount of calcium intake for an adult?
    A. 100 mg–300 mg daily.
    B. 400 mg–600 mg daily.
    Ⓒ. 800 mg or more daily.
    D. Don't know

23. How much milk must an adult drink to meet the recommended amount of calcium?
    A. 1/2 glass daily.
    B. 1 glass daily.
    Ⓒ. 2 or more glasses daily.
    D. Don't know

24. Which of the following is the *best reason* for taking a calcium supplement?
    A. If a person skips breakfast.
    Ⓑ. If a person does not get enough calcium from diet.
    C. If a person is over 45 years old.
    D. Don't know

43

Preoperative Self-Efficacy Scale

Developed by Sharon Oetker-Black

INSTRUMENT DESCRIPTION, ADMINISTRATION, AND SCORING GUIDELINES

Preoperative instruction about deep breathing and coughing, leg exercises/position change, ambulation, hydration, pain management, and knowledge about the procedures and processes related to surgery have been found to decrease postoperative complications and the length of hospitalization. Self-efficacy is hypothesized to be one of the mechanisms by which this effect is created.

The Preoperative Self-Efficacy Scale (PSES) measures behaviors important to postoperative self-care in four subscales established through factor analysis: deep breathing (items 1 to 3), turning (items 4 to 6), mobility (items 7 to 12), and pain relaxation (items 13 to 15) (Oetker-Black, 1996). Each subscale is summed and behaviorally specific. Increased self-efficacy is linked to an increased likelihood that patients will enact behaviors; therefore, patients with low self-efficacy may need additional patient teaching to increase their confidence in their ability to perform behaviors postoperatively. Patients took 10 to 15 minutes to complete the questionnaire (Oetker-Black, Hart, Hoffman, & Geary, 1992).

PSYCHOMETRIC PROPERTIES

The PSES was first tested with 68 patients undergoing cholecystectomy. Content validity was supported by professional experts' judgments about how each item fit the conceptual definitions of efficacy expectations and postoperative behaviors. Cronbach's α was .78. Scores were related significantly to deep breathing, ambulation, and recollection of preoperative events, which are postoperative behaviors designed to minimize complications and facilitate recovery, providing support for validity (Oetker-Black et al., 1992).

A second study (Oetker-Black & Taunton, 1994) involved 200 adult surgical patients excluding those undergoing open-heart and orthopedic procedures because of the potential limitations

318

of their postoperative activities. The best items were retained based on item means, standard deviations, ranges, item subscale score correlations, α if deleted, and factor loadings, with 16 items remaining. Cronbach's α was .74. Face validity was assessed with patients who found the scale clear and readable, content validity by experts in self-efficacy and nursing, and construct validity was assessed by testing the hypothesis that those patients who already had received preoperative instruction would score higher than those who had not. This hypothesis was not supported, perhaps, in part, because it was difficult to control for previous surgical experience.

A third study was carried out with 85 adult patients scheduled for unilateral knee replacements under general anesthesia. Means after completion of the hospital's routine preoperative teaching, ranged from 5.8 for turning self in bed every hour to 8.5 for remembering one third of preoperative activities. Most items had an optimal range of 10. These means indicate that patients were moderately confident (0 = no confidence, 10 = total confidence) about their ability to perform the postoperative behaviors listed on the questionnaire. Cronbach's αs for the four subscales were recalling activities self-efficacy (SE), .90; breathing deeply SE, .84; turning SE, .97; and mobility SE, .98 (Oetker-Black & Kauth, 1995).

A fourth study tested PSES with 75 women having total abdominal hysterectomies (Oetker-Black, 1996). Scores on the PSES after completion of routine preoperative instruction ranged from 4.9 for turning self every hour to 8.6 for ambulating 10 feet. Factor analysis showed the same factors as described previously, with Cronbach's αs of .94 for mobility, .97 for turning, .96 for relaxation techniques, and .95 for breathing.

CRITIQUE AND SUMMARY

Development of the PSES should enable nurses to more effectively assess patients' levels of need for preoperative teaching and to more systematically evaluate the effectiveness of preoperative teaching in preparing patients for the surgical experience (Oetker-Black & Taunton, 1994). Instructional techniques can be tailored to improving SE (use of mastery and vicarious experiences, modeling of desired behaviors, and persuasion) in the areas where a particular patient shows low SE.

Although norms have not been established, scores on items in the present version of the PSES were reported in study 3 summarized earlier. Studies using PSES have been carried out only on adults; socioeconomic or minority status were not reported, although mean educational level was 12 to 13.5 years. Further studies need to control for both the experience of past surgeries and determine whether the PSES is sensitive to the effects of instruction. In addition, more research is needed to determine what types of preoperative instruction will motivate postoperative patients to perform behaviors, especially those that cause pain. The authors also believe that new items that deal with relaxation techniques need to be written and tested. Although there is a core of behaviors that are common across surgeries (Oetker-Black & Kauth, 1995), it will be important to note whether the specific scale items match with those required of your patient.

REFERENCES

Oetker-Black, S. L. (1996). Generalizability of the Preoperative Self-Efficacy Scale. *Applied Nursing Research, 9*, 40–44.

Oetker-Black, S. L., & Kauth, C. (1995). Evaluating a revised self-efficacy scale for preoperative patients. *Association of Operating Room Nurses Journal, 62,* 244–250.

Oetker-Black, S. L., Hart, F., Hoffman, J., & Geary, S. (1992). Preoperative self-efficacy and postoperative behaviors. *Applied Nursing Research, 5,* 134–139.

Oetker-Black, S. L., & Taunton, R. L. (1994). Evaluation of a self-efficacy scale for preoperative patients. *Association of Operating Room Nurses Journal, 60,* 43–50.

PREOPERATIVE SELF-EFFICACY SCALE

DIRECTIONS: This questionnaire should take no more than 10–15 minutes to complete.

Each of the statements below is written so patients can describe their perceptions of their confidence in performing certain behaviors that they are commonly expected to do after surgery.

Please *circle the number* that identifies how confident you are *right now* of your ability to perform each of the behaviors. Remember there are no right or wrong answers but it is very important that you answer the questions honestly.

Example: How confident are you right now that you will be able to exercise your leg once every hour in bed the day of surgery?

0	1	2	3	4	5	6	7	8	9	10

No Confidence   Total Confidence

---

1. How confident are you right now that you will be able to do deep breathing exercises three times an hour after surgery?

0	1	2	3	4	5	6	7	8	9	10

No Confidence   Total Confidence

2. How confident are you right now that you will be able to do deep breathing excrcises six times an hour after surgery?

0	1	2	3	4	5	6	7	8	9	10

No Confidence   Total Confidence

3. How confident are you right now that you will be able to do deep breathing exercises ten times an hour after surgery?

0	1	2	3	4	5	6	7	8	9	10

No Confidence   Total Confidence

4. How confident are you right now that you will be able to turn yourself from side to side in bed every three hours the day of surgery?

0	1	2	3	4	5	6	7	8	9	10

No Confidence   Total Confidence

5. How confident are you right now that you will be able to turn yourself from side to side in bed every two hours the day of surgery?

0   1   2   3   4   5   6   7   8   9   10

No Confidence   Total Confidence

6. How confident are you right now that you will be able to turn yourself from side to side in bed every hour the day of surgery?

0   1   2   3   4   5   6   7   8   9   10

No Confidence   Total Confidence

7. How confident are you right now that you will be able to get into a chair with assistance one time the day of surgery?

0   1   2   3   4   5   6   7   8   9   10

No Confidence   Total Confidence

8. How confident are you right now that you will be able to get into a chair with assistance two times the day of surgery?

0   1   2   3   4   5   6   7   8   9   10

No Confidence   Total Confidence

9. How confident are you right now that you will be able to get into a chair with assistance three times the day of surgery?

0   1   2   3   4   5   6   7   8   9   10

No Confidence   Total Confidence

10. How confident are you right now that you will be able to walk 5 minutes with assistance the first day after surgery?

0   1   2   3   4   5   6   7   8   9   10

No Confidence   Total confidence

11. How confident are you right now that you will be able to walk 10 minutes with assistance the first day after surgery?

0   1   2   3   4   5   6   7   8   9   10

No Confidence   Total Confidence

12. How confident are you right now that you will be able to walk 15 minutes with assistance the first day after surgery?

0   1   2   3   4   5   6   7   8   9   10

No Confidence   Total Confidence

13. How confident are you right now that you will be able to do relaxation exercises one time when you experience pain?

0	1	2	3	4	5	6	7	8	9	10

No Confidence　　　　　　　　　　　　　　　　　　　　　　Total Confidence

14. How confident are you right now that you will be able to do relaxation exercises often when you experience pain?

0	1	2	3	4	5	6	7	8	9	10

No Confidence　　　　　　　　　　　　　　　　　　　　　　Total Confidence

15. How confident are you right now that you will be able to do relaxation exercises every time you experience pain?

0	1	2	3	4	5	6	7	8	9	10

No Confidence　　　　　　　　　　　　　　　　　　　　　　Total Confidence

Before finishing this questionnaire, please fill in all of the blank spaces in this section.

1. What is your age? _____

2. How many years of education have you completed? _____ _

3. What is your approximate annual family income before taxes? _____

4. Have you ever had surgery before? Yes ____ No ____

▼　*If yes, what type of surgery?* _____

▼　*If yes, did you receive information on how to care for yourself after surgery? (check one)*

　Yes ____　No ____

5. Have you received any information on how to care for yourself after surgery during this hospital visit?

　Yes ____　No ____

Thank you for completing this questionnaire.

Today's Date _____

Date of Scheduled Surgery _____

Home Address _____

_____

_____

_____

Home Phone Number _____

Work Phone Number _____

44

Chronic Obstructive Pulmonary Disease Knowledge Scale

Developed by Yvonne Krall Scherer

INSTRUMENT DESCRIPTION, ADMINISTRATION, AND SCORING GUIDELINES

This instrument was developed to assess the effectiveness of patient education in helping persons with chronic obstructive pulmonary disease (COPD) adjust to their disease process. Version I of the COPD Knowledge Scale consisted of 12 true-false items administered to 17 volunteers from 58 individuals enrolled in Help Yourself to Better Breathing Classes (Scherer, Janelli, & Schmieder, 1989). In Version II, 4 questions were added and administered to 24 volunteer participants before and after the Help Yourself to Better Breathing Classes. After the second study (Scherer, Janelli, & Schmieder, 1994), several questions were restructured to make them more grammatically correct. The volunteers involved were described as middle class, with a good level of social support.

The current version of the COPD Knowledge Scale may be found on pp. 326–327. Correct responses are scored as a 1 and incorrect responses as 0, with unsure responses scored as incorrect. The range of possible scores is 0 to 16; the higher the score, the greater is the knowledge level (Y. K. Scherer, personal communication, February, 1996).

PSYCHOMETRIC PROPERTIES

To address content validity, the scale was submitted to a panel of experts consisting of physicians and nurses who specialized in caring for individuals with COPD. Suggestions made by these experts were incorporated into the Scale. The Cronbach α for internal consistency was .89 for Version II (Y. K. Scherer, personal communication, 1996). Administration of Version II in the second study showed improvement in knowledge for most items before and after six 1-hour

324

classes including content in pathophysiology of COPD, proper breathing and exercise, respiratory irritants, energy conservation, medical management including medications and nutrition, and relaxation and stress control, and use of home equipment. Attendance at the classes did significantly improve pulmonary knowledge scores. The percentages of the group answering each item correctly before and after instruction may be found in Scherer, Janelli, and Schmieder (1994).

CRITIQUE AND SUMMARY

A sampling plan of items from domains of knowledge or outcome objectives could not be located in the description of tool development. Although not common, experts for purposes of establishing content validity should also include patients because their views of essential information are likely to differ from views of professionals. Thus, an explicit match between knowledge thought by various stakeholders to be essential for good adjustment and items in the scale would be helpful.

The COPD Knowledge Scale has been used to evaluate knowledge of small groups of volunteers before and after a patient education program. Individuals involved were older adults, most of whom had at least a high school education. In the reported research, no control groups were used, and the relationship of measures of coping or quality of life and knowledge were not reported. No other tests of validity were reported.

Although the scale is in initial stages of development, a knowledge test for COPD that can be shown to be predictive of a positive adjustment to the disease process would be helpful. Certain kinds of knowledge are usually necessary but not sufficient to yield the outcome of patient adjustment to a chronic disease.

REFERENCES

Scherer, Y. K., Janelli, L. M., & Schmieder, L. E. (1989). Chronic obstructive pulmonary disease—does participating in a Help Yourself to Better Breathing Program make a difference? *Journal Cardiopulmonary Rehabilitation, 9,* 492–496.

Scherer, Y. K., Janelli, L. M., & Schmieder, L. (1994). The effects of a pulmonary education program on quality of life in patients with chronic pulmonary disease. *Rehabilitation Nursing Research, 3,* 62–68.

COPD

Knowledge Quiz

The following questions deal with factual information about chronic obstructive lung disease.

INSTRUCTION: Please circle *one* number to indicate your answer to each question.

1 = True   2 = False   3 = Not Sure

		True	False	Not Sure
1.	The diaphragm is a muscle which does most of the work of breathing.	1	2	3
2.	Emphysema is a disease which primarily affects your air sacs (alveoli).	1	2	3
3.	"Pursed lip breathing" helps prevent collapsing of small airways.	1	2	3
4.	You can abruptly stop taking a steroid medication such as prednisone whenever you want without any ill effects.	1	2	3
5.	Changing the flow rate on your oxygen can be dangerous.	1	2	3
6.	Eating six small meals a day rather than three large ones may help to reduce shortness of breath during and after meals.	1	2	3
7.	Foods high in protein such as fish are an important part of your diet.	1	2	3
8.	Drinking water has no effect on the mucus in your lungs.	1	2	3
9.	One should rinse their mouth out after using a metered dose inhaler.	1	2	3
10.	When climbing up stairs, a person with lung disease should briefly hold their breath while they take a step up.	1	2	3
11.	The most efficient method of completing a task is to work quickly in short bursts with frequent rests.	1	2	3
12.	Someone with lung disease should exhale when they exert themselves during activities.	1	2	3
13.	When taking antibiotics, you should stop taking them when you feel better.	1	2	3

	True	False	Not Sure
14. In diaphragmatic breathing, your abdomen should pull in during inhalation.	1	2	3
15. Keeping your shoulder muscles relaxed is important in order to decrease the amount of oxygen used up for breathing.	1	2	3
16. A bronchodilator, such as Theodur, gets rid of infection.	1	2	3

Answers: (1, T; 2, T; 3, T; 4, F; 5, T; 6, T; 7, T; 8, F; 9, T; 10, F; 11, F; 12, T; 13, F; 14, F; 15, T; and 16, F).

G

Health Promotion, Disease Prevention, and Increasing Quality of Life

45

Health Motivation Assessment Inventory

Developed by Melanie McEwen

INSTRUMENT DESCRIPTION, ADMINISTRATION, AND SCORING GUIDELINES

The health motivation model, depicted in Figure 45.1, is a modification of the health belief model focusing on the motivation of health promotion behaviors. It guided the development of this inventory. Scoring guidelines may be found on page 333. It is important to note that because some items apply to only women, scores will reflect that difference.

PSYCHOMETRIC PROPERTIES

There are three parts to the Health Motivation Assessment Inventory (HMAI): Part I to discover behaviors and actions believed to promote health; Part II specifically to address actions, beliefs, and knowledge associated with cardiovascular disease; and Part III to capture aspects of the variable defined as a catalyst. Three nursing experts who had published work related to motivation and health were asked to match the item with the best subscale, and to comment on whether items were ambiguous, unclear, or not appropriate (McEwen, 1993).

HMAI was pilot tested with 100 adults at an industrial setting and then with a convenience sample of 285 working adults at two large manufacturing facilities in a city in the southern United States. This latter sample was largely white, and 60% were college graduates, with an average family income of $40,000 per year. The α coefficient for Part I was .89 and for Part II .71. Factor analysis identified six subscales. Their α coefficients are previous knowledge, .73; perceived susceptibility, .58; perceived severity, .56; perceived value of action, .76; internal aids/hindrances, .63; and external aids/hindrances, .60 (McEwen, 1993).

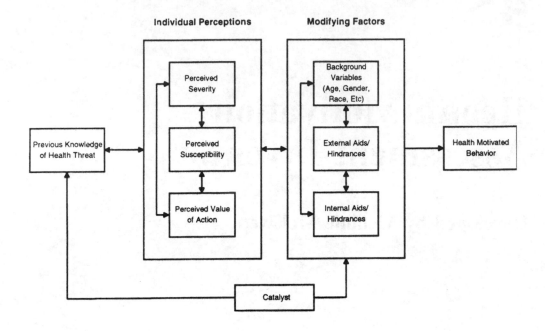

FIGURE 45.1   Health motivation model.

From McEwen, M. (1993). The Health Motivation Assessment Inventory. *Western Journal of Nursing Research, 15*(6), 770–779. Copyright 1993 by Sage Publications, Inc. Reprinted by permission of Sage Publications, Inc.

CRITIQUE AND SUMMARY

The author acknowledges that it is difficult to find research specifically directed at determining what produces health motivation. Additional validity studies are necessary as is rewording of present questions and writing new questions to improve α levels and substantiate the importance of each variable in health motivation (McEwen, 1993). Reliability levels for the subscales are modest.

It is not clear how the content for the inventory was determined, the content domains from which items were constructed and selected. Do the items represent the domains? Does HMAI adequately represent motivation for the health behaviors that would be most beneficial to most adults? Cardiovascular disease is represented by a subscale, whereas other common diseases are not. A basic assumption underlying the HMAI is that the Health Belief Model, on which it is based, is itself valid for predicting whether behaviors will be undertaken. Its performance in this regard is highly variable (Harrison, Mullen, & Green, 1992).

REFERENCES

Harrison, J. A., Mullen, P. D., & Green, L. W. (1992). A meta-analysis of studies of the health belief model with adults. *Health Education Research, 7,* 107–116.

McEwen, M. (1993). The Health Motivation Assessment Inventory. *Western Journal of Nursing Research, 15,* 770–779.

HEALTH MOTIVATION ASSESSMENT INVENTORY

Scoring Summary

The Health Motivation Assessment Inventory (HMAI) was designed in three parts in an attempt to capture the very complex nature of the concept of Health Motivation.

PART I of the HMAI is comprised of 17 questions (22 for women) in which the respondent is asked to complete a number of multiple choice questions to determine specific motivations for health-related actions. This section is to be used to determine behaviors and actions the respondent employs that are believed to promote health. This information can be used for statistical comparison with results obtained from the remainder of the instrument.

PART II of the HMAI is composed of Likert-style questions that were specifically designed to measure one of the variables identified as components of Health Motivation regarding actions, beliefs and knowledge associated with cardiovascular disease. The subscales and the corresponding question numbers are listed below. Questions 6, 13, 17, 20, 21, 22, 25, 28, 30, 33, 36, 38, and 39 did not factor out and should be re-written or discarded.

SUBSCALE	*ITEM NUMBERS*
PREVIOUS KNOWLEDGE	2, 7, 8, 12, 26, 40
PERCEIVED SEVERITY	19, 29, 32
PERCEIVED SUSCEPTIBILITY	1, 3, 10, 11
PERCEIVED VALUE OF ACTION	4, 5, 9, 14, 15, 34, 35
INTERNAL AIDS/HINDRANCES	16, 18, 31
EXTERNAL AIDS/HINDRANCES	23, 24, 27, 37

PART III of the HMAI was designed to capture aspects of the variable defined as "catalyst" and asks the respondent to describe an anecdote or incident in which he/she was motivated to engage in an action or behavior that was perceived as beneficial to health. These responses are examined independently of Parts I and II of the questionnaire. Answers can be categorized and analyzed to look for similarities, differences, and trends to explore health motivation from another angle.

HEALTH MOTIVATION ASSESSMENT INVENTORY

Part I—Please indicate your response by circling the most appropriate response to each question. There is no "right" or "wrong" answer. If more than one answer is appropriate, rank your choices—1st for the primary reason, 2nd, 3rd, etc. If you choose a response labeled "other," please specify.

1. I quit (would like to quit) smoking
   A. to improve my health.
   B. because it is expensive.
   C. because of pressure from my spouse or family.
   D. because of pressure felt at work and elsewhere.
   E. I have never smoked.

2. I smoke
   A. less than one pack of cigarettes per day.
   B. 1 to 2 packs of cigarettes per day.
   C. more than 2 packs of cigarettes per day.
   D. I don't smoke.

3. I drink alcoholic beverages
   A. never.
   B. less than once a month.
   C. less than once a week.
   D. once or twice each week.
   E. three or four times each week.
   F. daily.

4. I would like to lose weight
   A. to improve my appearance.
   B. to please my spouse.
   C. to improve my health.
   D. I am comfortable with my weight.
   E. Other _____

5. I would like to exercise regularly
   A. to lose/maintain weight.
   B. to improve/maintain cardiovascular fitness.
   C. to increase my energy level.
   D. to relieve stress.
   E. I don't desire regular exercise.
   F. Other _____

6. I exercise regularly for 20 minutes or more
   A. less than once each week.
   B. 1 or 2 times each week.
   C. 3 times each week.
   D. 4 or more times each week.

7. I believe my diet is
   A. excellent—I regularly eat fruits and vegetables; eat sparingly of fatty foods, salt and sweets; and eat three meals per day.

B.   good—I usually eat balanced meals and try to limit my intake of foods that have low nutritional value.

C.   fair—I occasionally eat well-balanced meals, but frequently eat foods with low nutritional value.

D.   poor—I rarely eat balanced meals.

8.   My diet needs improvement
A.   because I prefer to eat sweets such as candy, cakes, and doughnuts.
B.   because I prefer to eat meals that are convenient ("fast food" such as hamburgers, french fries, pizza, etc.).
C.   I frequently skip meals because I'm too busy.
D.   I am usually able to eat two or three balanced meals per day.
E.   Other _____

9.   With regard to my weight, I believe that I am
A.   about right.
B.   too low.
C.   less than 15 pounds overweight.
D.   15–30 pounds overweight.
E.   more than 30 pounds overweight.

10.   When I am sick, I usually
A.   don't go to the doctor because I know what's wrong and I will be well in a few days.
B.   don't go to the doctor because it's too expensive.
C.   don't go to the doctor because it's too much of a hassle and I don't have time.
D.   go to the doctor to find out what is wrong and seek treatment.
E.   Other _____

11.   I believe that knowing my cholesterol level
A.   is important because high cholesterol may contribute to heart disease.
B.   is important but I haven't had an opportunity to have mine checked.
C.   is not important for me because I don't believe that I will have a heart attack.
D.   is not important because a high cholesterol level is not a good indicator of risk of having a heart attack.
E.   is not important to me because I will eat what I want regardless of my cholesterol level.

12.   If I discovered my cholesterol level was high, I would
A.   see my doctor and follow his advice.
B.   do nothing.
C.   cut back on eating foods that are high in fat.
D.   have the test done again.
E.   Other _____

13.   I worry most about getting
A.   heart disease.
B.   cancer.
C.   AIDS.
D.   a chronic degenerative disease such as Alzheimer's Disease.
E.   I don't worry about getting ill.
F.   Other _____

14. I am concerned about the illness in question #13 because
    A.   I have a family history of the illness.
    B.   I have a close friend or family member that has had it and I know how it affected
         them.
    C.   I have some "risk factors" or symptoms associated with that illness.
    D.   I have heard and read about it frequently.
    E.   Not applicable.
    F.   Other _____

15. I wear my seatbelt because
    A.   it's required by law.
    B.   it will reduce or eliminate injury in case of an accident.
    C.   it's an example to my children.
    D.   I don't wear my seatbelt.

16. I wear my seatbelt
    A.   all of the time.
    B.   most of the time.
    C.   occasionally.
    D.   rarely.
    E.   never.

17. I sometimes don't take prescriptions as my doctor orders because
    A.   they may cause undesirable side effects.
    B.   they are too expensive.
    C.   I don't really understand what they are supposed to do and how long to take them.
    D.   the symptoms are gone, and I feel the medication is no longer necessary.
    E.   I always take prescriptions as ordered.

Questions 18–22 for women only.

18. Each month
    A.   I regularly examine my breasts to determine if there are any lumps or changes.
    B.   I usually don't examine by breasts because I am afraid that I may find a lump.
    C.   I usually forget to examine my breasts.
    D.   I don't examine my breasts because I don't know if it is important or I don't know
         how.

19. If I noticed a lump in my breast, I would
    A.   immediately make an appointment to see my doctor.
    B.   wait a few weeks to see if it remained and see a doctor if it did not go away.
    C.   put off going to the doctor because of fear of cancer.
    D.   ignore it.

20. I have had a mammogram because
    A.   it is a good way to recognize breast cancer early.
    B.   my doctor recommended it because of my age (over 40).
    C.   I had a lump in my breast.
    D.   I have never had a mammogram.

21. I have never had a mammogram
    A.   because of my age.

B.   because of the expense.
C.   because it has never been available or suggested to me.
D.   because I have never found a lump in my breast.
E.   I have had a mammogram.

22. I go to my doctor for a pap smear
A.   regularly each one to two years.
B.   only if I am experiencing a problem with my menstrual periods or menopause.
C.   I rarely go because it's too expensive or too time consuming.
D.   very rarely because I never have problems.
E.   I have never had a pap smear.

Part II—The following statements are related to Heart Disease (heart attack, angina), its risk factors (such as family history, high blood pressure, high cholesterol, obesity) and possible preventative actions (weight control, diet, exercise). Please answer each question by circling the appropriate letters indicating how you respond to the statement. Mark

"SA"   If you STRONGLY AGREE
"A"   if you AGREE
"N"   if you DON'T KNOW or NOT APPLICABLE
"D"   if you DISAGREE
"SD"   if you STRONGLY DISAGREE
        with the statement.
        Again, there are no "right" or "wrong" answers.

1.	I worry about having a heart attack.	SA	A	N	D	SD
2.	I am aware of risk factors that effect the development of heart disease.	SA	A	N	D	SD
3.	There is a history of heart disease in my family.	SA	A	N	D	SD
4.	I believe a regular exercise program improves cardiac fitness.	SA	A	N	D	SD
5.	Personal habits such as smoking and excessive alcohol intake have a strong effect on cardiac risk.	SA	A	N	D	SD
6.	I believe that coronary bypass surgery (open-heart surgery) can cure heart disease.	SA	A	N	D	SD
7.	I know my usual blood pressure.	SA	A	N	D	SD
8.	I know my cholesterol level.	SA	A	N	D	SD
9.	I believe that lowering personal stress levels can reduce chances of having a heart attack.	SA	A	N	D	SD
10.	High blood pressure (hypertension) runs in my family.	SA	A	N	D	SD
11.	Diabetes runs in my family.	SA	A	N	D	SD
12.	I know the symptoms of a heart attack.	SA	A	N	D	SD

13. I believe that my health will improve if I follow my doctor's recommendations.   SA   A   N   D   SD

14. My health is important to me.   SA   A   N   D   SD

15. I believe preventative actions are effective in reducing heart disease.   SA   A   N   D   SD

16. I find it hard to stay on a diet that is low in salt, fat, or calories, even if prescribed by my doctor.   SA   A   N   D   SD

17. I feel I have no control over the future.   SA   A   N   D   SD

18. I believe that my weight puts me at risk for a heart attack.   SA   A   N   D   SD

19. A heart attack would change my life drastically.   SA   A   N   D   SD

20. My employer provides health programs to help me learn about health and screen for problems.   SA   A   N   D   SD

21. I have health insurance that will pay for screenings and routine physical examinations.   SA   A   N   D   SD

22. I am optimistic about the future.   SA   A   N   D   SD

23. I don't have time to exercise regularly.   SA   A   N   D   SD

24. I don't enjoy exercising.   SA   A   N   D   SD

25. I know someone who has died from a heart attack.   SA   A   N   D   SD

26. I have read books and articles about heart disease and its causes and prevention.   SA   A   N   D   SD

27. I would like to lose weight, but my spouse (or _____) hinders me.   SA   A   N   D   SD

28. I have a convenient place to exercise.   SA   A   N   D   SD

29. I believe that a heart attack would endanger my career.   SA   A   N   D   SD

30. I believe that medical science can cure or manage heart disease once it occurs, through surgery or medication.   SA   A   N   D   SD

31. I would like to lose weight but I often can't resist sweets or foods not on my diet.   SA   A   N   D   SD

32. A heart attack would change how people treat me and act around me.   SA   A   N   D   SD

33. My spouse really helps and encourages me when I am dieting.   SA   A   N   D   SD

34. I believe changing personal habits such as stopping smoking, reducing alcohol intake, and regular exercise will improve my health.   SA   A   N   D   SD

35. I believe that eating a diet low in fat will improve my cholesterol level and improve my risk for heart disease.   SA   A   N   D   SD

36. Heart disease runs in my family, and I feel I will eventually have a heart attack no matter what precautions I take.   SA   A   N   D   SD

37. I would exercise more regularly but the weather is too hot in the summer and too cold in the winter.   SA   A   N   D   SD

38. I feel I have control over my life.   SA   A   N   D   SD

39. I don't believe that smoking will cause me to have a heart attack because my grandfather (father, mother, etc.) smoked for years and never had heart problems.   SA   A   N   D   SD

40. I know what foods to eliminate or reduce to lower my cholesterol.   SA   A   N   D   SD

41. What is your age? _____

42. Sex:
    A. male.
    B. f emale.

43. Race/ethnic group:
    A. white.
    B. African-American.
    C. Hispanic.
    D. Oriental.
    E. other _____

44. Education level:
    A. did not complete high school.
    B. high school diploma.
    C. some college.
    D. college graduate.
    E. post-graduate.

45. Family income level:
    A. less than $10,000 per year.
    B. 10,000–20,000.
    C. 20,001–30,000.
    D. 30,001–40,000.
    E. more than 40,000 per year.

46. Marital status:
    A. single (never married).
    B. married.
    C. divorced.
    D. separated.
    E. widowed.

Part III—For this section, think of a specific example of when you modified your normal lifestyle to do something to promote your health (for example: lose weight, start an exercise program, stop smoking). Briefly describe what caused you to take that particular action at that time (for example: you saw a picture of yourself in a swimsuit; a friend younger than you had a heart attack; you discovered your cholesterol level was too high).

Used with permission of Melanie McEwen, PhD, RN, CS.

46

Exercise Knowledge Test

Developed by Maryann Leslie and Pamela Schuster

INSTRUMENT DESCRIPTION, ADMINISTRATION, AND SCORING GUIDELINES

Patient education is an essential component of cardiac rehabilitation programs, which are designed to assist patients recovering from acute and chronic cardiac events in modifying or decreasing coronary risk factors. The Exercise Knowledge Test is based on American College of Sports Medicine Guidelines. These guidelines recommend that patients should show an ability to maintain their exercise prescription within the designated range and to recognize the signs and symptoms of exertion intolerance. At a minimum, patients should know pulse rate parameters and safety precautions required to monitor their activity and the basic components of their exercise prescription.

Although knowledge in no way guarantees adherence to the exercise regimen, it does correct misperceptions about ability to tolerate activity that may result either in overexertion or underexertion (Leslie & Schuster, 1991). The score on the Exercise Knowledge Test is the total number of correct responses.

PSYCHOMETRIC PROPERTIES

Items for the Exercise Knowledge Test were developed to assess knowledge of pulse-counting techniques, basic principles of the exercise prescription, and safety measures to be taken before, during, and after the exercise session including the patient's individualized pulse rate parameters. The test was reviewed by 12 cardiac rehabilitation professionals for clarity, content, and face validity; revised; and then administered to 97 cardiac patients. Revisions were again made, based on patient responses to test questions.

Twenty-eight patients referred for cardiac rehabilitation participated in a study to assess the effect of contingency contracting on patient attendance and on their knowledge of exercise. Those in the contingency-contracting group showed significantly greater gains on the Test (mean score from 6.6 to 14.0 at 8 weeks) than did those in the standard treatment (mean score from 6.5 to 10.3 at 8 weeks). Thus, the test showed sensitivity to an educational intervention. Test-retest reliability was .76 (Leslie & Schuster, 1991).

CRITIQUE AND SUMMARY

Because no description of full content domains was included in the report about the test, it is difficult to judge how well items represent these domains. There is also no sense of the criterion level of knowledge associated with safe exercise. The tool has been tested on a few predominantly male patients, with ethnic and class diversity unknown, and over a short time span.

REFERENCE

Leslie, M., & Schuster, P. A. (1991). The effect of contingence contracting on adherence and knowledge of exercise regimens. *Patient Education and Counseling, 18,* 231–241.

EXERCISE KNOWLEDGE TEST

Please answer these questions concerning exercise procedures. Circle the letter of each answer.

1. In order to develop and maintain fitness, what is the minimum number of days per week exercise should be done?
   A. One.
   B. Two.
   C. Three.
   D. Four.
   E. Don't know

2. Which of these factors is LEAST important to an exercise prescription?
   A. Current fitness level.
   B. Intensity and duration of exercise.
   C. Frequency and type of exercise.
   D. Body composition.
   E. Don't know

3. In order to maintain fitness, the length of each exercise session (not counting warm-up and cool-down periods)
   A. should be 5–10 minutes each session.
   B. should be 15–60 minutes each session.
   C. should be 65–70 minutes each session.
   D. should be 75–80 minutes each session.
   E. Don't know

4. The most important reason for keeping the heart rate within the target heart rate is to achieve
   A. muscular benefits.
   B. body composition benefits.
   C. physical fitness benefits.
   D. nonaerobic benefits.
   E. Don't know

5. Warm-up before exercise is important because it
   A. decreases the chance of heart and muscle injury.
   B. decreases the oxygen delivery to the working muscles.
   C. decreases the speed of contraction of muscles.
   D. decreases the muscle temperature.
   E. Don't know

6. The warm-up routine also helps to improve
   A. aerobic capacity.
   B. cardio-respiratory endurance.
   C. flexibility.
   D. cardiovascular power.
   E. Don't know

7. The cool-down phase
   A. increases blood pressure.
   Ⓑ. decreases heart rate gradually.
   C. increases the chance of skipped heart beats.
   D. decreases the chance of having a heart attack.
   E. Don't know

8. Which of the following is the BEST way to check the pulse during exercise?
   Ⓐ. Count the pulse for 10 seconds and multiply the number by 6.
   B. Count the pulse for 60 seconds.
   C. There is no need to count the pulse because the pulse rate does not have to be checked during exercise.
   D. Count the pulse for 15 seconds and multiply the number by 4.
   E. Don't know

9. When symptoms occur during exercise (chest discomfort, shortness of breath), what action should be taken?
   A. Heart rate should be kept in the heart rate range.
   B. The heart rate can be exceeded.
   Ⓒ. The exercise should be gradually discontinued.
   D. Exercise can be done even if symptoms occur.
   E. Don't know

10. All of the following symptoms indicate that the intensity of exercise should be decreased except
    A. chest discomfort.
    B. skipped heart beats.
    Ⓒ. flushed skin color.
    D. shortness of breath.
    E. Don't know

11. When should the pulse rate be counted?
    A. before and after each activity.
    B. before and during each activity.
    C. during and after each activity.
    Ⓓ. before, during, and after each activity.
    E. Don't know

12. In general, as the intensity of exercise increases
    A. blood pressure decreases.
    B. breathing slows.
    Ⓒ. heart rate increases.
    D. pulse rate decreases.
    E. Don't know

13. What is the highest heart rate (maximum heart rate) that you should not go above WHILE EXERCISING?

    _____ beats per minute

    _____ don't know

14. What is the lowest heart rate (minimum heart rate) that you should not go below WHILE EXERCISING?

    _____ beats per minute

    _____ don't know

15. What is the heart rate that you should not go above no matter what activity you do?

    _____ beats per minute

    _____ don't know

16. What is your (average) resting heart rate?

    _____ beats per minute

    _____ don't know

47

English/Spanish Self-Efficacy Scale for Breast Self-Examination

Developed by Judith T. Gonzalez and Virginia M. Gonzalez

INSTRUMENT DESCRIPTION, ADMINISTRATION, AND SCORING GUIDELINES

Women of color and from lower socioeconomic groups have higher rates of breast cancer deaths, a greater percentage of which are considered preventable by early detection. Prior study showed that among low-income Mexican-American women, self-efficacy was the most significant predictor of breast self-examination (BSE). Study of this population is important because self-efficacy may include not only skills specific to a particular task but also related behaviors, such as communication with the health care provider or educator, to learn the complex performance of BSE and ability or motivation to break down barriers of access to health care (Gonzalez & Gonzalez, 1990).

Scores are obtained by adding the Likert scores of the original items. Items are available in both English and Spanish. Rating scales are adjectives describing degrees of intensity, found to work better with this group than did a 100-point visual analogue scale used in other measures of self-efficacy (Gonzalez & Gonzalez, 1990).

PSYCHOMETRIC PROPERTIES

The scale was tested on a convenience sample of 106 low-income, primarily Spanish-speaking Mexican-American women attending a clinic in Tucson. Average years of schooling was 8.7. Although 62% reported having had a breast examination by a physician in the past year, and 39% reported they examined their own breasts at least once a month, few possessed adequate knowledge of correct procedure (Gonzalez & Gonzalez, 1990).

α coefficient was .79. Factor analysis showed three subdimensions of self-efficacy: BSE skill related items (items 1 to 3), communication skill related (items 4 to 7), and ability to surmount barrier to health care (items 8 to 11). Self-efficacy was significantly correlated with actual skill measures for BSE (although with low interrater reliability), English language proficiency, and reported frequency of BSE, providing some evidence of validity. The mean self-efficacy score for this group was 48, SD 8.7, and median 4.8 (Gonzalez & Gonzalez, 1990).

CRITIQUE AND SUMMARY

Little research has been conducted among Mexican Americans relating self-efficacy to health outcomes; further use of this scale can provide more evidence. The author notes the possibility that responses to the scale and the reported skill in performing BSE are indicative of a tendency others have noted of Mexican Americans to give socially desirable responses. Traditional views of the human body in Mexico consider touching of the breasts as a breach of decency. Test-retest reliability was not assessed. This measure should also be compared with other methods of assessing self-efficacy to reevaluate construct validity. It should also be tested in other settings, with Mexican-American females who do not receive regular medical care, and in research testing the amount of change in self-efficacy related to training interventions (Gonzalez & Gonzalez, 1990).

Although in an early stage of development, this scale is important, in part, because it addresses cross-cultural issues. Not only is it important to develop scales in appropriate language and response modes, it is also important to incorporate self-efficacy beliefs related to the central skill of BSE (communication and overcoming barriers), and essential to carrying out the appropriate health action.

REFERENCE

Gonzalez, J. T., & Gonzalez, V. M. (1990). Initial validation of a scale measuring self-efficacy of breast self-examination among low-income Mexican American women. *Hispanic Journal of Behavioral Sciences, 12,* 277–291.

ENGLISH/SPANISH SELF-EFFICACY SCALE

English Response Choices

(1)   uncertain
(2)   somewhat uncertain
(3)   neither certain nor uncertain
(4)   somewhat certain
(5)   certain

Spanish Response Choices

(1)   muy insegura
(2)   algo insegura
(3)   ni segura, ni insegura
(4)   algo segura
(5)   segura

1.   How certain are you that you can do a breast self-examination without anyone's help?
¿Hasta qué punto se siente segura de que puede hacerse la auto-examinación de los senos sin la ayuda de otra persona?

2.   How certain are you that you can find a lump on your breast when you do the breast self-examination without help?
¿Hasta qué punto se siente segura de que puede encontrar un bulto en el seno al hacerse la auto-examinación sin la ayuda de nadie?

3.   How certain are you that you can teach another woman how to examine her breasts?
¿Qué tan segura se siente de que puede enseñarle a otra mujer como examinarse los senos?

4.   How certain are you that you can ask the doctor the necessary questions to get the information that you need about your health condition?
¿Qué tan segura se siente de que puede hacerle al médico las preguntas necesarias para obtener la información que Ud. necesita respecto a su condición física?

5.   How certain are you that you can understand the doctor's explanation about your health condition?
¿Qué tan segura se siente de que puede comprender la explicación que le da el médico respecto a su condición física?

6.   How certain are you that you can understand what the doctor is doing when he/she examines you?
¿Hasta qué punto se siente segura de que puede comprender lo que está haciendo el médico cuando la examina?

7.   Sometimes it is necessary to explain to our friends and family the results of pap smear. How certain are you that you can explain the results to another person?
A veces es necesario explicarle a sus amigas y familia los resultados del examen de la cervix (Pap smear). ¿Hasta qué punto se siente segura de que puede explicarle los resultados a otra persona?

8.   If needed, how certain are you that you can get someone to help you with child care so that you can get to the doctor?
     Si fuera necesario, ¿qué tan segura se siente de que puede conseguir a alguien que le ayude con el cuidado de los niños para que Ud. pueda ir con el doctor?

9.   How certain are you that you can keep your next appointment with the doctor?
     ¿Qué tan segura se siente Ud. de que pudrá ir a su siguiente cita con el médico?

10. How certain are you that you can do what the doctor recommends for required follow-up care?
     ¿Qué tan segura se siente que Ud. puede hacer lo que recomienda el doctor/la doctora en cuanto el cuidado necesario después de su consulta?

11. If needed, how certain are you that you can get a friend or family member to give you a ride to the clinic?
     Si fuera necesario, ¿qué tan segura se siente de que puede conseguir que una amiga o un familiar la lleve a la clinica?

48

Falls Efficacy Scale

Developed by Mary E. Tinetti, Donna Richman, and Lynda Powell

INSTRUMENT DESCRIPTION, ADMINISTRATION, AND SCORING GUIDELINES

The Falls Efficacy Scale (FES) was developed to measure fear of falling defined as ''low perceived self-efficacy at avoiding falls during ten essential, nonhazardous activities of daily living.'' Fear of falling may result in a self-imposed decline in activity and function not necessitated by physical disability or injury. It occurs in 50% to 60% of elderly who have fallen as well as in those who have not, and deterioration in the physical ability to balance may result from activity restriction mediated through fear of falling (Powell & Myers, 1995). It is hoped that the scale may identify elderly persons likely to become dependent on family, friends or agencies. Falls are the most prevalent form of injury among old people; 30% of community elderly persons fall each year. Falls and their sequelae represent one group of potentially modifiable factors contributing to functional decline (Tinetti, Mendes de Leon, Doucette, & Baker, 1994), and fear or falling or low confidence may represent a remediable independent contributor to functional decline (Tinetti & Powell, 1993).

The FES score is the sum of item scores (range from 0 to 100), with a lower score reflecting lower efficacy (Tinetti, Richman, & Powell, 1990).

PSYCHOMETRIC PROPERTIES

Items were generated by asking physical therapists, occupational therapists, rehabilitation nurses, and physicians to name the most important activities essential to independent living that would be safe and nonhazardous to most elderly persons. The consensus established in identifying these activities supported the validity of the items. In two pretests, the FES was administered to a total of 74 persons, with an average age of 79 years. Test-retest reliability was .71. There was sufficient variability to suggest that the instrument may measure the continuum of self-imposed activity restriction among elderly fallers (Tinetti, Richman, & Powell, 1990).

The FES score was associated with a measure of relevant skills, such as gait, and with past experience, such as difficulty in getting up after a fall, both of which would be predicted by theory. Convergent validity of the instrument was suggested by the finding that total score increased progressively among respondents who denied fear of falling, who acknowledged fear but denied avoiding activities, and who reported avoiding activities. The same trend of increase in efficacy score was found among individual activities as well (Tinetti & Powell, 1993). In a second study of community-dwelling elderly, fall-related efficacy was a potent independent correlate of activities of daily living and physical functioning. This suggests that clinical programs should attempt simultaneously to improve physical skills and confidence (Tinetti et al., 1994).

Powell and Myers (1995) describe the development of the Activities-Specific Balance Confidence Scale, a more situation-specific measure of balance confidence than is the FES including a wider continuum of activity difficulty and more detailed activity descriptors. Items include "reach at eye level" and "escalator not holding rail." These authors found a Cronbach's α of .90 for the FES administered to an independent sample of community-living seniors. Scores on the FES in this sample were more variable than in the study by Tinetti et al. (1990), where the range was restricted. Utility of the FES as a discriminative index was also supported based on significantly different scores in the expected direction, for high- and low-mobility groups. Mean score on the FES was 26.9 (SD 18.6), similar to a previously found mean score of 25.11 (SD 12.26). Taking a bath or shower was the item associated with the lowest self-efficacy. Scalability analysis supported the hierarchical nature of the FES (Tinetti et al., 1990).

The FES has also been used in other studies including the multicenter trial Frailty and Injuries: Cooperative Studies of Intervention Techniques (FICSIT), modified to use a four-category scoring system because respondents had difficulty with the 10 levels of response categories (Buchner et al., 1993). FICSIT is a series of clinical trials of biomedical, behavioral, and environmental interventions to reduce the risks of frailty and fall-related injury among the elderly.

A study that is part of the FICSIT delivered a multifactorial intervention to reduce the risk of falling among elderly people living in the community. Because the risk of falling increased with the number of risk factors present, such a multifactorial strategy of risk abatement may decrease the risk of falling. After assessment of the risk factors, interventions including education about use of sedative-hypnotic agents, gait training, and training in transfer skills were given. The intervention group had significantly fewer falls with a longer time until the first fall than did the control group. The mean change in the scores on the FES differed significantly in favor of the intervention group. At reassessment 4 months later, a significantly smaller percentage of the intervention group than of the control group continued to use at least four prescription medications, to transfer unsafely to bathtub or toilet, or to have impairment in balance or gait—all being risk factors for falling. Thus, the FES was sensitive to an education program (Tinetti et al., 1995).

CRITIQUE AND SUMMARY

An accurate measure of self-efficacy to avoid falls, with good predictive validity, used as one element of an assessment and intervention program, could have enormous impact, simply because falls in the elderly are so common and costly. FES may identify persons likely to become dependent on family, friends, or agencies. Preliminary findings suggest that the FES can be used to measure the impact of fear of falling on behavior and function, and in monitoring response to therapy. A program of intervention would, no doubt, assure adequate transfer and gait skills, decrease fall risks, and increase fall self-efficacy. Neither falling nor fear of falling should be considered inevitable accompaniments of aging. The FES can also be useful in research to show whether depression, anxiety trait, physical ability, and fear of falling exert an independent effect on functional decline (Tinetti & Powell, 1993; Tinetti et al., 1990).

Powell and Myers (1995) found problems with a ceiling effect, particularly for higher mobility participants, perhaps because FES items are limited to relatively nonhazardous activities. Further evidence of both concurrent and predictive validity would be helpful.

REFERENCES

Buchner, D. M., Hornbrook, M. C., Kutner, N. G., Tinetti, M. E., Ory, M. G., Mulrow, C. D., Schechtman, K. B., Gerety, M. B., Fiatarone, M. A., Wolf, S. L., Rossiter, J., Artken, C., Kanten, K., Lipsitz, L. A., Sattin, R. W., DeNino, L. A., & the FICSIT Group. (1993). Development of the common data base for the FICSIT trials. *Journal of the American Geriatric Society, 41,* 297–308.

Powell, L. E., & Myers, A. M. (1995). The Activities-Specific Balance Confidence Scale. *Journal of Gerontology: Medical Sciences, 50A,* M28–M34.

Tinetti, M. E., Mendes de Leon, C. F., Doucette, J. T., & Baker, D. I. (1994). Fear of falling and fall-related efficacy in relationship to functioning among community-living elders. *Journals of Gerontology: Medical Sciences, 49,* M140–M147.

Tinetti, M. E., & Powell, L. (1993). Fear of falling and low self-efficacy: a cause of dependence on elderly persons [Special issue]. *Journals of Gerontology, 48,* 35–38.

Tinetti, M. E., Richman, D., & Powell, L. (1990). Falls efficacy as a measure of fear of falling. *Journals of Gerontology: Psychological Sciences, 45,* P239–P243.

Tinetti, M. E., Baker, D. I., McAvay, G., Claus, E. B., Garrett, P., Gottschalk, M., Koch, M. L., Trainor, K., & Horwitz, R. I. (1995). A multifactorial intervention to reduce the risk of falling among elderly people living in the community. *New England Journal of Medicine, 331,* 821–827.

FALLS EFFICACY (FE)

On a scale from 0 to 10 with zero meaning not confident/sure at all, 5 being fairly confident/sure, and 10 being completely confident/sure, how confident/sure are you that you can do each of the following without falling:

IF "R" PHYSICALLY UNABLE TO DO ACTIVITY CONTINUE TO PROBE FOR A RESPONSE AND ASK IF THEY WERE ABLE.

(REPEAT FOR EACH ACTIVITY) How confident/sure are you that you can (ASK ACTIVITY BELOW) without falling?

		Not confident/ sure at all				Fairly confident/sure				Completely confident/sure		REF	DK	
+	1.	Clean house (e.g., sweep or dust)	00	01	02	03	04	05	06	07	08	09	10	97	98	(8)
+	2.	Get dressed and undressed	00	01	02	03	04	05	06	07	08	09	10	97	98	(10)
+	3.	Prepare simple meals (not involving carrying hot or heavy objects)	00	01	02	03	04	05	06	07	08	09	10	97	98	(12)
+	4.	Take a bath or shower	00	01	02	03	04	05	06	07	08	09	10	97	98	(14)
+	5.	Simple shopping	00	01	02	03	04	05	06	07	08	09	10	97	98	(16)
+	6.	Get in and out of a chair	00	01	02	03	04	05	06	07	08	09	10	97	98	(18)
+	7.	Go up and down stairs	00	01	02	03	04	05	06	07	08	09	10	97	98	(20)
+	8.	Walk around the neighborhood	00	01	02	03	04	05	06	07	08	09	10	97	98	(22)
+	9.	Reach into cabinets or closets	00	01	02	03	04	05	06	07	08	09	10	97	98	(24)
+	10.	Hurry to answer the telephone	00	01	02	03	04	05	06	07	08	09	10	97	98	(26)

+Do not ask proxy and/or nursing home respondent.

Tinetti, M. E., Richman, D., & Powell, L. (1990). Falls efficacy as a measure of fear of falling. *Journals of Gerontology: Psychological Sciences, 45,* 239–243. Copyright, The Gerontological Society of America.

49

Incontinence Quiz

Developed by Laurence G. Branch, Laura A. Walker, Terrie T. Wetle, Catherine E. DuBeau, and Neil M. Resnick

INSTRUMENT DESCRIPTION, ADMINISTRATION, AND SCORING GUIDELINES

Among the elderly, urinary incontinence (UI) is prevalent, morbid, and costly; yet fewer than half of persons with these symptoms seek treatment from a health professional. One barrier to symptom reporting is misinformation or lack of information about UI and its treatment, leading older people to accept it as a normal consequence of aging (Branch, Walker, Wetle, DuBeau, & Resnick, 1994).

The Incontinence Quiz was developed to test knowledge of the causes, evaluation, and treatment of UI. It was used to evaluate the ability of mass education to improve knowledge of community-dwelling persons 65 years and older about UI. The quiz requires respondents to agree or disagree with 14 statements about incontinence. The items can be grouped loosely into four categories: causes of incontinence, treatments and effects of incontinence, the relationship of aging and incontinence, and physician-patient discussions about incontinence (Branch et al., 1994), although confirmation of this grouping by statistical procedures could not be located.

PSYCHOMETRIC PROPERTIES

The Incontinence Quiz items were devised from research and the authors' experience on the subject, with the practice guidelines on incontinence developed by the Agency for Health Care Policy and Research as the primary reference source. It was administered to a sample of 1,140 community-dwelling persons aged 65 years and older from two counties in Massachusetts; their demographic characteristics approximated the population of that age in the U.S. population except that they were better educated (Branch et al., 1994).

The quiz was administered to a large sample that showed considerable lack of knowledge in this important area, particularly about urine loss being a result of normal aging (58% incorrect), and that by age 85 most people lose control of their urine (42% incorrect) (Branch et al., 1994).

CRITIQUE AND SUMMARY

No estimates of reliability are given. Although content validity was addressed, definition of domains of content and their importance to patients was unclear. No evidence was provided for relationship between scores on the quiz and one or more criterion behaviors, such as seeking help from a health professional for appropriate symptoms, or for sensitivity of the instrument to instruction. The instrument seems most useful for assessment of population groups.

REFERENCE

Branch, L. G., Walker, L. A., Wetle, T. T., DuBeau, C. E., & Resnick, N. M. (1994). Urinary incontinence knowledge among community-dwelling people 65 years of age and older. *Journal of the American Geriatrics Association, 42,* 1257–1262.

INCONTINENCE QUIZ

Next, I'll read some general statements about urinary incontinence. Please tell me whether you agree or disagree with each statement. The (first/next) statement is (READ ITEM). Do you agree or disagree with this statement?

	Agree	Disagree	Refused	Don't Know	Professional Consensus Response
1. Involuntary loss of urine, often called a leaky bladder or urinary incontinence, is one of the results of normal aging.	1	2	7	8	DISAGREE
2. Most people will involuntarily or accidentally lose control of their urine on a regular basis by the time they reach age 85.	1	2	7	8	DISAGREE
3. Many common over-the-counter medications can cause involuntary urine loss.	1	2	7	8	AGREE
4. Other than pads, diapers, and catheters, little can be done to treat or cure involuntary urine loss.	1	2	7	8	DISAGREE
5. Once people start to lose control of their urine on a regular basis, they usually can never regain complete control over it again.	1	2	7	8	DISAGREE
6. Most people who currently have involuntary urine loss live normal lives.	1	2	7	8	AGREE
7. Most physicians ask their older patients whether they have bladder control problems.	1	2	7	8	DISAGREE

(continued)

INCONTINENCE QUIZ (*continued*)

	Agree	Disagree	Refused	Don't Know	Professional Consensus Response
8. Women are more likely than men to develop urinary incontinence.	1	2	7	8	AGREE
9. Most people with involuntary urine loss talk to their doctors about it.	1	2	7	8	DISAGREE
10. Involuntary urine loss is caused by only one or two conditions.	1	2	7	8	DISAGREE
11. Many people with involuntary urine loss can be cured and almost everyone can experience significant improvement.	1	2	7	8	AGREE
12. Involuntary loss of urine can be caused by several easily treatable medical conditions.	1	2	7	8	AGREE
13. The best treatment for involuntary urine loss is usually surgery.	1	2	7	8	DISAGREE
14. There are exercises that can help control urine if one leaks when they cough, sneeze, or laugh.	1	2	7	8	AGREE

From Branch, L. G., Walker, L. A., Wetle, T. T., DuBeau, C. E., & Resnick, N. M. (1994). Urinary incontinence knowledge among community-dwelling people 65 years of age and older. *Journal of the American Geriatrics Society, 42,* 1257–1262.

50

HIV Prevention Attitude Scale

Developed by Mohammad R. Torabi and William L. Yarber

INSTRUMENT DESCRIPTION, ADMINISTRATION, AND SCORING GUIDELINES

For the human immunodeficiency virus (HIV) infection and the acquired immunodeficiency syndrome, prevention education is a major control measure. Needs assessments and evaluation of educational programs require appropriate instruments, both for populations and individuals. Adolescents are believed to be particularly at risk because they underestimate their risk, miscalculate their vulnerability, or feel impervious to negative outcomes. Little research is available to guide program developers regarding the content, timing, or format for risk reduction interventions targeting teenagers (St. Lawrence, Jefferson, Alleyne, & Brasfield, 1995).

The HIV Prevention Attitude Scale is based on a multidimensional conception of attitude including cognitive (belief), affective (feeling), and conative (intention to act). Beliefs express one's perceptions of concepts toward an attitudinal object; feelings are described as an expression of liking or disliking relative to an attitudinal object; and intention to act is an expression of what the individual says he or she would do in a given situation. Average time to respond to the forms is 12 minutes. Scoring guidelines may be seen at the end of each form. Minimum and maximum possible points for each form are 15 to 75, with higher scores indicating more positive attitudes toward HIV and HIV prevention (Torabi & Yarber, 1992).

PSYCHOMETRIC PROPERTIES

Items were generated from a two-way table of specifications—the three components of attitude (belief, feeling, and intention to act) as the horizontal dimension, and nature of HIV and HIV transmission and prevention as the vertical dimension. This structure and items were developed from a review of the literature. Items were reviewed by a jury of health educators, students, measurement specialists, and federal government HIV officials, for clarity and content validity, and refined. The 50-item scale was administered to a representative sample of 210 students in intact classes, in a midwestern high school. The group was 18% minority. From the first administration, 30 maximally discriminating items with the highest internal consistency and that fulfilled the table of specifications were selected for alternative forms.

The revised alternative forms of 15 comparable items each were then administered to a sample of 600 students from midwestern high schools, with 95% being White. Item correlation with total scale scores ranged from .39 to .63. Alternative parallel forms are shown subsequently. The percentage distributions of the responses by alternatives for both forms were described as reasonably spread and comparable, with means and standard deviations for total and subscale scores practically the same. Average scores with this administration were about 59 points. Reliability coefficients using Cronbach's α and split-half methods were .78 and .76 for Form A, and .77 and .69 for Form B. Test-retest reliability for the alternative forms with a 1-week interval was .60. Factor analyses of both forms identified reasonably comparable factor structures of myths about transmission, myths about infected people, communication for prevention, and methods of prevention, supporting content validity and comparability. For Form A, mean total scores were 59 (SD = 7.7), and for Form B, the mean was 59.4 (SD = 7.7). The authors indicate that it is premature to use the factors as subscales (Torabi & Yarber, 1992).

St. Lawrence et al. (1994) administered the HIV Prevention Attitude Scale before and after a five-session HIV risk reduction intervention to substance dependent adolescents ($N = 19$) court referred into a residential drug treatment facility. The intervention was similar to that reported in St. Lawrence, Jefferson, Alleyne, and Brasfield (1995). No control group was available, and statistical analysis was not done. The scale showed a Cronbach's α of .82 for this sample, with score means and standard deviations of 55.4 and 8.6 preintervention, and 60.3 and 11.5 postintervention. Following intervention, the participants reporting sexual activity in high-risk contexts decreased as did record of sexually transmitted disease treatment. The durability of the changes is not known.

A subsequent study with 34 similarly situated adolescents (16% African American) found behavioral skills training superior to standard education presented didactically and through interactive game formats. The behavioral skills training included skill rehearsal in correct condom use, interpersonal communication skills, problem solving, and self-management strategies. [Group leaders modeled the specific skills and their use in situations that might arise post–behavior skills training (pretraining mean 55.4, posttraining mean 63.0, statistically significant change).] Cronbach's α was .82 for this sample (St. Lawrence et al., 1995).

CRITIQUE AND SUMMARY

This scale is focused on HIV prevention attitudes among adolescents and is intended as an evaluation tool for educational approaches to HIV control. The availability of alternative forms is especially useful for pretest-posttest evaluation models. Evidence of content validity came from a jury of experts, table of specifications, and factor analysis procedures. There is also evidence of form comparability and reliability (Torabi & Yarber, 1992).

The original evidence of validity and reliability was obtained from samples of predominantly white in-school students. The two studies of substance-dependent adolescents in a residential drug treatment facility provide information about the scale's performance with a different population, although with small sample sizes. Scores for all groups were generally in the same range. No data relating scale scores to behavior or practices are available (criterion-related validity). Data regarding concurrent validity were available. No predictive validity data could be located. There is consistent evidence of the scales' sensitivity to intervention with a larger response to behavioral skills training, theoretically consistent with the kind of intervention that should create attitude change.

REFERENCES

St. Lawrence, J. S., Jefferson, K. W., Alleyne, E., & Brasfield, T. L. (1995). Comparison of education versus behavioral skills training interventions in lowering sexual HIV-risk behavior of substance-dependent adolescents. *Journal of Consulting and Clinical Psychology, 63,* 154–157.

St. Lawrence, J. S., Jefferson, K. W., Banks, P. G., Cline, T. R., Alleyne, E., & Brasfield, T. L. (1994). Cognitive-behavioral group intervention to assist substance-dependent adolescents in lowering HIV infection risk. *AIDS Education and Prevention, 6,* 425–435.

Torabi, M. R., & Yarber, W. (1992). Alternate forms of HIV Prevention Attitude Scales for teenagers. *AIDS Education and Prevention, 4,* 172–182.

ALTERNATE FORMS OF HIV PREVENTION ATTITUDE SCALE

Form A

DIRECTIONS: Please read each statement carefully. *Record your immediate reaction to the statement by blackening the proper oval on the answer sheet.* There is no right or wrong answer for each statement, so mark your own response. Use the below key:

KEY:

A = strongly agree
B = agree
C = undecided
D = disagree
E = strongly disagree

Example: Doing something to prevent getting HIV is the responsibility of each person.

A   B   C   D   E

RECORD ANSWER ON COMPUTER ANSWER SHEET

1.   I would feel very uncomfortable being around someone with HIV.

2.   I feel that HIV is a punishment for immoral behavior.

3.   If I were having sex, it would be insulting if my partner insisted we use a condom.

4.   I dislike the idea of limiting sex to just one partner to avoid HIV infection.

5.   I would dislike asking a possible sex partner to get the HIV antibody test.

6.   It would be dangerous to permit a student with HIV to attend school.

7.   It is easy to use the prevention methods that reduce one's chance of getting HIV.

8.   It is important to talk to a sex partner about HIV prevention before having sex.

9.   I believe that sharing IV drug needles has nothing to do with HIV.

10.   HIV education in schools is a waste of time.

11.   I would be supportive of persons with HIV.

12.   Even if a sex partner insisted, I would not use a condom.

13.   I intend to talk about HIV prevention with a partner if we were to have sex.

14.   I intend not to use drugs so I can avoid HIV.

15.   I will use condoms when having sex if I'm not sure if my partner has HIV.

Scoring instructions: Calculate the total points for each form using the following point values:
Form A, for items number 7, 8, 11, 13, 14, 15, strongly agree = 5 points, agree = 4, undecided = 3, disagree = 2, strongly disagree = 1, for the remaining items of Form A use strongly agree = 1, agree = 2, undecided = 3, disagree = 4, strongly disagree = 5.

From Torabi, M. R., & Yarber, W. (1992). Alternate Forms of HIV Prevention Attitude Scales for Teenagers. *AIDS Education and Prevention, 4*, 172–182. Reprinted App. A—Alternate Forms of HIV Prevention Attitude Scale Form A with permission.

ALTERNATE FORMS OF HIV PREVENTION ATTITUDE SCALE

Form B

DIRECTIONS: Please read each statement carefully. *Record your immediate reaction to the statement by blackening the proper oval on the answer sheet.* There is no right or wrong answer for each statement, so mark your own response. Use the below key:

KEY:

A = strongly agree
B = agree
C = undecided
D = disagree
E = strongly disagree

Example: Doing something to prevent getting HIV is the responsibility of each person.

A   B   C   D   E

RECORD ANSWER ON COMPUTER ANSWER SHEET

1.   I am certain that I could be supportive of a friend with HIV.

2.   I feel that people with HIV got what they deserve.

3.   I am comfortable with the idea of using condoms for sex.

4.   I would dislike the idea of limiting sex to just one partner to avoid HIV infection.

5.   It would be embarrassing to get the HIV antibody test.

6.   It is meant for some people to get HIV.

7.   Using condoms to avoid HIV is too much trouble.

8.   I believe that AIDS is a preventable disease.

9.   The chance of getting HIV makes using IV drugs stupid.

10.   People can influence their friends to practice safe behavior.

11.   I would shake hands with a person having HIV.

12.   I will avoid sex if there is a slight chance that the partner might have HIV.

13.   If I were to have sex I would insist that a condom be used.

14.   If I used IV drugs, I would not share the needles.

15.   I intend to share HIV facts with my friends.

Scoring instructions: Calculate the total points for each form using the following point values:
For items number 1, 3, 8, 9, 10, 11, 12, 13, 14, 15, strongly agree = 5, agree = 4, undecided = 3, disagree = 2, strongly disagree = 1, for the remaining items of Form B use strongly agree = 1, agree = 2, undecided = 3, disagree = 4, strongly disagree = 5.

From Torabi, M. R., & Yarber, W. (1992). Alternate Forms of HIV Prevention Attitude Scales for Teenagers. *AIDS Education and Prevention, 4*, 172–182. Reprinted App. B—Alternate Forms of HIV Prevention Attitude Scale Form B with permission.

51

Self-Efficacy Scale for Battered Women

Developed by Filomena F. Varvaro and Mary Palmer

INSTRUMENT DESCRIPTION, ADMINISTRATION, AND SCORING GUIDELINES

Self-Efficacy Scale for Battered Women (SESFBW) was developed to assess the self-efficacy (SE) needs of women who come to the emergency department with injuries and self-reported current abuse. It contains items related to self-efficacy to self-disclose and ask for help (items 1 and 2), plan for safety (items 3 to 9), and attain psychosocial functioning (items 10 to 12). Confidence in her ability to direct her own life with safety and without fear of abuse is believed to be necessary for health. The instrument takes 5 to 12 minutes to complete when self-administered. A score is obtained by dividing the number of the point where the person's X intersects the analogue line by the length of the line, summing across items and dividing by 12 (Varvaro, personal communication, February, 1996).

PSYCHOMETRIC PROPERTIES

Forty-three women entering the emergency department, who reported their current injury was caused by abuse or that they had experienced abuse in the past, completed the SESFBW. Nearly half were African American.

Cronbach's α has been found to be .88 and .96 (Varvaro & Palmer, 1993). Mean scores for women abused or reporting a history of being abused were 76.7 on entering the emergency department, 71.1 on entering an ambulatory medical clinic, and 63.9 on entering a shelter for battered women. Actual scores on individual items ranged from 28 to 100. For assessment and subsequent teaching, the authors suggest that raw scores on an item of 72 or lower should be classified as lower SE; 73 to 89 as moderate range SE; and a score of 90 or better as higher range of SE (Varvaro, n.d.).

Construct validity is supported by significant positive relationships with Self-Mastery Scale ($r = .68$), Self-Esteem Scale ($r = .64$), and Psychological General Well-Being Index ($r = .53$).

Factor analysis showed two factors of efficacy expectation in battered women: having information of abuse and planning for safety, and decreasing fear to promote adaptive psychological functioning in daily living (Varvaro, n.d.).

Varvaro and Palmer (1993) summarize studies showing that education including mastery modeling can be associated with an increase in SE related to coping skills and defense against assaults, decreased vulnerability to assaults, and intrusive negative thinking. Their article includes a detailed plan for a teaching intervention, which was tested in a 12-week class designed as an educational support group for six battered women. The women showed a significant increase in SESFBW scores, giving evidence of the instrument's sensitivity to interventions.

CRITIQUE AND SUMMARY

The SESFBW is meant to measure a woman's perceived ability to take positive steps in dealing with an abusive situation. It would be used along with other direct measurements, such as interview and history taking. It can form the basis for developing an individualized teaching plan to increase SE (Varvaro, n.d.).

It would be useful to determine whether increased SESFBW scores are related to improvement of behavioral consequences of abuse, such as anxiety, loss of self-esteem, feelings of loss, and grief. In addition, the tool has been used with a small group of mostly White women. Establishment of content validity was described as informal, based on a literature search and on clinical experience of the authors (Varvaro & Palmer, 1993). A more formal description of relevant content domains and how items were chosen from them would be helpful.

REFERENCES

Varvaro, F. F., & Palmer, M. (1993). Promotion of adaptation in battered women: A self-efficacy approach. *Journal of the American Academy of Nurse Practitioners, 5,* 264–270.

Varvaro, F. F. (n.d.). *Manual for the Self-Efficacy Scale for Battered Women.* Author. Pittsburgh: University of Pittsburgh.

SELF-EFFICACY SCALE FOR BATTERED WOMEN (SESFBW)

A population-specific assessment tool
to measure self-efficacy ability in battered women

Directions: We would like to know how sure you can do with the following behaviors. To indicate how sure you are, mark an X on the line that best reflects your level of sureness.

Example: I can be in control of my own life.

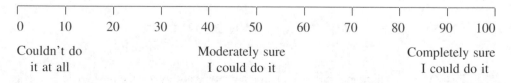

1. I can ask for help by talking to the nurse or doctor about my abusive situation.

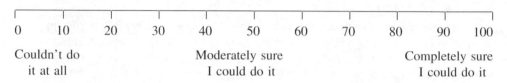

2. I can spend time telling someone such as a close friend/counselor the facts about my abusive situation.

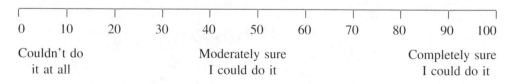

3. I can ask for help by calling a shelter hotline for abused women.

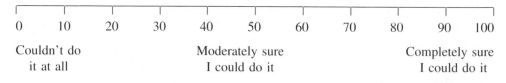

4. I can plan ahead to ensure safety when and if I choose to leave the abusive relationship.

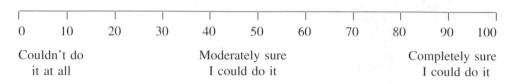

5. I can do things I normally enjoy without fear of being abused.

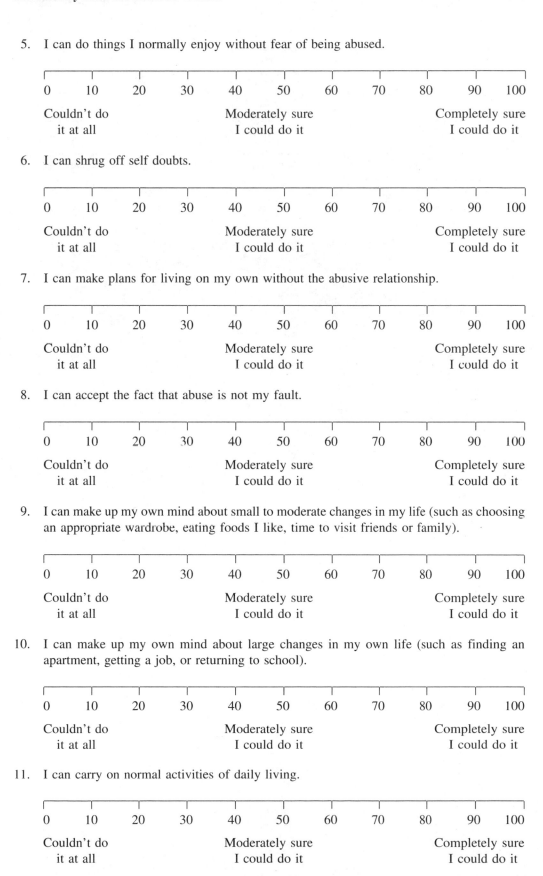

| 0 | 10 | 20 | 30 | 40 | 50 | 60 | 70 | 80 | 90 | 100 |

Couldn't do   Moderately sure   Completely sure
  it at all   I could do it   I could do it

6. I can shrug off self doubts.

| 0 | 10 | 20 | 30 | 40 | 50 | 60 | 70 | 80 | 90 | 100 |

Couldn't do   Moderately sure   Completely sure
  it at all   I could do it   I could do it

7. I can make plans for living on my own without the abusive relationship.

| 0 | 10 | 20 | 30 | 40 | 50 | 60 | 70 | 80 | 90 | 100 |

Couldn't do   Moderately sure   Completely sure
  it at all   I could do it   I could do it

8. I can accept the fact that abuse is not my fault.

| 0 | 10 | 20 | 30 | 40 | 50 | 60 | 70 | 80 | 90 | 100 |

Couldn't do   Moderately sure   Completely sure
  it at all   I could do it   I could do it

9. I can make up my own mind about small to moderate changes in my life (such as choosing an appropriate wardrobe, eating foods I like, time to visit friends or family).

| 0 | 10 | 20 | 30 | 40 | 50 | 60 | 70 | 80 | 90 | 100 |

Couldn't do   Moderately sure   Completely sure
  it at all   I could do it   I could do it

10. I can make up my own mind about large changes in my own life (such as finding an apartment, getting a job, or returning to school).

| 0 | 10 | 20 | 30 | 40 | 50 | 60 | 70 | 80 | 90 | 100 |

Couldn't do   Moderately sure   Completely sure
  it at all   I could do it   I could do it

11. I can carry on normal activities of daily living.

| 0 | 10 | 20 | 30 | 40 | 50 | 60 | 70 | 80 | 90 | 100 |

Couldn't do   Moderately sure   Completely sure
  it at all   I could do it   I could do it

12.   I can say what I think and feel without fear.

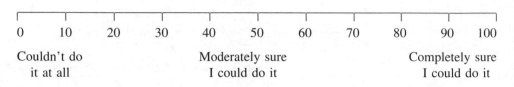

Couldn't do   Moderately sure   Completely sure
   it at all   I could do it   I could do it

Filomena F. Varvaro, PhD, RN, Assistant Professor, Acute/Tertiary Nursing Department, University of Pittsburgh, School of Nursing.

52

Levels of Institutionalization Scales for Health Promotion Programs: A Measure of How Well Established a Health Promotion Program Is in an Institution

Developed by Robert M. Goodman, Kenneth R. McLeroy, Allan B. Steckler, and Rick H. Hoyle

INSTRUMENT DESCRIPTION, ADMINISTRATION, AND SCORING GUIDELINES

In optimum circumstances, innovations, such as health promotion programs, are conceived, born, and nurtured within host organizations, mature, produce desired outcomes, and live for a long and productive period. They settle into their host organizations through mutual adaptation. An innovation need not be novel but merely new to the innovating organization.

Adoption and implementation of innovative programs have been much better studied than has institutionalization (the attainment of longevity); therefore, one is left without guidelines for positioning meritorious programs for survival so that their benefits will be available to clients. Different tasks distinguish these phases. Implementation focuses on immediate programmatic needs, such as client recruitment; institutionalization is more politically oriented, such as seeking permanent funding (Goodman & Steckler, 1989). Patient education programs are examples of innovations that must progress through institutionalization. The reasons that some of them fail to thrive have been neither well documented nor understood (Goodman & Steckler, 1989).

A model for the institutionalization of health promotion programs was developed from theory and a study of multiple programs in schools in Virginia. Institutionalization involves passages

| Dimensions | | Degrees | |
Subsystems	Passages	Routines	Niche Saturation
Production			
Maintenance			
Supportive			
Managerial			

FIGURE 52.1　Level of institutionalization matrix.

From Goodman, R. M., McLeroy, K. R., Steckler, A. B., & Hoyle, R. H. (1993). Development of Levels of Institutionalization Scales for Health Promotion Programs. *Health Education Quarterly, 20,* 161–178.

in procedure or structure, such as transition from outside to local funding and standardization of program job descriptions, and cycles survived, such as the number of budget cycles. A program achieving four or fewer passages and cycles was rated as low for institutionalization, 5 to 8 as low to moderate, 9 to 12 as moderate to high, and more than 12 as a highly institutionalized program (Goodman & Steckler, 1989).

Passages and cycles occurred within a context of six factors associated with program institutionalization: (a) standard operating routines, such as regular reports to supervisors about the program that provided people with enough information to assess the program's costs and benefits; (b) critical precursor conditions, such as awareness of and concern for a problem, receptivity to change, availability of solutions, and adequacy of program resources; (c) mutual adaptation of actors' aspirations—if the program supported their aspirations they became advocates for it; (d) development of a coalition of program advocates whose aspirations are being supported by the program and presence of a broker positioned at the middle to upper levels of the organization with good intuitive and negotiating skills who brings the coalition together; (e) mutual adaptation of program and organizational norms; and (f) fit with the host organization's mission and core operations (Goodman & Steckler, 1989).

Such a model suggests interventions to facilitate institutionalization as well as what should be measured to determine if institutionalization has occurred.

The Levels of Institutionalization Scales for Health Promotion programs (LoIn) were developed in a second study of dissemination of health promotion programs in junior high schools in North Carolina. Building on the exploratory model described earlier, LoIn measures the degree to which an innovation is integrated into four subsystems of an organization (production, managerial, maintenance, and supportive) through three stages (passages, routines, and niche saturation). A passage might be the first time an innovation is actually implemented; routines might be included in the annual budget, surviving turnover of staff; niche saturation is defined as the maximum feasible expansion of an innovation within an organization. Figure 52.1 depicts this model. One might say that the more cells that a particular health program occupies, the more embedded into these subsystems and the more institutionalized the program becomes. Scoring guidelines may be found on pages 380–382; no total scores in published sources could be located (Steckler, Goodman, McLeroy, Davis, & Koch, 1992).

PSYCHOMETRIC PROPERTIES

The LoIn was developed from a theoretical base in which relationships between the concepts are specified, important for construct validity. As a result of review by five experts in fields of organizational theory, health care administration, and health education research, the original 32-item instrument was revised to 15 three-part items. A study of 322 health promotion programs provided data for a confirmatory factor analysis. It supported the hypothesis of an eight-factor model: four factors concern how routinized the program was in each subsystem (more highly correlated with program longevity), and four factors concern the degree of program niche saturation within each subsystem (more highly correlated with managers' perceptions of program permanence). Because the factor analysis did not control for age of programs, further testing is needed to assure that the scale is applicable regardless of the age of a program. Details of the factor analysis may be found in Goodman, McLeroy, Steckler, and Hoyle (1993). Subscale α coefficients ranged from .44 to .86. Neither estimates of predictive validity nor of sensitivity to change could be located.

CRITIQUE AND SUMMARY

It is first important to affirm that not all programs deserve to be institutionalized. They may not have been successful in reaching their goals, or there may be little demand for them. For those that are serving their clients well, however, it is important to be able to measure the likelihood that they will be sustained and to take action to protect them. LoIn may eventually be helpful in this regard.

The LoIn helps one to retain the perspective that program institutionalization is largely a political endeavor that entails trade-offs and compromises among key members of the organization in which a program operates. LoIn is based both on organizational theory and empirical research of health promotion programs in organizations. It offers insights both for staff trying to institutionalize a program as well as for funders seeking innovative programs in which their investment will last. The LoIn has recently been used in a study of diabetes education programs (Redman & Barab, 1997).

Penha-Walton and Pichert (1993) compare diabetes foot care educational programs in two Veteran Administration medical centers, using the conceptual framework from the LoIn. Although no formal hypothesis testing was carried out, differences between the program that survived and the one that did not were replacement of the champion who had left and use of institutional funds for start-up as opposed to use of grant funds (the program ceased when the grant funds ran out). This and others studies suggest that important elements to identify or develop in a patient education program include presence of a well-placed program champion, placing the program in an institution with strong subsystems to provide program support, fitting the program to the host institution's mission and establishing appropriate periods to sustain the program through institutionalization. The usual three years of funding for a start-up program is insufficient to reach this goal (Steckler & Goodman, 1989).

The relationship between LoIn score and program survival in an institution is still unclear. Perhaps the present usefulness of this tool is more as a checklist for those trying to institutionalize meritorious programs or not institutionalize poor ones. Yet, although LoIn is in early stages of development, no other tools measuring this construct for health programs could be located.

Scheier (1993) points out that the items in each factor do not always seem to match the factor's conceptual definition raising issues of content validity; questions whether the eight scales are measuring independent dimensions of institutionalization (discriminant validity); and questions whether another respondent from the same agency would respond similarly (interrater reliability). She believes that the scales may not yet be ready for widespread use in research projects not focused on measurement development or by practitioners as diagnostic indicators of their organization's progress toward institutionalization of a program. The LoIn authors disagree. Clearly, there is more work to be done on the scale.

REFERENCES

Goodman, R. M., McLeroy, K. R., Steckler, A. B., & Hoyle, R. H. (1993). Development of level of institutionalization scales for health promotion programs. *Health Education Quarterly, 20,* 161–178.

Goodman, R. M., & Steckler, A. (1989). A model for the institutionalization of health promotion programs. *Family and Community Health, 11*(4), 63–78.

Penha-Walton, M. L. I., & Pichert, J. W. (1993). Institutionalizing patient education programs. *Journal of Nursing Administration, 23*(6), 36–41.

Redman, B. K., & Barab, S. (1997). Diabetes education infrastructure and capacity in hospitals and home health agencies in Maryland and Pennsylvania. *The Diabetes Educator, 23*(4): 1–13.

Scheirer, M. A. (1993). Are the Level of Institutionalization Scales ready for "prime time"? A commentary on "Development of Level of Institutionalization (LoIn) Scales for Health Promotion Programs." *Health Education Quarterly, 28,* 179–182.

Steckler, A., & Goodman, R. M. (1989). How to institutionalize health promotion programs. *American Journal of Health Promotion, 3*(4), 34–44.

Steckler, A., Goodman, R. M., McLeroy, K. R., Davis, S., & Koch, G. (1992). Measuring the diffusion of innovative health promotion programs. *American Journal of Health Promotion, 6,* 214–225.

LEVELS OF INSTITUTIONALIZATION (LoIn) SCALES
FOR HEALTH PROMOTION PROGRAMS
PRODUCTION SUBSYSTEM

1a.   Have the program's goals and/or objectives been put into writing?

      (1) ＿＿ Yes   (2) ＿＿ No   (3) ＿＿ Not sure/not applicable

        ↓   ↓

1b.   If yes, for how   Go to Question 2
many years have
written goals and
objectives actual-
ly been followed?

      ＿＿＿ Year(s)

        ↓   ↓

1c.   Of all the aspects of this program that could have written goals and objectives, what
is your best estimate of the proportion which actually have written goals and objectives?

No aspects of this program have written goals and objectives.	Few aspects of this program have written goals and objectives.	Most aspects of this program have written goals and objectives.	All aspects of this program have written goals and objectives.
1	2	3	4

2a.   Have any of the plans or procedures used for implementing this program been put
in writing?

      (1) ＿＿ Yes   (2) ＿＿ No   (3) ＿＿ Not sure/not applicable

        ↓   ↓

2b.   If yes, for how   Go to Question 3
many years have
such written plans
or procedures actu-
ally been fol-
lowed?

      ＿＿＿ Year(s)

        ↓   ↓

2c.   Of all the aspects of this program that could have written plans or procedures, what
is your best estimate of the proportion which actually have written plans or procedures?

No aspects of the program have written plans or procedures.	Few aspects of the program have written plans or procedures.	Most aspects of the program have written plans or procedures.	All aspects of the program have written plans or procedures.
1	2	3	4

3a.   Has a schedule (e.g., timetable, plan of action) used for implementing program activ-
      ities been put in writing?

      (1) _____ Yes   (2) _____ No   (3) _____ Not sure/not applicable

         ↓   ↓

3b.   If yes, for how   Go to Question 4
      many years have
      such written sched-
      ules actually been
      followed?

      _____ Year(s)

       ↓   ↓

3c.   Of all the aspects of this program that could have written schedules, what is your
      best estimate of the proportion which actually have written schedules?

No aspects of this program have writ-ten schedules.	Few aspects of this program have written schedules.	Most aspects of this program have written schedules.	All aspects of this program have writ-ten schedules.
1	2	3	4

4a.   Have the strategies for implementing this program been adapted to fit local circum-
      stances?

      (1) _____ Yes   (2) _____ No   (3) _____ Not sure/not applicable

         ↓   ↓

4b.   If yes, for how   Go to Question 5
      many years have
      locally adapted
      strategies actually
      been followed?

      _____ Year(s)

       ↓   ↓

4c.   Of all the aspects of this program that could be adapted to fit local circumstances,
      what is your best estimate of the proportion which have actually been adapted?

No aspects of this program have been adapted.	Few aspects of this program have been adapted.	Most aspects of this program have been adapted.	All aspects of this program have been adapted.
1	2	3	4

5a.   Has a formal evaluation of the program been conducted?

      (1) _____ Yes   (2) _____ No   (3) _____ Not sure/not applicable

         ↓   ↓

                                        Go to Question 6

5b. If yes, for how
     many times has
     the program been
     formally
     evaluated?

          _____ Year(s)

               ↓   ↓

5c. Of all the aspects of this program that could be formally evaluated, what is your
     best estimate of the proportion which have been formally evaluated?

No aspects of this program have been evaluated.	Few aspects of this program have been evaluated.	Most aspects of this program have been evaluated.	All aspects of this program have been evaluated.
1	2	3	4

MANAGERIAL SUBSYSTEM

6a. Has a supervisor (e.g., section chief, department head) been formally assigned to
     oversee this program?

          (1) ____ Yes   (2) ____ No   (3) ____ Not sure/not applicable

               ↓   ↓

6b. If yes, for how   Go to Question 7
     many years has
     such a supervisor
     actually been for-
     mally assigned to
     oversee the pro-
     gram?

          _____ Year(s)

               ↓   ↓

6c. Of all the aspects of this program that could receive supervision, what is your best
     estimate of the proportion which actually receives such supervision?

No aspects of this program receive supervision.	Few aspects of this program receive supervision.	Most aspects of this program receive supervision.	All aspects of this program receive supervision.
1	2	3	4

7a. Have formalized job descriptions been written for staff involved with this program?

          (1) ____ Yes   (2) ____ No   (3) ____ Not sure/not applicable

               ↓   ↓

                                                    Go to Question 8

7b.   If yes, for how
      many years have
      formalized job de-
      scriptions actually
      been followed?

         _____ Year(s)

              ↓   ↓

7c.   What is your best estimate of the number of staff involved with this program who
      have written job descriptions?

None of the staff involved with this program have written job descriptions.	Few of the staff involved with this program have written job descriptions.	Most of the staff involved with this program have written job descriptions.	All of the staff involved with this program have written job descriptions.
1	2	3	4

8a.   Are *evaluation reports* of this program done on a schedule similar to evaluation re-
      ports for most other programs in your organization?

         (1) ___ Yes   (2) ___ No   (3) ___ Not sure/not applicable
              ↓   ↓

8b   If yes, for how   Go to Question 9
      many years have
      evaluation reports
      actually been pro-
      duced on a sched-
      ule similar to such
      reports for most
      other programs in
      your organization?

         _____ Year(s)

              ↓   ↓

8c.   What is your best estimate of the extent that evaluation reports for this program are
      produced on a schedule similar to evaluation reports for most other programs in
      your organization?

No evaluation reports are produced on a similar schedule.	Few evaluation reports are produced on a similar schedule.	Most evaluation reports are produced on a similar schedule.	All evaluation reports are produced on a similar schedule.
1	2	3	4

MAINTENANCE SUBSYSTEM

9a. Have any permanent staff been assigned to implement this program?

(1) ____ Yes (2) ____ No (3) ____ Not sure/not applicable

↓ ↓

9b. If yes, for how many years have permanent staff been assigned to implement the program?

Go to Question 10

____ Year(s)

↓ ↓

9c. What is your best estimate of the number of staff who implement the program that are in permanent positions?

No staff involved are in permanent positions.	Few staff involved are in permanent positions.	Most staff involved are in permanent positions.	All staff involved are in permanent positions.
1	2	3	4

10a. Has an *administrative-level* individual within your organization been actively involved in advocating for this program's continuation?

(1) ____ Yes (2) ____ No (3) ____ Not sure/not applicable

↓ ↓

10b. If yes, for how many has this *administrative-level* individual actively advocated for this program's continuation?

Go to Question 11

____ Year(s)

↓ ↓

10c. What is your best estimate of how active this administrative-level individual has been in advocating for the program's continuation?

Not active at all	Minimally active	Moderately active	Very active
1	2	3	4

11a. Do staff in your organization, other than those actually implementing the program, actively contribute to the program's operations?

(1) ____ Yes (2) ____ No (3) ____ Not sure/not applicable

↓ ↓

Go to Question 12

11b. If yes, for how
many years have
such staff in your
organization ac-
tively contributed
to the program's
operation?

      _____ Year(s)

      ↓   ↓

11c. Of all the staff in your organization who could contribute to the operation of this
program, what is your best estimate of the proportion that actually contribute to it?

None of the staff contribute to the program's operation.	Few of the staff contribute to the program's operation.	Most of the staff contribute to the program's operation.	All of the staff contribute to the program's operation.
1	2	3	4

SUPPORTIVE SUBSYSTEM

12a. Has the program made a transition from trial or pilot status to permanent status in
your organization?

    (1) ___ Yes   (2) ___ No   (3) ___ Not sure/not applicable

       ↓   ↓

12b. If yes, for how   Go to Question 13
many years has
this program had
permanent status?

      _____ Year(s)

       ↓   ↓

12c. What is your best estimate of how permanent this program is in your organization?

Not permanent at all	Minimally perma-nent	Moderately perma-nent	Very permanent
1	2	3	4

13a. Has the program been assigned permanent physical space within your organization?

    (1) ___ Yes   (2) ___ No   (3) ___ Not sure/not applicable

       ↓   ↓

                                           Go to Question 14

13b. If yes, for how many years has it maintained such permanent space?

_____ Year(s)

↓   ↓

13c. Of all the permanent space that this program needs, what is your best estimate of the proportion of permanent space it currently occupies?

This program does *not* occupy any permanent space.	This program occupies only a *small* amount of the permanent space that it needs.	This program occupies *most* of the permanent space that it needs.	This program occupies *all* of the permanent space that it needs.
1	2	3	4

14a. Is this program's source of funding similar to the funding sources for other established programs within your organization?

(1) ___ Yes   (2) ___ No   (3) ___ Not sure/not applicable

↓   ↓

                                    Go to Question 15

14b. If yes, for how many years has this program's funding sources been similar to those for other established programs within your organization?

_____ Year(s)

↓   ↓

14c. In your best estimate, how permanent is the program's source of funding?

Not permanent at all	Minimally permanent	Moderately permanent	Very permanent
1	2	3	4

15a. Is the staff most closely associated with this program's implementation hired from a stable funding source?

(1) ___ Yes   (2) ___ No   (3) ___ Not sure/not applicable

↓

15b. If yes, for how
      many years has
      the staff most
      closely associated
      with this pro-
      gram's implemen-
      tation been hired
      from a stable fund-
      ing source?

            _____ Year(s)

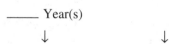

15c. What is your best estimate of how permanent the funding is for the staff most close-
      ly associated with this program's implementation?

Not permanent at all	Minimally permanent	Moderately permanent	Very permanent
1	2	3	4

From Goodman, R. M., McLeroy, K. R., Steckler, A., Hoyle, R. H. (1993). Development of Institutionalization (LoIn) Scales for Health Promotion Programs: Health Education Quarterly, RO(2), 161–178. Reprinted by permission of Sage Publications, Inc.

Definitions for Organizational Subsystems and Degrees of Program Penetration

*Subsystems**

Production: Concerned with "throughput," or those activities which are product directed.

Managerial: Concerned with coordinating the operations of the other subsystems.

Maintenance: Concerned with personnel issues and continuity of production in areas such as recruitment, indoctrination or socialization, rewarding, sanctioning and procurement of resources.

Supportive: Concerned with hospitable environmental conditions by establishing legitimacy and favorable organizational relationships.

Degrees

Passages: The first degree of program institutionalization which is signified by one-time sentinel events such as the formalization of program plans, the shift from soft to hard sources of funding, and the program's inclusion on the organizational chart.

Routines: The second degree of program institutionalization which is signified by the habituation, or routinization of program passages, such as the continued inclusion of the program in the organization's formal plans, annual renewal of stable funding, and continued inclusion of the program in new versions of the organizational chart.

Niche
saturation: The third degree of program institutionalization which is signified by the maximum feasible expansion of the program within the host organization's subsystems, such as the optimum realization of the programs plans, the achievement of optimum levels of funding, and the inclusion of the program in a core (versus peripheral) location on the organizational chart.

---

*The definitions for the subsystems are adapted from Katz and Kahn (1978).

+The definitions for the degrees are adapted from Yin (1979).

Scoring the LoIn Scale

The grid on the next page can be used to score the LoIn Scale in conjunction with the following directions:

Each question has three sub-questions (a, b, and c). Sub-questions "a" and "b" are scored together, resulting in one score for the two sub-items, and sub-question "c" forms is scored separately.

For all "a" and "b" sub-questions, score as follows:

- if you checked "No" or "Not sure/not applicable" for "a," then the score for the sub-item = 0;
- if you checked "Yes" for "a" *and* wrote "0" or "1" for "b," then the score for the sub-item = 1;
- if you checked "Yes" for "a" *and* wrote "2" or "3" for "b," then the score for the sub-item = 2;
- if you checked "Yes" for "a" *and* wrote "4" or "5" for "b," then the score for the sub-item = 3;
- if you checked "Yes" for "a" *and* wrote "6" or more for "b," then the score for the sub-item = 4

For all "c" sub-questions, score them as the number that you circled for that item (e.g., if you circled a "2" then the score for that item = 2).

Each three-part item represents one of the following organizational sub-systems: production (items 1–5), managerial (items 6–8), maintenance (items 9–11), supportive (items 12–15). Using the grid on the next page, add the scores for all sub-items "a" and "b" as indicated and divide by the number listed on the grid. Follow the same procedure for all "c" sub-items.

For sub-items "a" and "b":

- if the mean score is "1" or less then institutionalization is low;
- if the mean score is greater than "1" but less than or equal to "3" then institutionalization is low to moderate;
- if the mean score is greater than "3" but less than or equal to "5" then institutionalization is moderate to high;
- if the mean score is greater than "5" then institutionalization is high.

For sub-items "c":

- if the mean score is less than or equal to "2" then institutionalization is low;
- if the mean score is greater than "2" but less than or equal to "3" then institutionalization is moderate;
- if the mean score is greater than "3" then institutionalization is high.

*In which subsystems did you score **low**? What can you do to increase the institutionalization score for that subsystem?*

SCORE SHEET FOR PROGRAM INSTITUTIONALIZATION ITEMS "A" AND "B"

Subsystem	Item	Item Score	Mean Score		
PRODUCTION	1 "a" and "b"				
	2 "a" and "b"				
	3 "a" and "b"				
	4 "a" and "b"				
	5 "a" and "b"				
		Item sum =	Item sum/5 =		
MANAGERIAL	6 "a" and "b"				
	7 "a" and "b"				
	8 "a" and "b"				
		Item sum =	Item sum/3 =		
MAINTENANCE	9 "a" and "b"				
	10 "a" and "b"				
	11 "a" and "b"				
		Item sum =	Item sum/3 =		
SUPPORT	12 "a" and "b"				
	13 "a" and "b"				
	14 "a" and "b"				
	15 "a" and "b"				
		Item sum =	Item sum/4 =		

SCORE SHEET FOR PROGRAM INSTITUTIONALIZATION ITEM "C"

Subsystem	Item	Item Score	Mean Score		
PRODUCTION	1c				
	2c				
	3c				
	4c				
	5c				
		Item sum =	Item sum/5 =		
MANAGERIAL	6c				
	7c				
	8c				
		Item sum =	Item sum/3 =		
MAINTENANCE	9c				
	10c				
	11c				
		Item sum =	Item sum/3 =		
SUPPORT	12c				
	13c				
	14c				
	15c				
		Item sum =	Item sum/4 =		

Appendix: Summary of Tools

Author (language)	What is measured	Time to complete	Readability, grade	Scoring guide	Validity Content	Validity Construct	Sensitive to intervention	Reliability Int. consist.	Reliability Other
Anderson	A		10	Y		Y		0.63–0.71	
Austin	A/C			Y		Y		0.8	
Bartholomew	SE		6	Y	Y	Y		0.73–0.88	
Bernier	L				Y				
Biggs	K/A/C	20 min		Y					
Branch	K				Y				0.52
Callahan	A	10–15 min		Y		Y		0.68	
Degeling	L				?				
Devins (Fr)	K		9	Y	Y	Y	Y	0.85, 0.94	
Edworthy	K		8	Y	Y	Y	Y	0.72–0.84	
Ferrell	K			Y	Y	Y	Y	0.81	0.92
Fife	A			Y	Y	Y		0.81	
Froman	SE			Y	Y	Y		0.98	
Galloway	K	20 min		Y	Y	Y		0.93	
Galloway/ Bubela	L	20 min		Y	Y	Y		0.95–0.97	
Gattuso	SE			Y		Y	Y	0.90, 0.92	
Gibson	A	10 min		Y	Y	Y		0.82	0.83, 0.84
Gonzalez (Sp)	SE			Y		Y		0.79	
Goodman	L			Y		Y		0.44–0.86	
Gross	SE	5 min		Y	Y	Y	Y	0.95	0.87
Gupton	L			Y	Y	Y		0.82	0.67
Hickey	SE			Y	Y	Y		0.90	0.86–0.87
Hill	K			Y	Y	Y	Y	0.72	0.81
Hodnett (Da, Fr, He, Sp, Sw)	T	10 min		Y		Y	Y	0.91–0.98	

Appendix: Summary of Tools (*Continued*)

Author (language)	What is measured	Time to complete	Readability, grade	Scoring guide	Validity Content	Construct	Sensitive to intervention	Reliability Int. consist.	Other
Hussey	K			Y	Y		Y	0.85	
Ingersoll	QOL			Y	Y	Y		0.82–0.85	
Janofsky	L		6	Y		Y			0.95[a]
Kim	A	20 min		Y		Y		0.71–0.82	0.52–0.84
	SE			Y		Y		0.90	
	K			Y		Y		0.69	
Leslie	K			Y	Y		Y		0.76
Levin	A			Y		Y		0.63	
Levinson (Fr)	SE	10 min		Y	Y	Y	Y	0.73	
Lorig (Du, Sp, Sw)	SE			Y	Y	Y	Y	0.76–0.92	0.81–0.91
Lowe	SE		7–8	Y	Y	Y		0.86–0.95	0.46–0.76
McEwen	L			Y	Y			0.89, 0.71	
Mesters	K			Y	Y		Y	0.81	
	A			Y	Y		Y	0.33, 0.59	
	SE			Y	Y		Y	0.93	
	A			Y	Y		Y	0.92	
Oetker-Black	SE	10–15 min		Y	Y	Y		0.84–0.98	

Appendix: Summary of Tools (*Continued*)

Author (language)	What is measured	Time to complete	Readability, grade	Scoring guide	Validity Content	Construct	Sensitive to intervention	Reliability Int. consist.	Other
Polonsky	L			Y	Y	Y		0.95	
Pridham	L			Y		Y		0.85	
Reece	SE	10 min		Y	Y	Y		0.86–0.91	
Richards	A					Y		0.71–0.87	
Scherer	K			Y	Y		Y	0.89	
Schuster	K			Y	Y			0.84	
Shiloh	K	5 min	<6	Y	Y		Y	0.62	
Spirito	K		7–9	Y	Y	Y		0.62–0.78	0.75–0.80
Teti	SE			Y	Y	Y		0.79–0.86	
Tinetti	SE			Y	Y	Y	Y	0.90	0.71
Torabi	A	12 min		Y	Y	Y	Y	0.77–0.82	0.69, 0.76
Varvaro	SE	5–12 min		Y		Y	Y	0.88–0.96	
Vega (Sp)	K/C			Y			Y	0.51, 0.80	0.73, 0.76
Weinrich	K			Y			Y	0.69	0.65

Note. A, attitude/belief/behavior; C, for children; K, knowledge; L, learning assessment/instructional design or delivery; QOL, quality of life; SE, self-efficacy; T, theoretical model; Da, Danish; Du, Dutch; Fr, French; He, Hebrew; Sp, Spanish; Sw, Swedish; Int. Consist., internal consistency for full scale (unless all that was reported was for subscales).

[a]Represents interobserver reliability; all others in this column are test-retest reliability.

Index

Entries followed by f refer to figures.

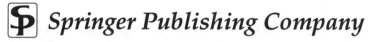 *Springer Publishing Company*

Planning, Implementing, and Evaluating Critical Pathways

A Guide for Health Care Survival into the 21st Century

Patricia C. Dykes, MA, RN
Kathleen Wheeler, PhD, CS, APRN, Editors
Foreword by **Karen Zander,** RN, MS, CS, FAAN

This is a practical guide to developing critical pathways for a multitude of settings — acute care, ambulatory, home care, rehabilitation, and long-term care. The book takes the reader from the very first steps of critical pathway design, through the ins-and-outs of implementation, and then assists the reader with evaluating patient and systems outcomes, and improving practice. Concrete examples are given of how to adapt pathways to meet the needs of individual institutions and how to incorporate them into a continuous quality improvement process.

Specific legal concerns are addressed in a chapter by attorneys who are also nurses and an entire chapter is devoted to the computerization of pathways. Students, educators, administrators and clinicians will find this an essential resource for providing quality care, efficient case management, and a sound outcomes management program.

Contents:

1997   184pp   0-8261-9790-6   hardcover

536 Broadway, New York, NY 10012-3955 • (212) 431-4370 • Fax (212) 941-7842

℠ *Springer Publishing Company*

Nursing Management of Diabetes Mellitus, 4th Edition
A Guide to the Pattern Approach

Diana W. Guthrie, RN, PhD, ARNP, FAAN, CDE, LMFT, CHN, and **Richard A. Guthrie,** MD, FAAP, CDE, FACE with contributors

This fourth edition continues to provide readers with a sound understanding of current and
established information on diabetes and its
practical management. Topics include physical and emotional effects; patient and family
education; self management, including
glucose monitoring, dietary management, and
exercise; and also acute and long term care.
This new edition provides an explanation of
the revised classification categories — "insulin dependent" and
"noninsulin dependent" instead of "juvenile and mature onset";
the latest glucose monitoring and insulin pump devices, and
more. The appendix includes a detailed education program for
patients. The authors, a nurse-physician team, bring a multidisciplinary perspective to this complex topic. Contributors come
from the fields of nursing, nutrition, exercise, sex therapy, and
marriage and family therapy.

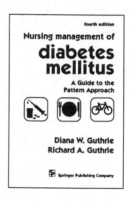

Partial Contents: Definition, Facts, and Statistics • Diagnosis • Physiology of
Glucose Metabolism • Child • Young and Middle Adult • The Older Adult
• Meal Plan • Insulin • Oral Hypoglycemic Agents • Psychosocial Consid-
erations • Self-Monitoring of Blood Glucose • Hygiene • Exercise • Acute
Complications • Chronic Complications • Stress and Diabetes Management
• Effects on Sexual Function • Pregnancy • Surgery • Drugs and Alcohol •
Development of an Education Program • Assessment of Patient's Education

1997   480pp   0-8261-7261-X   hardcover

536 Broadway, New York, NY 10012-3955 • (212) 431-4370 • Fax (212) 941-7842

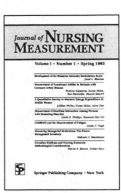

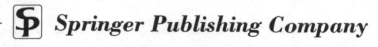

SP *Springer Publishing Company*

Nursing Leadership Forum

Barbara Stevens Barnum, RN, PhD, FAAN, Editor

Nursing Leadership Forum is a quarterly journal designed for the nurse who practices, or aspires to, leadership in a variety of settings — in working with patients, families, and nursing staff, as well as with health care or academic institutions, or in the larger community. Within this broad context, the journal explores the ethics, values, and theories underlying the exercise of nursing leadership, as well as innovative ideas for leadership effectiveness.

Each issue of the journal features a wide range of articles, from research presentations, to papers written in a scholarly style, to thought-provoking personalized accounts. Some articles in the journal are role-related while others deal with concepts and trends that apply in various settings. Book reviews, interviews with colleagues, and a letter column are also vital parts of each issue.

Sample Articles:

- Life Transition Theory: It Works for the Unemployed Nurse Executive as Well as for Patients, *E. Barba & F. Selder*

- Shifting Paradigms: An Approach to Teaching in an Era of Rapid Change, *J.P. Flynn*

- Nursing Leadership With the Pen: Two Peas in a Pod, *H. Forman*

- Preparing the Nurse Executive of the Future, *H. Feldman*

- Spirituality in Nursing: Everything Old Is New Again, *B.S. Barnum*

Volume 4, 1997-98 • 4 issues annually • ISSN 1076-1632

536 Broadway, New York, NY 10012-3955 • (212) 431-4370 • Fax (212) 941-7842